Logansport Cass County Public Library

LOGANSPORT LIBRARY

1501 9100 262 013 1

616.075 SHA

Medical tests sourcebook :

Healthy Heart Sourcebook for Women

Heart Diseases & Disorders
  Sourcebook, 2nd Edition

Household Safety So...

Immune System Dis...

Infant & Toddler He...

Infectious Diseases Sourcebook

Injury & Trauma Sourcebook

Kidney & Uri...
  Disorders S...

Learning Disa...
  2nd Edition

Leukemia Sou...

Liver Disorde...

Lung Disorde...

Medical Tests Sourcebook, 2nd Edition

Men's Health Concerns Sourcebook,
  2nd Edition

Mental Health Disorders Sourcebook,
  2nd Edition

Mental Retardation Sourcebook

Movement Disorders Sourcebook

Obesity Sourcebook

Osteoporosis Sourcebook

Pain Sourcebook, 2nd Edition

Pediatric Cancer Sourcebook

Physical & Mental Issues in Aging
  Sourcebook

Podiatry Sourcebook

Pregnancy & Birth Sourcebook,
  2nd Edition

Prostate Cancer

Public Health Sourcebook

Reconstructive & Cosmetic Surgery
  Sourcebook

Rehabilitation Sourcebook

Respiratory Diseases & Disorders
  Sourcebook

Sexually Transmitted Diseases
  Sourcebook, 2nd Edition

Skin Disorders Sourcebook

Sleep Disorders Sourcebook

Sports Injuries Sourcebook, 2nd Edition

...ated Disorders Sourcebook

...urcebook

...e Abuse Sourcebook

Surgery Sourcebook

T........... ......urcebook

...urcebook

...ok

...ncerns Sourcebook,

.... Safety Sourcebook

...ourcebook

D0908363

Teen Health Series

Cancer Information for Teens

Diet Information for Teens

Drug Information for Teens

Fitness Information for Teens

Mental Health Information
  for Teens

Sexual Health Information
  for Teens

Skin Health Information
  for Teens

Sports Injuries Information
  for Teens

Medical Tests
SOURCEBOOK

Second Edition

Health Reference Series

Second Edition

Medical Tests
SOURCEBOOK

*Basic Consumer Health Information
about Medical Tests, Including Age-Specific
Health Tests, Important Health Screenings
and Exams, Home-Use Tests, Blood and
Specimen Tests, Electrical Tests, Scope Tests,
Genetic Testing, and Imaging Tests,
Such as X-Rays, Ultrasound, Computed
Tomography, Magnetic Resonance Imaging,
Angiography, and Nuclear Medicine*

*Along with a Glossary and Directory of
Additional Resources*

Edited by
Joyce Brennfleck Shannon

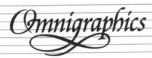

Omnigraphics

615 Griswold Street • Detroit, MI 48226

Logansport Cass County Public Library

Bibliographic Note

Because this page cannot legibly accommodate all the copyright notices, the Bibliographic Note portion of the Preface constitutes an extension of the copyright notice.

Edited by Joyce Brennfleck Shannon

Health Reference Series

Karen Bellenir, *Managing Editor*
David A. Cooke, MD, *Medical Consultant*
Elizabeth Barbour, *Permissions Associate*
Dawn Matthews, *Verification Assistant*
Laura Pleva Nielsen, *Index Editor*
EdIndex, Services for Publishers, *Indexers*

* * *

Omnigraphics, Inc.

Matthew P. Barbour, *Senior Vice President*
Kay Gill, *Vice President—Directories*
Kevin Hayes, *Operations Manager*
Leif Gruenberg, *Development Manager*
David P. Bianco, *Marketing Director*

* * *

Peter E. Ruffner, *Publisher*

Frederick G. Ruffner, Jr., *Chairman*

Copyright © 2004 Omnigraphics, Inc.

ISBN 0-7808-0670-0

Library of Congress Cataloging-in-Publication Data

The Cataloging in Publication record (CIP data) for *Medical Tests Sourcebook, 2ⁿᵈ Ed.* was not available at the time of manufacturing.

To obtain a copy of the CIP data for this book, visit www.omnigraphics.com/cataloging, or contact Omnigraphics' Customer Service department at 800-234-1340.

Electronic or mechanical reproduction, including photography, recording, or any other information storage and retrieval system for the purpose of resale is strictly prohibited without permission in writing from the publisher.

The information in this publication was compiled from the sources cited and from other sources considered reliable. While every possible effort has been made to ensure reliability, the publisher will not assume liability for damages caused by inaccuracies in the data, and makes no warranty, express or implied, on the accuracy of the information contained herein.

This book is printed on acid-free paper meeting the ANSI Z39.48 Standard. The infinity symbol that appears above indicates that the paper in this book meets that standard.

Printed in the United States

624682

Table of Contents

Logansport Cass County Public Library

Part III: Screenings and Diagnostic Tests for Specific Concerns

Part IV: Home-Use Tests and Assessments

Part: V: Testing of Blood, Body Fluids, and Specimens

Part VII: Electrical Tests

Part VIII: Scope Tests

Part IX: Genetic Testing

Part X: Additional Information

Preface

About This Book

Medical tests open a window through which the functions of the human body can be viewed and evaluated. They provide the patient and the doctor with vital information about general health, current symptoms, or the silent start of a health problem. Timely colonoscopy, mammography, and cardiac catheterization, for example, are credited with extending many lives. Scope tests can even replace some surgeries. Regular check-ups that include recommended screening tests for heart disease, diabetes, and cancer are a key to maintaining or improving health.

Medical tests have limits and risks, however. Patients can get the best results from medical tests by:

- carefully following test preparation instructions,
- making sure that the doctor is aware of all current medications and health information,
- asking questions and sharing any concerns with the doctor.

This *Sourcebook* provides health information about medical tests and laboratory services. Readers will learn about tests used for specific health screenings and disease diagnosis. Other tests presented include age-specific health tests, screenings for disease prevention, home-use tests, blood and specimen tests, imaging tests, electrical tests, scope tests, and genetic tests. A glossary and a directory of additional resources are also included.

How to Use This Book

This book is divided into parts and chapters. Parts focus on broad areas of interest. Chapters are devoted to single topics within a part.

Part I: Essential Patient Information about Medical Tests explains why medical tests are necessary and suggests questions to ask about the tests. It offers tips on finding quality lab services and examines health insurance issues, including medical necessity, denied requests, and insurance for children.

Part II: Age-Specific Health Screenings, Preventive Tests, and Exams describes the recommended guidelines for preventive care for newborns, children, teens, and adult men and women.

Part III: Screenings and Diagnostic Tests for Specific Concerns explains health exams used to screen for and diagnose many of the top causes of death in the U.S., including cardiovascular disease, cancer, and diabetes. Other common health exams for such problems as osteoporosis, asthma and lung disease, vision changes, hearing loss, infertility, and sexually transmitted diseases are also described.

Part IV: Home-Use Tests and Assessments discusses the large market of home-use tests available in the U.S. It explains the pros and cons and offers a physician's perspective on home-use test results. Tests described include cholesterol, drug use, fecal occult blood, HIV, pregnancy, and fertility tests. Online screening tools for mental illness, alcohol abuse, and other assessments are also described.

Part V: Testing of Blood, Body Fluids, and Specimens gives the specifics of blood tests, including lipid profiles, liver function tests, thyroid function tests, and cancer markers. It also details strep cultures, sweat tests, urine tests, stool tests, lumbar punctures, and biopsies. Test procedures and results are explained.

Part VI: Imaging Tests describes x-ray, ultrasound, computed tomography (CT), magnetic resonance imaging (MRI), angiography, and nuclear medicine tests. Basic information about the procedures and specifics of common imaging tests are presented.

Part VII: Electrical Tests deals with evaluations of the cardiac, nervous, and brain systems. Individual chapters explain brain wave tests, nerve conduction velocities, cardiovascular tests of the heart, and sleep patterns.

Part VIII: Scope Tests describes tests that give doctors invaluable information about internal conditions or diseases. These include bronchoscopy, cardiac catheterization, colonoscopy, sigmoidoscopy, and endoscopy.

Part IX: Genetic Testing presents when and why genetic testing may be helpful in family planning and disease prevention, how to order genetic testing, and cautions regarding discrimination by health insurance companies based on genetic information.

Part X: Additional Information includes a glossary of important terms related to medical testing and a directory of organizations able to provide additional information.

Bibliographic Note

This volume contains documents and excerpts from publications issued by the following U.S. government agencies: Agency for Healthcare Research and Quality (AHRQ); Centers for Disease Control and Prevention (CDC); National Cancer Institute (NCI); National Center for Health Statistics (NCHS); National Eye Institute; National Heart, Lung, and Blood Institute (NHLBI); National Human Genome Research Institute; National Institute of Allergy and Infectious Diseases (NIAID); National Institute of Child Health and Human Development (NICHD); National Institute of Diabetes and Digestive and Kidney Diseases (NIDDK); the National Institutes of Health's Warren Grant Magnuson Clinical Center, the U.S. Department of Health and Human Services (HHS); and the U.S. Food and Drug Administration (FDA).

In addition, this volume contains copyrighted documents from the following organizations and individuals: A.D.A.M, Inc.; Al-Anon Family Group Headquarters; Alcohol Research Group; Amarillo Medical Specialists, L.L.P.; American Academy of Allergy; American Academy of Ophthalmology; American Association for Clinical Chemistry; American Gastroenterological Association; American Heart Association; American Speech-Language-Hearing Association; A.S.M Systems, Inc.; Asthma and Immunology; Beth Israel Deaconess Medical Center–Department of Radiology; Cardiology Associates; Children's Hospital and Regional Medical Center and University of Washington; Cincinnati Children's Hospital Medical Center; Cystic Fibrosis Foundation; Ernst & Mattison Law Corporation; Florida Cardiovascular Institute; Dr. Wayne K. Goodman; Healthcheck USA; Illinois Department of Insurance; International Osteoporosis Foundation; Joint Commission on Accreditation of Healthcare Organizations (JCAHO); Mater Imaging;

Medical University of South Carolina–Digestive Disease Center; Muscular Dystrophy Association–USA; National Council on Alcoholism and Drug Dependence, Inc.; National Mental Health Association; National Newborn Screening and Genetics Resource Center; Nemours Foundation; Osteoporosis and Related Bone Diseases–National Resource Center; RESOLVE: National Infertility Association; Society of American Gastrointestinal Endoscopic Surgeons; Society of Interventional Radiology; Society of Nuclear Medicine; Society of Radiologists in Ultrasound; St. Joseph Sleep Disorders Center; University of Chicago Asthma Center; University of Pittsburgh Medical Center; University of Washington/Hall Health Center Women's Clinic; WebMD Corporation; and World Health Organization (WHO).

Full citation information is provided on the first page of each chapter. Every effort has been made to secure all necessary rights to reprint the copyrighted material. If any omissions have been made, please contact Omnigraphics to make corrections for future editions.

Acknowledgements

Special thanks go to the many organizations, agencies, and individuals who have contributed materials for this *Sourcebook* and to the managing editor Karen Bellenir, medical consultant Dr. David Cooke, permissions specialist Liz Barbour, verification assistant Dawn Matthews, indexer Edward J. Prucha, and document engineer Bruce Bellenir.

Note from the Editor

This book is part of Omnigraphics' *Health Reference Series*. The *Series* provides basic information about a broad range of medical concerns. It is not intended to serve as a tool for diagnosing illness, in prescribing treatments, or as a substitute for the physician/patient relationship. All persons concerned about medical symptoms or the possibility of disease are encouraged to seek professional care from an appropriate health care provider.

Our Advisory Board

The *Health Reference Series* is reviewed by an Advisory Board comprised of librarians from public, academic, and medical libraries. We would like to thank the following board members for providing guidance to the development of this series:

Dr. Lynda Baker,
Associate Professor of Library and Information Science,
Wayne State University, Detroit, MI

Nancy Bulgarelli,
William Beaumont Hospital Library, Royal Oak, MI

Karen Imarisio,
Bloomfield Township Public Library, Bloomfield Township, MI

Karen Morgan,
Mardigian Library, University of Michigan-Dearborn,
Dearborn, MI

Rosemary Orlando,
St. Clair Shores Public Library, St. Clair Shores, MI

Medical Consultant

Medical consultation services are provided to the *Health Reference Series* editors by David A. Cooke, MD. Dr. Cooke is a graduate of Brandeis University, and he received his M.D. degree from the University of Michigan. He completed residency training at the University of Wisconsin Hospital and Clinics. He is board-certified in Internal Medicine. Dr. Cooke currently works as part of the University of Michigan Health System and practices in Brighton, MI. In his free time, he enjoys writing, science fiction, and spending time with his family.

Health Reference Series *Update Policy*

The inaugural book in the *Health Reference Series* was the first edition of *Cancer Sourcebook* published in 1989. Since then, the *Series* has been enthusiastically received by librarians and in the medical community. In order to maintain the standard of providing high-quality health information for the layperson the editorial staff at Omnigraphics felt it was necessary to implement a policy of updating volumes when warranted.

Medical researchers have been making tremendous strides, and it is the purpose of the *Health Reference Series* to stay current with the most recent advances. Each decision to update a volume will be made on an individual basis. Some of the considerations will include how much new information is available and the feedback we receive from people who use the books. If there is a topic you would like to see added to the update list, or an area of medical concern you feel has not been adequately addressed, please write to:

Editor
Health Reference Series
Omnigraphics, Inc.
615 Griswold Street
Detroit, MI 48226
E-mail: editorial@omnigraphics.com

Part One

Essential Patient Information about Medical Tests

Chapter 1

Quick Tips when Getting Medical Tests

The single most important way you can stay healthy is to be an active member of your own health care team. One way to get high quality health care is to find and use information and take an active role in all of the decisions made about your care. This information will help you when making decisions about medical tests.

Doctors order blood tests, x-rays, and other tests to help diagnose medical problems. Perhaps you do not know why you need a particular test or you don't understand how it will help you. Here are some questions to ask:

- How is the test done?
- What kind of information will the test provide?
- Is this test the only way to find out that information?
- What are the benefits and risks of having this test?
- How accurate is the test?
- What do I need to do to prepare for the test? (What you do or don't do may affect the accuracy of the test results.)
- Will the test be uncomfortable?
- How long will it take to get the results, and how will I get them?

This chapter includes, "Quick Tips–When Getting Medical Tests," Agency for Healthcare Research and Quality, AHRQ Publication No. 01-0040b, May 2002; and "Speak Up, Help Prevent Errors in Your Care," © Joint Commission on Accreditation of Healthcare Organizations, 2003. Reprinted with permission.

Logansport Cass County Public Library

- What's the next step after the test?

One study found that anywhere from 10 percent to 30 percent of Pap smear test results that were called normal were not normal. Errors such as this can lead to a wrong or delayed diagnosis. You want your tests to be done the right way, and you want accurate results.

What Can You Do?

- For tests your doctor sends to a lab, ask which lab he or she uses, and why. You may want to know that the doctor chooses a certain lab because he or she has business ties to it. Or, the health plan may require that the tests go there.

- Check to see that the lab is accredited by a group such as the College of American Pathologists (800-323-4040) or the Joint Commission on Accreditation of Healthcare Organizations (telephone, 630-792-5800; website, http://www.jcaho.org).

- If you need a mammogram, make sure the facility is approved by the Food and Drug Administration. You can find out by checking the certificate in the facility. Or, call 800-422-6237 (4-CANCER) 9:00 a.m.–4:30 p.m. EST to find out the names and locations of certified facilities near you.

What about the Test Results?

- Do not assume that no news is good news. If you do not hear from your doctor, call to get your test results.

- If you and your doctor think the test results may not be right, have the test done again.

Remember, quality matters, especially when it comes to your health.

Speak Up: Help Prevent Errors in Your Care

Everyone has a role in making health care safe—physicians, health care executives, nurses, and technicians. Health care organizations across the country are working to make health care safety a priority. You, as the patient, can also play a vital role in making your care safe by becoming an active, involved, and informed member of your health care team.

An Institute of Medicine (IOM) report has identified the occurrence of medical errors as a serious problem in the health care system. The IOM recommends, among other things, that a concerted effort be made to improve the public's awareness of the problem.

The "Speak Up" program, sponsored by the Joint Commission on Accreditation of Healthcare Organizations, urges patients to get involved in their care. Such efforts to increase consumer awareness and involvement are supported by the Centers for Medicare and Medicaid Services. This initiative provides simple advice on how you, as the patient, can make your care a positive experience. After all, research shows that patients who take part in decisions about their health care are more likely to have better outcomes. To help prevent health care errors, patients are urged to "Speak Up."

Speak up if you have questions or concerns, and if you don't understand, ask again. It's your body and you have a right to know.

- Your health is too important to worry about being embarrassed if you don't understand something that your doctor, nurse, or other health care professional tells you.

- Don't be afraid to ask about safety. If you're having surgery, for example, ask the doctor to mark the area that is to be operated upon, so that there's no confusion in the operating room.

- Don't be afraid to tell the nurse or the doctor if you think you are about to receive the wrong medication.

- Don't hesitate to tell the health care professional if you think he or she has confused you with another patient.

Pay attention to the care you are receiving. Make sure you're getting the right treatments and medications by the right health care professionals. Don't assume anything.

- Tell your nurse or doctor if something doesn't seem quite right.

- Expect health care workers to introduce themselves when they enter your room and look for their identification badges. A new mother, for example, should know the person to whom she is handing her baby. If you are unsure, ask.

- Notice whether your caregivers have washed their hands. Hand washing is the most important way to prevent the spread of infections. Don't be afraid to gently remind a doctor or nurse to do this.

- Know what time of day you normally receive a medication. If it doesn't happen, bring this to the attention of your nurse or doctor.

- Make sure your nurse or doctor confirms your identity, that is, checks your wristband or asks your name, before he or she administers any medication or treatment.

Educate yourself about your diagnosis, the medical tests you are undergoing, your treatment plan, and exactly what is covered by your health plan.

- Ask your doctor about the specialized training and experience that qualifies him or her to treat your illness (and be sure to ask the same questions of those physicians to whom he or she refers you).

- Gather information about your condition. Good sources include your doctor, your library, respected websites, and support groups.

- Write down important facts your doctor tells you, so that you can look for additional information later. And ask your doctor if he or she has any written information you can keep.

- Ask whether your health plan dictates standardized procedures for certain diseases or medical conditions.

- Be sure you know what procedures are covered or excluded under your health plan and whether your plan will cover your expenses if you schedule a visit with a doctor or hospital outside the network.

- Thoroughly read all medical forms and make sure you understand them before you sign anything. If you don't understand, ask your doctor or nurse to explain them.

Ask a trusted family member or friend to be your advocate.

- Your advocate can ask questions that you may not think of while you are under stress.

- Be sure that you and your advocate know what your rights and responsibilities are under your health plan.

- Ask this person to stay with you, even overnight, when you are hospitalized. You will be able to rest more comfortably and your advocate can help to make sure you get the right medications and treatments.

- Your advocate can also help remember answers to questions you have asked, and speak up for you if you cannot.

- Make sure this person understands your preferences for care and your wishes concerning resuscitation and life support.

- Review consents for treatment with your advocate before you sign them and make sure you both understand exactly what you are agreeing to.

- Make sure your advocate understands the type of care you will need when you get home. Your advocate should know what to look for if your condition is getting worse and whom to call for help.

Know what medications you take and why you take them. Medication errors are the most common health care mistakes.

- Ask about the purpose of the medication and ask for written information about it, including its brand and generic names. Also, inquire about the side effects of the medication.

- If you do not recognize a medication, verify that it is for you. Ask about oral medications before swallowing, and read the contents of bags of intravenous (IV) fluids. If you're not well enough to do this, ask your advocate to do this.

- If you are given an IV, ask the nurse how long it should take for the liquid to run out. Tell the nurse if it doesn't seem to be dripping properly (that it is too fast or too slow).

- Whenever you are going to receive a new medication, tell your doctors and nurses about allergies you have, or negative reactions you have had to medications in the past.

- If you are taking multiple medications, ask your doctor or pharmacist if it is safe to take those medications together. This holds true for vitamins, herbal supplements, and over-the-counter drugs, too.

- Make sure you can read the handwriting on any prescriptions written by your doctor. If you can't read it, the pharmacist may not be able to either.

Use a health plan, hospital, clinic, surgery center, or other type of health care organization that has undergone a rigorous

on-site evaluation against established, state-of-the-art quality and safety standards, such as that provided by JCAHO.

- Ask about the health plan's experience with participants who have your type of illness. The type of health plan you choose may depend upon your medical history and present medical condition.

- If you have more than one hospital or other facility to choose from, ask your doctor which one offers the best care for your condition.

- Before you leave the hospital or other facility, ask about follow-up care and make sure that you understand all of the instructions.

- Go to *Quality Check* at www.jcaho.org to find out whether your health plan and the sites where you will receive care are accredited.

Participate in all decisions about your treatment. You are the center of the health care team.

- You and your doctor should agree on exactly what will be done during each step of your care.

- Know who will be taking care of you, how long the treatment will last, and how you should feel.

- Understand that more tests or medications may not always be better. Ask your doctor what a new test or medication is likely to achieve.

- Keep copies of your medical records from previous treatments or tests and share them with your health care team. This will give them a more complete picture of your health history.

- Don't be afraid to seek a second opinion. If you are unsure about the nature of your illness and the best treatment, consult with one or two additional specialists. The more information you have about the options available to you, the more confident you will be in the decisions made.

- Understand your health plan's appeal and grievance process. This information will be important if a course of treatment is recommended and coverage is denied under your health plan.

- Ask to speak with others who have undergone the procedure you are considering. These individuals can help you prepare for the days and weeks ahead. They also can tell you what to expect and what worked best for them as they recovered.

Additional Information

Joint Commission on Accreditation of Healthcare Organizations
One Renaissance Blvd.
Oakbrook Terrace, IL 60181
Phone: 630-792-5800
Fax: 630-792-5005
Website: www.jcaho.org
E-mail: customerservice@jcaho.org

Chapter 2

Why Doctors Order Lab Tests

A laboratory test is a medical procedure in which a sample of blood, urine, or other tissues or substances in the body is checked for certain features. Such tests are often used as part of a routine checkup to identify possible changes in a person's health before any symptoms appear. Laboratory tests also play an important role in diagnosis when a person has symptoms.

Some laboratory tests are precise, reliable indicators of specific health problems. Others provide more general information that simply gives doctors clues to possible health problems. Information obtained from laboratory tests may help doctors decide whether other tests or procedures are needed to make a diagnosis. The information may also help the doctor develop or revise a patient's treatment plan. All laboratory test results must be interpreted in the context of the overall health of the patient and are generally used along with other exams or tests. The doctor who is familiar with the patient's medical history and current condition is in the best position to explain test results and their implications. Patients are encouraged to discuss questions or concerns about laboratory test results with the doctor.

This chapter includes "Interpreting Laboratory Test Results," Fact Sheet 5.27, National Cancer Institute (NCI), reviewed January 2003; and "Lab Tests," Center for Devices and Radiological Health, U.S. Food and Drug Administration, updated April 2003.

11

Why Does Your Doctor Use Lab Tests?

Your doctor uses laboratory tests to help:

- identify changes in your health condition before any symptoms occur,
- diagnose a disease or condition before you have symptoms,
- plan your treatment for a disease or condition,
- evaluate your response to a treatment, or
- monitor the course of a disease over time.

How Are Lab Tests Analyzed?

After your doctor collects a sample from your body, it is sent to a laboratory. Laboratories perform tests on the sample to see if it reacts to different substances. Depending on the test, a reaction may mean you do have a particular condition or it may mean that you do not have the particular condition. Sometimes laboratories compare your results to results obtained from previous tests to see if there has been a change in your condition.

What Do Lab Tests Show?

Lab tests show whether or not your results fall within normal ranges. Normal test values are usually given as a range, rather than as a specific number, because normal values vary from person to person. What is normal for one person may not be normal for another person.

Some laboratory tests are precise, reliable indicators of specific health problems, while others provide more general information that gives doctors clues to your possible health problems. Information obtained from laboratory tests may help doctors decide whether other tests or procedures are needed to make a diagnosis or to develop or revise a previous treatment plan. All laboratory test results must be interpreted within the context of your overall health and should be used along with other exams or tests.

What Factors Affect Your Lab Test Results?

Many factors can affect test results, including:

- sex

- age
- race
- medical history
- general health
- specific foods
- drugs you are taking
- how closely your follow preparatory instructions
- variations in laboratory techniques
- variation from one laboratory to another

How Can You Get More Information about Lab Tests?

The American Association for Clinical Chemistry (AACC) and other prominent laboratory associations have created a detailed website about clinical lab testing. You can use this website to learn general information about lab tests as well as specific information about lab tests your doctor may prescribe.

American Association for Clinical Chemistry (AACC)
Website: www.labsonline.org

Chapter 3

Identifying Quality Laboratory Services

Selecting quality health care services for yourself, a relative, or friend requires special thought and attention. The Joint Commission on Accreditation of Healthcare Organizations has prepared this information to assist you in making your selection. Knowing what to look for and what to ask will help you choose a laboratory that provides quality care and best meets your needs.

Although you may not always have the opportunity to choose the laboratory where your tests are processed, you can obtain some important information about the laboratory. By doing so, you'll have confidence that your tests will be performed properly.

Begin by asking your physician why he/she selected the laboratory(ies) and the quality improvement processes the laboratory has in place.

Questions to Ask Your Doctor about a Laboratory

About the Laboratory

- Do you know the name and location of the laboratory where your tests are being processed?

- Does the doctor verify the accuracy of the tests? What criteria does the doctor use to choose the laboratory?

"Helping You Identify Quality Laboratory Services," © Joint Commission on Accreditation of Healthcare Organizations, 2003. Reprinted with permission.

- Does the laboratory notify the doctor if a specimen is incorrectly collected? What is the follow-up procedure?

- Has the doctor ever received an incorrect result from the laboratory? How did the doctor handle the situation?

- Can the doctor explain how complaints about inaccurate test results are handled?

About Sample Collection

- Does the laboratory provide the doctor with guidelines outlining the proper collection procedures for specimens? Is this information included in the office staff's orientation and training materials? Is it periodically updated?

- Is the specimen labeled with your full name at the time it is collected? If it's a Pap smear, are the slides sealed at the time they are collected to prevent mislabeling or contamination?

- Were you informed about how to prepare for the lab test (e.g., no eating, drinking)?

- If you are collecting the specimen yourself, did you receive adequate instructions for appropriate collection?

About the Test Results

- Were you told how soon you can expect to learn the test results?

- Were you told how you will be informed of test results? Will there be a personal call if there was an abnormal test result?

- Is there a number you can call if you have questions?

About Accreditation

- Is the laboratory accredited by a nationally recognized accrediting body such as the Joint Commission on Accreditation of Healthcare Organizations? Joint Commission accreditation means the organization voluntarily sought accreditation and met national health and safety standards.

Founded in 1951, the Joint Commission on Accreditation of Healthcare Organizations is an independent, not-for-profit organization that evaluates and accredits nearly 18,000 health care organizations and programs, including ambulatory care centers, behavioral health care organizations, health plans, home care organizations, hospitals, laboratories, long term care facilities, and long term care pharmacies.

Additional Information

Joint Commission on Accreditation of Healthcare Organizations (JCAHO)
One Renaissance Blvd.
Oakbrook Terrace, IL 60181
Phone: 630-792-5000
Fax: 630-792-5005
Website: www.jcaho.org
E-mail: customerservice@jcaho.org

Quality Check™ of JCAHO
Toll-Free Office of Quality Monitoring: 800-994-6610
Customer Service Center: 630-792-5800
Website: www.jcaho.org/qualitycheck/directry/directry.asp
E-mail: complaint@jcaho.org

To find out if the laboratory you are considering is accredited by the Joint Commission, see Quality Check™. Quality Check™ is a comprehensive guide to all Joint Commission accredited health care organizations. It includes an organization's name, address, telephone number, accreditation decision, and accreditation date as well as website and e-mail links, if available.

Quality Check™ also provides performance reports that include information on the organization's overall performance level and how it compares to other organizations nationally in specific performance areas. If a report is not available on Quality Check™ or you would like a printed copy, please call the Customer Service Center.

Chapter 4

Health Insurance

Chapter Contents

Section 4.1

What Is Medical Necessity?

"Illinois Insurance Facts: Medical Necessity," is reprinted
with permission from the Illinois Department of Insurance,
http://www.ins.state.il.us. © 2003 State of Illinois.

Editor's Note: This information was written for citizens of Illinois.
Please contact your state insurance department for local rules about
medical necessity.

Whether you submit a claim after treatment or attempt to pre-
certify a proposed treatment, insurance companies and HMOs will review that claim or pre-certification request to determine if the services
are medically necessary. If the insurance company or HMO determines
the service is not medically necessary, they will deny the claim or pre-
certification request.

Almost all insurance companies and HMOs pay claims based upon
the concept of medical necessity. This section explains what medical
necessity means and how to appeal adverse decisions by your insurer
or HMO.

What Is Medical Necessity?

A sample definition of *Medically Necessary* contained in an insurance policy is:

> *Medically Necessary means that a service, supply, or medicine is*
> *necessary and appropriate and meets the standards of good*
> *medical practice in the medical community for the diagnosis or*
> *treatment of a covered illness or injury, as determined by the in-*
> *surance company.*

If you are a member of an HMO, your primary care physician is
responsible for deciding if a proposed treatment or service is medically necessary. However, the HMO may require the primary care
physician to obtain approval from its medical director.

Examples of hospitalizations and other health care services and supplies that are not considered medically necessary include:

- Inpatient hospitalizations for treatment that could be safely and adequately provided on an outpatient basis;
- Continued inpatient hospital care, when the patient's medical symptoms and condition no longer required a continued stay in the hospital;
- Cosmetic surgery;
- Treatment provided for the convenience of the patient, such as an elective caesarean section;
- An advanced procedure or treatment provided without first trying less invasive, less expensive treatments.

Insurance companies and HMOs exclude coverage for treatment that is not medically necessary because they do not want to pay for unnecessary treatment. The problem is that medical necessity is a judgment call. Just because your doctor prescribes a treatment or procedure, it does not mean the insurance company or HMO will agree it is medically necessary.

Most major medical policies and all HMOs require that you pre-authorize elective inpatient hospital stays and major surgical procedures. Failure to pre-authorize the service can result in a penalty or denial of the claim. If your policy requires pre-authorization, follow the proper procedure so you know whether or not coverage is available. If your policy does not require pre-authorization of the service, you will not know if it is covered until the claim is submitted.

Note: Preauthorization by an insurance company is not a guarantee that benefits will be paid. All policy provisions, such as preexisting condition waiting periods apply. Additionally, benefits are only payable if you are eligible for coverage on the date the service is provided.

How to Appeal a Denial Due to Medical Necessity

If an insurer or HMO denies a pre-authorization request or a claim due to lack of medical necessity, you may appeal the decision.

For HMOs: Appeal procedures for HMOs are set forth within the *Managed Care Reform and Patient Rights Act.* You or your physician can file an oral or written appeal with the HMO. The Act requires an

HMO to render a decision on an appeal for urgently needed treatment within 24 hours after submission of the appeal. All other appeals must be handled within 15 business days of receipt of all necessary information. If the appeal is denied, you are entitled to an external independent review. You, your physician, and the HMO select the independent reviewer jointly. The decision of the independent reviewer is final.

For insurance companies: There are no state laws or rules governing appeals to insurance companies. The federal ERISA regulations do provide some appeals procedure requirements. To find out if your plan is protected by those regulations, refer to your plan document. Most companies have an appeal procedure that requires a medical director to review appeals of medical necessity denials. You should ask your doctor to write a letter to the company explaining why the treatment is medically necessary. The appeal should include pertinent medical records. State law does not require an insurance company to grant you an external independent review. If your appeal is denied, you may contact the Department of Insurance for assistance. Although the Department of Insurance is unable to review your medical records and make medical determinations, we can contact the company and request the highest level of review of the claim or pre-authorization request. If the matter is not resolved through this process, it is possible you may have to seek remedy through the legal system where a judge can make the decision.

Section 4.2

Insure Kids Now Initiative

This section includes "Insure Kids Now! A National Initiative to Linking Families to Low-Cost Insurance Programs," 2003; and "Questions and Answers," found at www.insurekidsnow.gov, Health Resources and Services Administration, U.S. Department of Health and Human Services, 2003.

Your Children May Be Eligible for Free or Low-Cost Health Insurance

You work hard to provide for your children and want to make sure they grow up strong, smart, and healthy. But like many parents whose children don't have health insurance, you worry about taking care of them.

Now, you may have one less thing to worry about. Your state, and every state in the nation, has a health insurance program for infants, children, and teens. The insurance is available to children in working families, including families that include individuals with a variety of immigration status. (Materials are available that explain more about immigration and children's health insurance.)

For little or no cost, this insurance pays for:

- doctor visits,
- hospitalizations, and
- prescription medicines,
- much more.

Kids that do not currently have health insurance are likely to be eligible, even if you are working. The states have different eligibility rules, but in most states, uninsured children 18 years old and younger, whose families earn up to $34,100 a year (for a family of four) are eligible.

Questions and Answers about the Insure Kids Now Initiative

I need health insurance for my children. What are my options?

Call 877-543-7669 or go to www.insurekidsnow.gov on the Internet. When you call the free and confidential hotline, you will be directly

23

connected to your state's program that provides either free or low-cost health insurance for children. The states have different eligibility rules, but in most states, uninsured children 18 years old and younger whose families earn up to $34,100 a year (for a family of four) are eligible.

Is there a limit on the amount of time my child can remain enrolled?

Your child can stay on the program as long as he or she qualifies. Although there is no limit on the amount of time your child can remain on the program, you will need to renew their coverage periodically, generally every 6 to 12 months. As long as your children continue to meet the eligibility criteria established by your state, they can remain on the program.

What services does the insurance cover?

For little or no cost, this insurance pays for doctor visits, prescription medicines, hospitalizations, and much more. Most states also cover the cost of dental care, eye care, and medical equipment.

Is this program new?

In 1997 Congress passed legislation that allows states to provide health insurance to more children in working families. These programs build on the Medicaid program that started covering children and adults in the mid-1960s.

Is this a welfare program?

Children's health insurance programs are not welfare programs. Everyone has a stake in making sure America's children are healthy. These programs are designed to support working families and low-income families alike in providing health insurance to their children.

Why is health insurance for children and teens important?

Children who have health insurance generally have better health throughout their childhood and into their teens. They are more likely to:

- Receive needed shots that prevent disease;
- Get treatment for recurring illnesses such as ear infections and asthma;

- Get preventative care to keep them well;
- Get sick less often; and
- Get the treatment they need when they are sick.

How does having health insurance affect my child's ability to learn?

Children who have health insurance have a better chance of being healthy. Having health insurance will allow you to give them the medical care necessary for them to stay healthy and focus on their studies. Children with health insurance are less likely to miss school because they are sick. By helping them go to school every day ready to learn, you can help boost your child's performance in school today and in the future.

How will having insurance help my child stay healthy?

You'll be able to pick a doctor for your child and see that doctor every time your child gets sick, without having to worry about how you are going to pay for it. Your child can get immunizations and well-child visits required to attend school and play sports. If your child gets sick, you can get prescription medicines to help him or her get better fast. Finally, you won't have to sit for hours in the emergency room when your child has an illness that could be easily treated in your doctor's office.

How much does it cost?

Health insurance provided to children through these programs is free or low-cost. The costs are different depending on the state and your family's income, but when there are charges they are minimal.

Who pays for these health insurance programs?

Your tax dollars fund these state and federally sponsored programs. The state and federal governments want to help working families like yours protect their children's health and future. In some states you may need to pay a premium or co-payment for your children's health insurance.

Who can qualify for health insurance?

Most states cover children up to their nineteenth birthday with family incomes of up to $34,100 a year (for a family of four). Some states cover children whose families have higher incomes. Your income and family size will determine whether or not your children qualify.

Is coverage available for my entire family?

Depending on your income and the state you live in, it may be possible for your entire family to receive health insurance.

I have teenagers. Are they eligible, too?

Yes! In most states, children from birth until their nineteenth birthday can receive free or low-cost health insurance. Remember each state has its own program name.

I have a job. Can my children still qualify?

Children's health insurance is not a welfare program. The majority of children covered by this health insurance come from working families. Many working families, who cannot afford or whose children are not covered by the employer sponsored health insurance or other private health insurance, may be eligible.

Who can apply for health insurance for my child?

In addition to parents, in many states, grandparents and legal guardians can also enroll children in their care for free or low-cost health insurance.

What if my children are covered by Medicaid already?

If your children are currently on Medicaid, they already have comprehensive health insurance. If you are having trouble seeing a doctor or getting a needed service, please contact your caseworker or call your state's Medicaid line.

What if my state tells me that my children are eligible for Medicaid but I don't want to enroll them in Medicaid? Can I qualify for another insurance program?

Children eligible for Medicaid are not eligible to enroll in the newly developed state program. Medicaid provides comprehensive health benefits for children. If you think your child may qualify for Medicaid, please call the toll-free hotline 1-877-KIDS NOW to discuss your questions and concerns with someone from your state.

How do I apply?

In most states, you can complete a short application and send it through the mail.

Is it hard to apply?

Most states have made it very easy to apply for health insurance for your children, often the application is very short. In most states you can complete the application through the mail or over the phone without having to take time off of work. If you have trouble filling out the application, you can ask for help by calling 1-877-KIDS NOW.

Do I have to give my Social Security number to get health insurance for my child?

No. Parents and other household members cannot be required to give their social security numbers to get health insurance for their children. You may be asked to provide social security numbers for your children that are applying for coverage.

Do I have to give information about my immigration status in order to get health insurance for my children?

No. Parents and other household members do not have to give any information about their immigration status to get health insurance for their children. You may be asked to list the people in your household. This information is used to determine the size of your family. You will only have to provide immigration status information for those children that are applying for coverage.

What other information will I have to provide to get health insurance for my children?

Even if you don't have to give information about your immigration status or your Social Security number, you still will have to give information about your family's income. In some states, you also may be asked to provide proof of your family's income, your costs for childcare, or when your child was last covered by health insurance.

I'm applying to become a U.S. citizen. Can I still apply for health insurance for my children without affecting my chances of becoming a citizen or my children's chances?

Yes, you can apply for health insurance for your children without affecting either your chances or your child's chances of becoming a U.S. citizen. Government medical benefits that pay for your child's immunizations, doctor and clinic visits, short-term hospital care, prescriptions, and many other health needs will not be considered by immigration officers.

Section 4.3

How to Handle Denied Requests for Insurance Coverage

This section includes "My Insurance Claim Was Denied; What to Do" and "Types of Insurance Denials." Reprinted with permission from the website of Ernst & Mattison, Inc., www.ernst-mattison.com. Copyright 2002. Ernst & Mattison, a Law Corporation.

Types of Insurance Denials

Insurance companies deny paying benefits for a variety of reasons that are sometimes misleading, often incorrect, and occasionally done in bad faith. You usually learn that your insurance claim has been denied by a form called an Explanation of Benefits (EOB). The EOB will usually contain an itemization of covered and noncovered charges as well as a set of corresponding codes that refer you to a guide either on the bottom or the back of the form. These so-called explanations are difficult to interpret, even by those in the field, and should not necessarily be taken at face value or as the final word.

Although insurance companies are required to provide meaningful and understandable information on claim denials by law, often the first time you learn that your claim has not been paid is when the hospital contacts you to pay the entire bill. In that case it is always important to find out exactly what the hospital has been told as the reason the insurance will not pay the claim.

Don't overlook the possibility that a simple error took place, i.e., inappropriate medical code assigned to your case, dates of coverage don't match the dates of service, misstated service, accounting errors, etc.

The following seem to be the most common reasons claims are denied and they can often be challenged:

- Not medically necessary
- Preexisting conditions
- Noncovered benefit
- Termination of coverage
- Failure to obtain preauthorization
- Out of network provider
- Could have been provided at a lesser level of care

Not Medically Necessary

This reason is often given by insurance companies even though the person that supposedly reviewed your claim has never seen the patient and quite often is not a licensed physician or other medical practitioner. Variations on this theme include "treatment could have been provided in a less restrictive setting" or "treatment could have been performed at a lesser level of care." All these really say is that a third party reviewer (not to be confused necessarily with "independent") in some distant office, usually being compensated by the insurance company, has determined that the treating physician was somehow incorrect in his treatment course. The proper response to such a denial is to write an appeal letter outlining the reasons this treatment was medically necessary stressing the fact that this decision was made by a doctor personally familiar with the patient and based on the individual circumstances of your case. If unsuccessful, you may wish to seek legal action.

Preexisting Condition

This frequently used explanation to deny a claim is often incorrect when compared to the actual language of the preexisting clause of the policy. These clauses vary dramatically from policy to policy, sometimes going back six to twelve months while others apply lifetime.

Another distinction is that some policies require that the condition actually be diagnosed and treated in order to trigger the clause, while others simply require the existence of symptoms that would cause a reasonable person to seek treatment. Legal analysis of your policy language in light of the facts of your particular case may be required in order to determine if the preexisting clause is applicable. In any event, an insurance company may have the right to rescind a policy, before or after a claim arises, if the applicant/insured failed to disclose material facts relating to the risk of which she or he had knowledge. (Ins. Code Sections 331, 338, 359.) An applicant is only required to answer questions to the best of his/her knowledge. How do you know what is important? Answer this: if the company had been aware of the circumstances, would they have issued the policy?

Noncovered Benefit

Insurance policies all contain a list and description of items that are covered as well as a list of those that are excluded. The definitions used in the actual policy language are often so vague to be of no practical use. Many courts have held that overly broad and vague descriptions of policy exclusions cannot be used to deny claims. Legal involvement may be needed in evaluating the legal impact of the medical terms your company uses compared to your actual situation.

Termination of Coverage

We often see this explanation in the context of extended hospitalizations for treatment of mental conditions and substance abuse. Frequently an employer will learn that an employee had previously sought treatment for such a condition or supposedly related and attempt to retroactively terminate their coverage. This would have to be based upon a falsification of the initial application. Here the carrier must show that they detrimentally relied upon an incorrect application response and would not have issued coverage or would have made it a preexisting exclusion. When coverage is terminated back to its inception many times all premiums paid must be refunded. Oftentimes carriers try to relate employment back to the last day the person was physically present at work. This is sometimes done without the knowledge of the employee and when the hospital telephones the insurance company to verify coverage, it is told that the person is covered. Depending on the federal circuit, the hospital would have a right to enforce coverage according to the benefits it relied upon during the admissions process. The location of the hospital, the employer, the employee, and the insurance company are all relevant in determining which federal circuit or circuits would apply in such a circumstance and if this has happened to you, legal intervention may enforce payment of the claim.

Failure to Obtain Preauthorization

These days many insurance companies require either the individual or the hospital to call an 800 number on the insurance card in order to obtain prior authorization of a particular treatment. Occasionally, this cannot be done due to an emergency situation, which can be a subjective term. A potential problem is communication difficulties between your doctor and the insurance company's representative. Treatment cannot always be delayed while waiting for busy medical professionals to reach each other on the telephone. Usually there is no reason why a claim for a particular treatment cannot be evaluated after the fact to determine its medical appropriateness and eligibility for coverage.

Even when claims are paid, penalties are often applied when preauthorization was not obtained. If the failure to obtain precertification was due to either a medical emergency or other problems that are not the fault of you or your doctor, these penalties can usually be waived. When requesting a retrospective review of a claim it is always important to explain the circumstances surrounding it, taking care to point out information that might not be evident by simply reading the claim forms and medical record.

Out of Network Provider

This is usually encountered in situations involving a medical emergency or when the appropriate type of specialist or specialized treatment cannot be provided in a particular locale. The policy itself may have definitions that come into play in determining what is a medical emergency and what is required when the type of treatment you are seeking is not available in a particular location. When the practicality of a situation prevents you from seeking treatment from a provider on your plan's list, it must be pointed out to your insurance company. Again, penalties and reduced coverage to the provider should be fought when they are inappropriate, and often the policy's own language can be used against the insurance company if it is too vague to understand or if they have failed to adhere to their own contract.

Could Have Been Provided at a Lesser Level of Care

Normally associated with mental health providers. Normally all charges are paid as contracted except for the facility. The psychiatrist is paid but the hospital is not. Nor is the hospital paid for therapies or medications that would have been utilized even at a lower level of care. This is often a catch-all denial where the insurer is not comfortable with denying it for medical necessity reasons which could easily be overturned.

My Insurance Claim Was Denied

If you have a policy, know it. Read your evidence of coverage (which is your contract with your insurance provider) and carefully assess how the plan could be interpreted in your favor or in your insurance provider's favor. Be familiar with any appeals process. Make sure you have the entire policy or coverage booklet and all of the endorsements. Now read them. Increasingly, these documents are written in language an average person can follow. You will often find that your claim is covered under the policy for some reason which had not occurred to you. If you don't have these documents, the company must provide them.

Request an explanation from your insurance provider for any denial—and get it in writing. Make the call. Some experts say that up to half of the claims initially rejected are paid upon review. The Insurance Code requires that the company must give you the basis for the denial of your claim in writing. Demand that they do so and compare the reasons given with the policy or coverage booklet. Often the solution to your problem will become obvious at this point. Many errors are corrected at this stage by, for example, providing a letter from your doctor or other evidence which might cause the claims adjuster to change his or her mind. The company must provide you with any personal information, like lab tests or medical records, they relied on in denying your claim.

Carefully document everything. Good notes help you remember what was said, will aid anyone who tries to help you, and can be used to support your case in the event you need legal assistance. Keep notes of each telephone conversation or other contact you have with the people working on your claim. Keep track of the date, time, identity, and title of each person involved. This will avoid having to tell the story twice, personalizes your case, and helps make sure you're speaking with someone who has the power to help you. Always keep correspondence and put your communications in writing so the company cannot ignore you or pretend that you have not pressed your claim. If you are given an opinion, request that it be provided in writing. Follow-up all oral contacts with the company with a letter ("As we discussed today..."). Send everything by certified mail. This will avoid the possibly of a company saying the correspondence was not received.

Educate yourself about your condition. Ask your doctor(s) for support and assistance. Don't be shy. A denial may be something as simple as an incorrect medical code assigned to your file. Request your doctor write a letter for you explaining why the claim should be covered, or why the company's reason for denying the claim is incorrect.
Remember:

- State your questions/requests clearly and concisely; don't allow a misunderstanding to come between you and what you want.

- Stick to the subject at hand; no one cares about what happened during your Aunt Tilly's operation.

- Remain firm, don't be intimidated. If your claim has been rejected, you have a right to find out why.

Additional Information

Center for Health Care Rights
520 S. Lafayette Park Place
Suite 214
Los Angeles, CA 90057
Toll-Free: 800-824-0780
Phone: 213-383-4519
Fax: 213-383-4598
Website: www.healthcarerights.org
E-mail: center@healthcarerights.org

Citizen Action
1730 Rhode Island Ave. N.W.
Suite 403
Washington, DC 20036
Phone: 202-775-1580
Fax: 202-296-4054

Consumer Insurance Advocates Association
402 Edgemere
Garland, TX 75043
Phone: 972-613-9432
Website: www.ciaaoftexas.com
E-mail: consultants@ciaaoftexas.com

Ernst & Mattison, A Law Corporation
1020 Palm Street, San Luis Obispo, CA 93401
P.O. Box 1327
San Luis Obispo, CA 93406
Phone: 805-541-0300
Fax: 805-541-5168
Website: www.ernst-mattison.com

Families USA Foundation
1334 G St. N.W., Suite 300
Washington, DC 20005
Phone: 202-628-3030
Fax: 202-347-2417
Website: www.familiesusa.org
E-mail: info@familiessusa.org

National Committee for Quality Assurance
2000 L St. N.W., Suite 500
Washington, DC 2003
Toll-Free: 888-275-7585
Phone: 202-955-3500
Website: www.ncqa.org/index.asp

State, County, and City Government Consumer Protection Offices
Website: pueblo.gsa.gov/crh/state.htm

Chapter 5

Self-Ordered Tests

Contents

Section 5.1

Ordering Your Own Lab Tests

This section includes excerpts from "FAQs," reprinted with permission of HealthcheckUSA. © 2003 HealthcheckUSA. All rights reserved. For additional information, visit www.healthcheckusa.com. Also, an excerpt from "Home Diagnostic Tests: The Ultimate House Call?" *FDA Consumer*, November-December 2001, U.S. Food and Drug Administration.

Frequently Asked Questions about Self-Ordered Lab Tests

What is a laboratory test?

A laboratory test is a health screening service that can determine many things about your health that may otherwise go undetected. The tests that you order are the same medically accepted lab tests ordered by physicians. A small sample of your blood is tested by a fully accredited medical reference laboratory, and then analyzed for the tests that have been requested by you or your doctor.

Why are these tests useful?

A regular physical examination helps to determine your level of health that a doctor can see, hear, or touch, such as vision, hearing, weight, respiratory functions, etc. A laboratory test provides additional information about your health that cannot be measured in such a way. Test results keep you and your doctor informed about health issues that may otherwise be overlooked.

Will my insurance pay for this test?

Some insurance plans will reimburse you if it is written in the plan as a preventive coverage with no doctor's script. Other insurance plans will reimburse you if you have a doctor's written script. Call your insurance company's toll-free number to find out in advance.

Are these tests covered by Medicare/Medicaid?

No. Only the laboratory that performs the analysis can be reimbursed by Medicare. If you are a Medicare patient, you must have a doctor's order, your doctor must have a Medicare number, and your doctor must provide a diagnostic code accepted by Medicare.

I am healthy—why do I need a test?

Knowledge of your blood's chemistry is your best defense against degenerative disease. A simple blood test can indicate what is happening long before any symptoms of disease occur. Similar to a warning indicator on your automobile, your blood profile is one of the best warning indicators now known to medicine. When blood tests reveal abnormalities, it is urgent to reverse the warnings as quickly as possible to avert the danger of degenerative disease. Even a test result that is normal is useful: not only does it help to rule out potential problem areas, it establishes a baseline of normal ranges against which future tests can be monitored. When you understand these tests and the role blood plays in your body, you can keep your test values within normal ranges through diet, exercise, and proper nutrition. When you visit your physician, a history of laboratory reports that you have kept can often provide the clue to a proper diagnosis.

Are these tests accurate?

Yes—a fully accredited medical reference laboratory analyzes all test results.

Why do I need a complete blood count (CBC)?

A CBC is the most frequently performed lab test. It provides a great deal of information about the three kinds of cells in the blood—red blood cells, white blood cells, and platelets. It is most frequently used as a screening test, as an anemia check, and as a test for infection, but it is also used to aid in the diagnosis and treatment of a large number of other conditions. Included in the CBC are hematocrit, hemoglobin, red blood cell count, red blood cell indices, white blood cell count, white blood cell differential, and platelet count.

Why do I need a thyroid profile?

The thyroid is one of the most important glands in the body. This hormone regulates the metabolism of the body by increasing the rate of the reactions taking place in the body's cells. The test is used to evaluate the symptoms of excess (hyperthyroidism) such as unexplained weight loss, tremor, nervousness, rapid heart rate, diarrhea, or the sensation of always being too hot. Symptoms of too little thyroid hormone (hypothyroidism) are unexplained weight gain, tiredness, dry skin, or the sensation of always being too cold.

How do I take a test?

Choose which lab test you wish to take from those offered through online or mail-order services, select the most convenient laboratory location, fill out the client information profile, and select your method of payment. You will be sent a personalized requisition form by first class mail to take to your selected laboratory location. The technician at the laboratory will draw a small sample of your blood for testing. As you have prepaid for this service, no further payment will be required at the laboratory.

Do I need to fast before taking a test?

To ensure absolute accuracy, a ten-hour fast is recommended. Black coffee and water are permitted during your period of fast.

How can I contact someone if I have questions about my test results?

Any questions regarding significant findings or abnormal levels should be discussed with your doctor.

Can I take the results to my doctor for a diagnosis?

Yes—the tests that you order are the same medically accepted lab tests ordered by physicians, and your doctor will be able to discuss them with you. Your doctor will use these results in conjunction with your history and may even decide to order additional tests to confirm the results of any abnormalities.

What do abnormal test results mean?

Abnormalities should be considered as an early warning system alerting you that it is necessary to reverse the condition immediately. To bring your test values back to within normal ranges, your doctor may suggest a change in diet, exercise, and nutrition.

How does the physician interpretation work?

Once you have your blood drawn, your results are sent directly to you as usual. If you elect to have your results reviewed by a board certified physician, you will also receive instructions on how to access the interpretation of your results. By calling a toll-free number and using your user identification number and personal identification number (provided with instructions), you will have access to your personal interpretation. Interpretations are usually available 72 hours after your blood draw.

What is the proper use of drug screenings?

Self-ordered drug tests are for screening purposes only. Positives have not been confirmed for legal use and specimens have not been collected under legal guidelines for secure collection, therefore, results cannot be used for employment or other legal reasons. Although a negative result indicates no drugs were detected above the method's cutoff level, other methods may be used to detect lower levels of the drugs in the urine. Results can also be affected by the amount of urine excreted, weight or body type of person taking drug, acidity or alkalinity (pH) of urine, and frequency of drug taken.

Home Diagnostic Tests: The Ultimate House Call?

See Your Doctor, Too

While convenience, confidentiality, and the cost-saving benefits of self-ordered or home testing cannot be overlooked, doctors are concerned about the availability of medical tests that encourage self-diagnosis because of the possibility that the results could be mis-interpreted and treatment might be delayed.

Those who rely on self-ordered or home tests also miss out on pre- and post-test counseling, which offer information, support, competence, interpretation, and follow-up advice to consumers that only a health care professional can give. The benefit of having a health care professional involved in a test or screening procedure is that the results can be evaluated within the context of the whole health picture, not just one test. Furthermore, receiving news of potential pregnancy, illness, or infection over the phone, or from the color of a test strip, can be devastating.

"The first 72 hours following a positive result for an illness as serious as HIV is when people are most likely to hurt themselves," says

Edward Geraty, a licensed clinical social worker with Behavioral Science Associates in Baltimore. Geraty says it's important to have a face-to-face relationship when delivering the news of a positive HIV test. Without it, he says, "there's a psychological component of the person's illness that is completely left out of the process."

Bob Barret, Ph.D., agrees. A professor of counseling at the University of North Carolina at Charlotte, Barret believes that self-ordered or home test kits, particularly for HIV, "are best used only by those who are well-educated about the disease, and who are in touch with their emotions and have a good support system around them."

Section 5.2

Whole Body Scanning Using Computed Tomography

"Whole Body CT Screening—Should I or Shouldn't I Get One?" Center for Devices and Radiological Health, U.S. Food and Drug Administration, updated April 2002.

Whole-body CT screening—should I or shouldn't I get one?

If you have no symptoms of illness but are considering getting a whole-body CT screening exam, you may be thinking either or both of the following:

- "For my peace of mind, I just want to know that I don't have any diseases now."

- "If I have a disease, I want to know about it now so that I can do something about it."

What you may not realize is that getting a whole-body CT screening exam may not accomplish either of these goals. In particular, an abnormal finding may not be a serious finding at all. And a normal finding may be inaccurate. We will consider these one at a time, but before we do, the good news is that if you have no symptoms of illness the probability is high that there is nothing seriously wrong with you—and this is true without your ever getting a whole-body CT screening exam.

Should you be screened? Like any other medical procedure, there are risks involved. Before undergoing this exam, be sure to read about the procedure. Consider further that the FDA has never approved CT for screening any part of the body for any specific disease, let alone for screening the whole body when there are no specific symptoms of disease at all. No manufacturer has submitted data to FDA to support the safety and efficacy of screening claims for whole-body CT screening.

What is a screening exam?

A screening exam is a medical exam that is performed on individuals who are at risk for a particular disease or condition, but who lack any signs or symptoms of the disease or condition, to determine if the disease or condition is present. Common examples of screening procedures are:

- mammography for breast cancer in women over 40 years of age
- Pap smear for cervical cancer in women over 18 or sexually active
- colonoscopy for colon cancer in men and women over 50
- blood pressure measurement for hypertension in anyone
- measuring blood sugar for diabetes in anyone

As the examples illustrate, screening exams are generally done to look for a particular disease or condition, and they should generally be done only when clinical studies have demonstrated that screening exams may do more good than harm.

Is CT the best way to screen for any disease or condition?

At this time, no—although there are trials currently in process to determine if:

1. spiral CT might be a useful method to screen for lung cancer in smokers of particular ages,

2. CT virtual colonoscopy is as good as colonoscopy in men and women over 50, and

41

3. CT coronary calcium scoring is effective in predicting heart disease.

Some diseases that do have effective treatments can be found early enough with tests other than CT. For example, though this has again become controversial, screening mammography has been shown to find breast cancer early enough in many cases to be curable, but CT has not been found to have such capability. Similar results have been found for Pap smears for cervical cancer and colonoscopy for colon cancer. There are also diseases and conditions, other than cancer, for which early treatment, even if the disease were identified, would be no more effective than when treated later, at least with treatments currently available. And there are significant diseases that cannot be seen on CT, such as diabetes and hypertension.

When is screening beneficial?

Screening tests can be extremely beneficial, but only under the following conditions:

- when the test is for a particular disease or condition, rather than for just anything that can be found,

- when the test is for a disease or condition that is curable or manageable if found early enough, but life-threatening by the time symptoms arise,

- when the test can find that disease or condition early enough to be curable or manageable,

- when the test doesn't reveal too many findings that resemble the disease or condition which in reality would not hurt you,

- when the test doesn't miss too many cases of the disease or condition,

- when the test itself doesn't harm you significantly, and

- when the treatment for the disease or condition doesn't cause more harm than the disease or condition itself.

As mentioned, examples of such screening tests are mammography, Pap smears, colonoscopy, and blood pressure measurement. Although there are ongoing clinical studies of CT to see if there is more benefit than harm for some diseases and conditions, at this time, there is no disease for which CT has been shown to satisfy the preceding conditions.

When is CT beneficial?

CT can be extremely beneficial when a person has signs or symptoms of some particular disease or condition. CT can help to diagnose or rule out the disease or condition. Furthermore, in someone diagnosed with some particular disease or condition, CT can be extremely helpful in determining the extent of disease and in monitoring the effects of treatment. Such diagnostic use of CT in people with signs or symptoms differs from the use of CT in screening of people with no signs or symptoms. People with symptoms have a much higher probability of having the disease or condition than people without symptoms. Also, people with symptoms probably have more advanced disease than someone without symptoms, which makes it easier to find the disease on CT. The result is that in a group of people with signs or symptoms, the probability of a true finding of actual disease is much higher, while the probability of a finding of something harmless that is mistaken for disease is much lower.

What are the risks and benefits of whole-body CT screening?

Many people believe incorrectly that a medical test always distinguishes between the abnormal and the normal, the sick and the well, or the diseased and the non-diseased. Every test does this only in some cases, and you can rely on the fact that every test, including CT, gives incorrect results a certain portion of the time.

To understand the risks and benefits of whole-body CT screening, it is perhaps easiest to divide the results of the exam into two possible outcomes, normal and abnormal.

If your CT examination result is interpreted as normal, either

- you may really have nothing significant wrong with you, or

- you may have a hidden disease that fails to show up on a CT image or is missed or misinterpreted by the radiologist.

If your CT examination result is interpreted as abnormal, either

- the abnormal interpretation may be incorrect or you may have nothing significant wrong with you, or

- you may really have a life-threatening disease for which there may or may not be a cure and, if a cure exists, there may or may not be time to do something that can cure it.

43

Consider these possibilities one at a time. If you receive a normal report and there really is nothing significant wrong with you, then you might go away with peace of mind, but you will have exposed yourself to radiation and its associated risks. The radiation exposure of a CT exam can be several hundred times that of a chest x-ray. Not only might this amount of radiation exposure give you a slightly increased chance of getting cancer, but also, if large numbers of healthy people now start to receive radiation exposure from whole-body CT screening for questionable benefit, the overall effect on public health could be detrimental. This would be detrimental all the more so if people were to receive this examination repeatedly, on a regular basis.

If you receive a normal report but a life-threatening disease is really present, then you will have received false reassurance that could interfere with your recognizing symptoms or getting appropriate screening tests later. In addition, you will have exposed yourself to radiation from which you derived no benefit.

If your CT screening result is interpreted as abnormal and there really is nothing significant wrong with you, then you may be subjected to still further tests or treatments, all of which have their own risks. For example, further tests may bring about additional radiation exposure and the small chance of toxicity from contrast material needed for visualization, or the bleeding, infection, and potential disfigurement associated with biopsy or exploratory surgery. And treatments may include surgery, radiation, chemotherapy, or medicines, each with its own small risks of injury, toxicity, or even death. The surprising fact about a CT interpretation of abnormality when there is nothing significant wrong is that it is far more likely to happen to you than the finding of any actual life-threatening disease, since the likelihood that you actually have any deadly disease is so small to begin with.

Finally, if your CT is interpreted as abnormal and the abnormality represents an actual hidden, life-threatening disease, then you may have benefited. The benefit will be real only if:

- the disease has an effective treatment, and

- it is found early enough to benefit from this treatment.

Many life-threatening diseases do not have effective treatments, or, if they do, the period in which the treatment might have worked may have passed already.

In summary, when possible risks are compared to the possible benefits, the harms currently appear to be both far more likely and in some cases may not be insignificant. These harms are:

1. radiation exposure which has a small risk of cancer induction for an individual CT procedure, and

2. the possibility of either a false finding of an abnormality or a true finding of an insignificant abnormality, either of which could lead to further harm.

So, if you are apparently healthy, the good news is that the probability is already high that there is nothing seriously wrong with you, without ever getting a whole-body CT screening exam.

Part Two

Age-Specific Health Screenings, Preventive Tests, and Exams

Chapter 6

Genetic and Metabolic Screening of Newborn Infants

Newborn Screening

Newborn screening is recognized internationally as an essential, preventive public health program for early identification of disorders in newborns that can affect their long term health. Early detection, diagnosis, and treatment of certain genetic, metabolic, or infectious congenital disorders can lead to significant reductions of death, disease, and associated disabilities.

History

Newborn screening programs in the U.S. began with the work of Dr. Robert Guthrie, who in the 1960s developed a screening test for phenylketonuria. When Dr. Guthrie also introduced a system for collection and transportation of blood samples on filter paper, cost effective wide-scale genetic screening became possible.

The federal Maternal and Child Health Bureau (MCHB), a branch of the Health Resources and Services Administration (HRSA) has been involved in the evolution of newborn screening from the beginning,

---

This chapter includes "Overview of National Newborn Screening," © 2003 and "U.S. National Screening Status Report," © 2003 which are reprinted with permission from the National Newborn Screening and Genetics Resource Center (NNSGRC). For more information, contact the NNSGRC at 1912 W. Anderson Lane, Suite 210, Austin, TX 78757, 512-454-6419, or visit their website at http://genes-r-us.uthscsa.edu.

and it now funds many different activities dedicated to strengthening and expanding newborn screening programs.

Current Status and Scope

States routinely test blood spots collected from newborns for up to thirty metabolic and genetic diseases of which the four most commonly included are phenylketonuria (PKU), congenital hypothyroidism (CH), galactosemia (GAL), and sickle cell disease (SS, SC, etc.). Many states are also tasked with providing follow-up to infants identified through newborn screening programs, including ensuring appropriate diagnosis, treatment, and ongoing evaluation. In many cases, education (professional and consumer) is also a program responsibility along with counseling and provision of other ancillary services.

The panel of newborn disorders screened for varies from state to state, and decisions for adding or deleting tests involve many complex social, ethical, and political issues. Usually, newborn population screening disorders are tied to issues such as disorder prevalence, detectability, treatment availability, outcome, and overall cost effectiveness. It is possible to screen for many disorders at birth and soon more will be possible. Currently, improvements in tandem mass spectrometry screening procedures allow detection of up to 30 additional metabolic disorders.

The role and scope of newborn screening is expanding. While traditional newborn screening was only concerned with a few inborn errors that led to mental retardation, programs now include disorders that can cause premature death, infectious diseases, hearing disorders, and even heart problems.

Future Challenges

In the last decade many technological changes have occurred that have the potential for improving the sensitivity, specificity, and scope of newborn screening services. DNA research and the human genome project have the potential for allowing genotyping, not only as a secondary confirmation of many newborn screening conditions as is now the case, but also as a routine primary screen. It may also soon be possible to detect many adult onset disorders at birth.

As technology improves, the definition of screening shifts closer to diagnosis and in the wake of these advances, it is essential that public health policy makers take advantage of opportunities for newborn screening program improvement in a timely and effective way. To that end, a National Newborn Screening Task Force, organized by the

American Academy of Pediatrics and funded by the Health Resources and Services Administration, was convened to review the issues and challenges faced by newborn screening programs, and to offer recommendations to strengthen and standardize these programs.

Routine Disorders Included in Newborn Screening (Listed in Alphabetical Order)

Biotinidase Deficiency

Biotinidase deficiency is caused by the lack of an enzyme called biotinidase, resulting in an inability to liberate biotin from a bound form so that it can be used by the body. Without sufficient biotin, several other critical enzyme systems are unable to function properly. Biotinidase deficiency can lead to seizures, developmental delay, eczema, and hearing loss. Newborns with the disorder appear normal, but develop critical symptoms after the first weeks or months of life. Symptoms include hypotonia, ataxia, seizures, developmental delay, hair loss, seborrheic dermatitis, hearing loss, and optic nerve atrophy. Metabolic acidosis can result in coma and death. Biotinidase deficiency is treated with daily biotin supplement, and with early diagnosis and treatment, all symptoms can be prevented.

Congenital Adrenal Hyperplasia (CAH)

CAH is a group of disorders caused by the deficiency of an adrenal enzyme resulting in decreased cortisol (and sometimes aldosterone) production. Without sufficient cortical and aldosterone the affected newborn may appear normal, but can quickly develop symptoms including lethargy, vomiting, muscle weakness, and dehydration. In severe cases, death may occur within a few weeks if left untreated. Infants with milder forms of the disorder are at risk for reproductive and growth difficulties. If detected early and maintained on appropriate doses of medication, infants diagnosed with CAH should have normal growth and development.

Congenital Hypothyroidism (CH)

CH is the result of an inability to produce adequate amounts of thyroid hormone. Left untreated, this congenital deficiency of thyroid hormone can result in mental retardation and stunted growth. Newborns may appear normal up to three months of age. If detected early (before three weeks) and maintained on appropriate levels of thyroid hormone medication, infants diagnosed with CH should have normal growth and development.

Congenital Toxoplasmosis

Congenital toxoplasmosis is caused by infection of the fetus with the protozoan parasite *Toxoplasma gondii*, typically by active infection of the mother during pregnancy. The mothers can become infected by eating raw or undercooked contaminated meat, or by accidentally ingesting cat oocysts in feces or in contaminated soil or unwashed vegetables. Signs of congenital infection may be present at birth or develop over the first few months of life. Newborns may show signs of central nervous system disorders, enlargement of the liver and spleen, blindness, and mental retardation. Early diagnosis and drug therapy will greatly reduce the risk of serious complications.

Cystic Fibrosis (CF)

CF results from an altered synthesis of a protein involved in the transport of chloride ions. The major clinical consequences are the production of abnormally thickened mucous secretions in the lungs and digestive systems of affected newborns. With early detection and lifelong comprehensive treatment plans, infants diagnosed with CF can be expected to live longer and in a better state of health than in the past.

Galactosemia (GAL)

GAL results from a deficiency in the enzyme needed to metabolize galactose in milk sugar. Newborns typically appear normal, however, within a few days to two weeks after initiating milk feedings, vomiting, diarrhea, lethargy, jaundice, and liver damage develops. Untreated, the disorder may result in developmental retardation, hepatomegaly, growth failure, cataracts, and in severe cases death. With early detection and strict adherence to a galactose-free diet, infants diagnosed with GAL can be expected to achieve satisfactory general health. However, since some galactose can be produced in the body and cause negative effects, close developmental monitoring and assessment is recommended.

Homocystinuria

This disorder is caused by an enzyme deficiency that blocks the metabolism of homocysteine to cystathionine. The major clinical features include optical dislocation (affecting 80% of homocystinurics by age 15), mental retardation, osteoporosis, and thromboembolism (causing death in 50% of homocystinurics by age 20, and 75% by age 30). With early detection, strict dietary management, and vitamin supplements, growth and development should be normal.

Maple Syrup Urine Disease (MSUD)

MSUD is a disorder due to a deficiency of the branched-chain ketoacid decarboxylase enzyme affecting the metabolism of amino acids. Newborns typically appear normal, but by the first week of life can present with feeding difficulties, lethargy, and failure to thrive. Left untreated, the disorder can lead to progressive neurological problems, acidosis, seizures, and sudden apnea that can rapidly lead to coma and death. Treatment consists of strict dietary management and supplements along with close developmental monitoring and assessment. With early detection and treatment, infants diagnosed with MSUD can avoid many of the severe effects of the disease and lead normal lives.

Medium-Chain Acyl-CoA Dehydrogenase Deficiency (MCAD)

MCAD is a rare hereditary disease that results from the lack of an enzyme required to convert fat to energy. Complications typically arise when the affected infants have long periods between meals, requiring the body to use its own fat reserves to produce energy. When this action is blocked by the lack of the necessary enzyme, serious life threatening symptoms and even death can occur. MCAD causes no apparent symptoms at birth, but low blood sugar, seizures, brain damage, cardiac arrest, and serious illness can occur very quickly in infants who are not feeding well. Treatment for the disorder requires close monitoring of the infant to determine safe time periods between meals, and adhering to a strict feeding schedule. With early detection and monitoring, and avoidance of fasts, children diagnosed with MCAD can lead normal lives particularly as the safe time between meals expands as they mature.

Phenylketonuria (PKU)

PKU is the result of an inability to break down the amino acid, phenylalanine, which is found in the protein of foods. Infants may appear normal in the first few months of life, but left untreated, PKU can cause mental and motor retardation, microcephaly, poor growth rate, and seizures. With early detection and proper dietary treatment, growth and development should be normal.

Sickle Cell Diseases (SCD)

Sickle cell diseases are inherited abnormalities in the function of hemoglobin. Sickling is the term referring to changes in the red blood cells causing them to become hard, sticky, and crescent shaped. These changes prevent them from moving smoothly through the body. The most catastrophic abnormal hemoglobin conditions are sickle cell anemia and sickle beta thalassemia. Affected newborns will appear normal, but anemia develops in the first few months of life, followed by increased susceptibility to infection, slow growth rates, and the possibility of life threatening splenic sequestration. With appropriate medical care including penicillin prophylaxis, appropriate vaccinations, and long term management, the complications of sickle cell disease can be minimized. Note: Infants identified with sickle cell trait typically will have few or no clinical symptoms.

U.S. National Screening Status Report

The U.S. National Screening Status Report (shown in Table 6.1) lists the status of newborn screening in the United States. The disorder must be a requirement of the state in order for an asterisk (*) to be added. An asterisk in brackets [*] indicates that MS/MS is used for detecting the analyte of interest.

Table 6.1. Status of Newborn Screening in the United States

State	PKU	CH	GAL	MSUD	HCY	Bio	SCD	CAH	MS/MS	Other
Alabama	*	*	*				*	*		
Alaska	*	*	*	*		*	*	*		
Arizona	*	*	*	*	*	*	*	*		
Arkansas	*	*	*				*			
California	*	*	*				*			
Colorado	*	*	*			*	*	*		2
Connecticut	*	*	*	*	*	*	*	*	c	2a, 4
D.C.	[*]	*	*	[*]	[*]		*			5

Table 6.1. Status of Newborn Screening in the United States

State	PKU	CH	GAL	MSUD	HCY	Bio	SCD	CAH	MS/MS	Other
Delaware	[*]	*	*	[*]	[*]		*	*	*	
Florida	*	*	*				*	*		
Georgia	*	*	*	*	*	*	*	*	c	3
Hawaii	[*]	*	*	[*]	[*]	*	*	*	*	
Idaho	[*]	*	*	[*]	[*]	*			*	
Illinois	[*]	*	*	[*]	[*]	*	*		*	
Indiana	[*]	*	*	[*]	[*]	*	*	*	*	
Iowa	[*]	*	*	[*]	[*]	*	*	*	*	
Kansas	*	*	*				*			
Kentucky	*	*	*				*			
Louisiana	*	*	*			*	*			
Maine	[*]	*	*	[*]	[*]	*	*	*	*	
Maryland	[*]	*	*	[*]	[*]	*	*	*	*	[3]
Massachusetts	[*]	*	*	[*]	[*]	*	*	*	*	1, 2b
Michigan	[*]	*	*	[*]		*	*	*	*	
Minnesota	[*]	*	*	[*]	[*]		*	*	*	
Mississippi	[*]	*	*	[*]	[*]	*	*	*	*	2, 3
Missouri	*	*	*	c	c	c	*	*	c	5c
Montana	*	*	*			a	*	a	a	2a
Nebraska	[*]	*	*	[a]	[a]	*	*		*	
Nevada	[*]	*	*	[*]	[*]	*	*	*	*	
New Hampshire	[*]	*	*	[*]	[*]		a			1
New Jersey	[*]	*	*	[*]		*	*	*	*	2
New Mexico	*	*	*			*	*	*		
New York	[*]	*	*	[*]	[*]	*	*	*	*	2, 4
North Carolina	[*]	*	*	[*]	[*]		*	*	*	
North Dakota	[*]	*	*	[b]	[*]	*	*	*	*	
Ohio	[*]	*	*	[*]	[*]		*	*	*	
Oklahoma	*	*	*				*			
Oregon	[*]	*	*	[*]	[*]	*	*	*	*	
Pennsylvania	[*]	*	*	[*]	[a]	a	*	*	a	2a, 5a
Rhode Island	[*]	*	*	[*]	[*]	*	*	*	*	

Table 6.1. Status of Newborn Screening in the United States

State	PKU	CH	GAL	MSUD	HCY	Bio	SCD	CAH	MS/MS	Other
South Carolina	[*]	*	*	c	c	c	*	*		
South Dakota	[*]	*	*	[a]	[a]		a		a	
Tennessee	*	*	*			*	*	*		
Texas	*	*	*				*	*		
Utah	*	*	*				*			
Vermont	[*]	*	*	[*]	[*]	*	*			
Virginia	*	*	*	*	*	*	*	*	c	
Washington	*	*					*	*		
West Virginia	*	*	*				*			
Wisconsin	[*]	*	*	[*]	[*]	*	*	*	*	2
Wyoming	*	*	*			*	*			2

PKU = Phenylketonuria, **CH** = Congenital Hypothyroidism, **GAL** = Galactosemia, **MSUD** = Maple Syrup Urine Disease, **HCY** = Homocystinuria, **BIO** = Biotinidase, **SCD** = Sickle Cell Disease, **CAH** = Congenital Adrenal Hyperplasia, **MS/MS** = Tandem Mass Spectrometry Screening

Other: a = (not mandated) selected populations, limited pilot programs, or by request, **b** = (not mandated) universal pilot, **c** = testing mandated but not implemented

1 = Toxoplasmosis, **2** = Cystic Fibrosis, **3** = Tyrosinemia, **4** = HIV, **5** = G-6-PD Deficiency

Chapter 7

Child Health Guide: Checkup Visits, Tests, and Exams

Working with the doctor, nurse, or other health care provider to keep your child well is as important as getting treatment when he or she is sick. This chapter briefly explains preventive care for children—such as checkup visits, immunizations, and tests and exams—and provides guidance on related issues.

To get the most from your child's health care:

- Be an active member of your child's health care team. Ask your health care provider any questions that you may have.

- Use records to keep track of the immunizations (shots), tests, exams, and other types of health care that your child receives. Use these records to remind you when your child needs to be seen next.

- Keep the records in a safe place. Check often to make sure your child is getting the preventive care that he or she needs. Keep the records up-to-date.

Checkup Visits

Checkup visits are important because they allow your health care provider to review your child's growth and development, perform tests, or give shots. To help your provider get a complete picture of your

Excerpts from "Put Prevention into Practice: Child Health Guide," Agency for Healthcare Research and Quality (AHRQ), Publication No. APPIP 98-0026, reviewed January 2003.

child's health status, bring your child's health record and a list of any medications your child is taking to each visit.

Checkup visits are a time for parents to ask questions. Bring a list of concerns you have. For example:

- My child is not sleeping through the night yet.
- I don't think my child is eating enough.
- My child seems uncoordinated and is always walking into things.

Some authorities recommend checkup visits at ages 2–4 weeks; 2, 4, 6, 9, 12, 15, and 18 months; 2, 3, 4, 5, 6, 8, 10, 12, 14, 16, and 18 years. Some children may need to be seen more often, others less. Ask your clinician how often your child will need to be seen.

Immunizations

This information on immunizations is based on recommendations issued by the Advisory Committee on Immunization Practices, the American Academy of Pediatrics, and the American Academy of Family Physicians.

Your child needs immunizations. Immunizations (shots) protect your child from many serious diseases. Following is a list of immunizations and the ages when your child should receive them. Immunizations should be given at the recommended ages—even if your child has a cold or illness at the time. Ask your health care provider when your child should receive these important shots. Ask also if your child needs other immunizations.

- Polio (IPV): At 2 months, 4 months, 6–18 months, and 4–6 years.
- Diphtheria-Tetanus-Pertussis (DTaP): At 2 months, 4 months, 6 months, 15–18 months, and 4–6 years. Tetanus-Diphtheria (Td) at 11–16 years.
- Measles-Mumps-Rubella (MMR): At 12–15 months and 4–6 years or as soon thereafter as possible.
- Haemophilus influenzae type b (Hib): At 2 months, 4 months, 6 months, and 12–15 months; or 2 months, 4 months, and 12–15 months, depending on the vaccine type.
- Hepatitis B: At birth–2 months, 1–4 months, and 6–18 months. If missed, get 3 doses starting at age 11 years.
- Chickenpox (Varicella): At 12–18 months or under 13 years.

- Hepatitis A (in selected areas): At 24 months–18 years; second dose 6–12 months after first dose.

- Pneumococcal disease (Prevnar™): At 2 months, 4 months, 6 months, and 12–15 months. If missed, talk to your health care provider.

- Influenza (children at high risk for chronic diseases): 6 months–18 years. Two doses at least 1 month apart for children aged 6 months–under 9 years who receive influenza vaccine for the first time.

Periodically, the recommended timing for immunizations changes.

Tests and Exams

Newborn Screening

Certain blood tests should be done before your baby is 7 days old. They are usually done just before your baby leaves the hospital. If the blood tests were done earlier than 24 hours after birth, a repeat test at 1 to 2 weeks of age is recommended. Common newborn screening tests include those for PKU, thyroid, and sickle cell disease.

Blood Pressure

Your child should have blood pressure measurements regularly, starting at around 3 years of age. High blood pressure in children needs medical attention. It may be a sign of underlying disease and, if not treated, may lead to serious illness. Check with your child's health care provider about blood pressure measurements.

Lead

Lead can harm your child, slowing physical and mental growth and damaging many parts of the body. The most common way children get lead poisoning is by being around old house paint that is chipping or peeling. Read the following questions. Any yes answers may mean that your child may need to be tested for lead.

Has your child:

- Lived in or regularly visited a house built before 1950? (This could include a day care center, preschool, the home of a baby-sitter or relative, etc.)

- Lived in or regularly visited a house built before 1978 (the year lead-based paint was banned for residential use) with recent, ongoing, or planned renovation or remodeling?

- Had a brother or sister, housemate, or playmate who has been followed or treated for lead poisoning?

Vision and Hearing

Your child's vision should be tested before starting school, at about 3 or 4 years of age. Your child may also need vision tests as he or she grows. Some authorities also recommend hearing testing beginning at 3 to 4 years of age.

If at any age your child has any of the vision or hearing warning signs listed below, be sure to talk with your health care provider.

Vision Warning Signs

- Eyes turning inward (crossing) or outward.
- Squinting.
- Headaches.
- Not doing as well in school work as before.
- Blurred or double vision.

Hearing Warning Signs

- Poor response to noise or voice.
- Slow language and speech development.
- Abnormal sounding speech.

Special Warning: Listening to very loud music, especially with earphones, can permanently damage your child's hearing.

Additional Tests

Your child may need other tests to prevent health problems. Some common tests are:

Anemia (Blood) Test—Your child may need to be tested for anemia when he or she is still a baby (usually around the first birthday). Children may also need this test as they get older. Some children are more likely to get anemia than others. Ask your health care provider about anemia testing.

Tuberculosis (TB) Skin Test—Children may need this test if they have had close contact with a person who has TB, live in an area where TB is more common than average (such as a Native American reservation, a homeless shelter, or an institution), or have recently moved from Asia, Africa, Central America, South America, the Caribbean, or the Pacific Islands.

Growth and Development

Children grow and develop at different rates. Your child's health care provider will measure your child's height and weight regularly. These measurements will help you and your health care provider know if your child is growing properly.

The following information shows the ages by which most young children develop certain abilities. It is normal for a child to do some of these things later than the ages noted here. If your child fails to do many of these at the ages given, or you have questions about his or her development, talk with your child's health care provider.

2 Months

- Smiles, coos.
- Watches a person, follows with eyes.

4 Months

- Laughs out loud.
- Lifts head and chest when on stomach, grasps objects.

6 Months

- Babbles, turns to sound.
- Rolls over, supports head well when sitting.

9 Months

- Responds to name, plays peek-a-boo.
- Sits alone, crawls, pulls self up to standing.

1 Year

- Waves bye-bye, says mama or dada.

- Walks when holding on, picks up objects with thumb and first finger.

18 Months

- Says three words other than mama or dada, scribbles.
- Walks alone, feeds self using spoon.

2 Years

- Puts two words together, refers to self by name.
- Runs well, walks up stairs by self.

3 Years

- Knows age, helps button clothing, washes and dries hands.
- Throws ball overhand, rides tricycle.

4 Years

- Knows first and last name, tells a story, counts four objects.
- Balances on one foot, uses children's scissors.

5 Years

- Names 4 colors, counts 10 objects.
- Hops on one foot, dresses self.

Additional Information

American Academy of Pediatrics
141 Northwest Point Boulevard
Elk Grove Village, IL 60007-1098
Phone: 847-434-4000
Fax: 847-434-8000
Website: www.aap.org
E-mail: kidsdocs@aap.org

Immunizations

Centers for Disease Control and Prevention
NIP Public Inquiries
Mailstop E-05
1600 Clifton Rd., NE
Atlanta, GA 30333

Centers for Disease Control and Prevention (continued)

Toll-Free: 800-232-2522
Toll-Free Spanish: 800-232-0233
Fax: 888-232-3299
Website: www.cdc.gov/nip
E-mail: NIPINFO@cdc.gov

Vaccine Adverse Event Reporting System

P.O. Box 1100
Rockville, MD 20849-1100
Toll-Free: 800-822-7967
Website: www.vaers.org
E-mail: info@vaers.org

Health Resources and Services Administration (HRSA) Information Center

U.S. Department of Health and Human Services
Parklawn Building
5600 Fishers Lane
Rockville, MD 20857
Toll-Free: 888-275-4772
Website: www.ask.hrsa.gov
E-mail: ask@hrsa.gov

Chapter 8

Teen Wellness Exam

Medical Care and Your 13- to 18-Year-Old

By meeting yearly with your teen, the doctor can keep track of changes in her physical, mental, and social development, and offer advice against unhealthy behaviors, such as smoking and drinking. The doctor can also help your child understand the importance of choosing a healthy lifestyle that includes good nutrition, proper exercise, and safety measures. The more teens understand about their physical growth and sexual development, the more they will recognize the importance of active involvement in their own health care.

What Happens at the Doctor's Office?

Teens should visit their doctors annually. At least three of these visits should include a complete physical examination: one performed during early adolescence (ages 11 to 14), one during middle adolescence (ages 15 to 17), and one during late adolescence (ages 18 to 21). If your child has a chronic medical condition or if certain clinical signs or symptoms are present, more frequent examinations may be indicated.

This information was provided by KidsHealth, one of the largest resources online for medically reviewed health information written for parents, kids, and teens. For more articles like this one, visit www.KidsHealth.org, or www.TeensHealth.org. © 2003 The Nemours Center for Children's Health Media, a division of The Nemours Foundation.

Medical care should include screenings for high blood pressure, obesity, and other eating disorders, and, if indicated, hyperlipidemia (an excess of cholesterol and/or other fats in the blood). A tuberculin (PPD) test may be administered if your teen is at risk for tuberculosis.

Your teen's doctor will also check her teeth for tooth decay, abnormal tooth development, malocclusion (abnormal bite), dental injuries, and other problems.. Your teen should also continue to have regular checkups with her dentist.

Vision and hearing will be checked.

Teens will also be checked for scoliosis (curvature of the spine).

Teens should receive a diphtheria and tetanus booster (Td) 10 years after their last childhood booster (usually at age 4 to 6 years) and every 10 years thereafter. They should have already completed their other immunizations, including varicella (if they have not had chicken pox); measles, mumps, and rubella (MMR); and the hepatitis B series (Hep B). If your teen will be living in an institutional setting, such as a college dormitory, speak with her doctor about receiving the meningococcal meningitis vaccine.

As your child goes through puberty, issues of sexual health will be addressed. Your child's doctor will teach your daughter how to perform a monthly breast exam. The doctor may also perform (or refer her to a gynecologist for) a gynecologic exam and a Pap smear to check for cervical cancer. Males will be checked for hernias and testicular cancer and taught to perform a testicular self-examination.

Teens should be asked about behaviors or emotional problems that may indicate depression or the risk of suicide. The doctor should also provide counseling about risky behaviors and other issues, including:

- sexual activities that may result in unintended pregnancy and sexually transmitted diseases (STDs), including HIV

- emotional, physical, and sexual abuse

- use of alcohol and other substances, including anabolic steroids

- use of tobacco products, including cigarettes and smokeless tobacco

- use of alcohol while driving

- use of safety devices, including bicycle helmets, seat belts, and protective sports gear

- how to resolve conflicts without violence, including how to avoid the use of weapons

- learning problems or difficulties at school
- appropriate warm-ups before exercise and importance of regular physical activity

What Should I Do if I Suspect a Medical Problem?

Parents or other caregivers should receive health guidance at least once during early, middle, and late adolescence from their teen's doctor. During these sessions, the doctor will provide information about normal development, including signs and symptoms of illness or emotional distress and methods to monitor and manage potentially harmful behaviors.

If you suspect that your teen has a physical disorder, a psychological problem, or a problem with drugs or alcohol, contact your child's doctor immediately.

Typical Medical Problems

Issues involving puberty and sexual development are typical concerns for this age group. Doctors who establish a policy of confidentiality can serve as a valuable resource for a teen by answering questions and providing guidance during this period of physical and emotional changes. Teens should be reassured that anything they discuss with their doctor will be kept confidential, unless their health or the health of others is endangered by the situation.

Sports injuries are common concerns. Osgood-Schlatter's disease, painful inflammation of the area just below the front of the knee, is particularly common in the early teen years. Knee pain is also a frequent complaint. Your teen's doctor should evaluate any severe or persistent pain of the joints, muscles, or other areas of the body.

Chapter 9

Personal Health Guide for Adults: Preventive Tests and Exams

Overview of Preventive Services for Normal-Risk Adults Recommended by the U.S. Preventive Services Task Force

Screening

- Blood pressure, height, and weight: Periodically, 18 years and older.
- Cholesterol:
    - Men—every 5 years, 35 years and older.
    - Women—every 5 years, 45 years and older.
- Diabetes: Periodically, adults with hypertension or hyperlipidemia.
- Pap smear: Women—every 1 to 3 years, 18–65 years.
- Chlamydia: 18–25 years.
- Mammography: Every 1 to 2 years, 40 years and older.

This chapter includes "Clinical Preventive Services for Normal-Risk Adults Recommended by the U.S. Preventive Services Task Force. Put Prevention into Practice," Agency for Healthcare Research and Quality, January 2003; "Personal Health Guide: Put Prevention into Practice," Agency for Health Care Policy and Research, Pub. No. APPIP 98-0027, April 1998, updated in November 2003 by Dr. David A. Cooke, MD, Diplomate, American Board of Internal Medicine; and "American Heart Association Updates Heart Attack, Stroke Prevention Guidelines," *AHA Journal* Report 07/15/2002. Reproduced with permission from the American Heart Association World Wide Web Site, www.american heart.org. © 2003. Copyright American Heart Association.

- Colorectal cancer: Periodically, 50 years and older.
- Osteoporosis: Women—routinely, over 65 years or over 60 years at increased risk for fractures.
- Alcohol use: Periodically, 18 years and older.
- Vision, hearing: Periodically, 65 years and older.

Immunization

- Tetanus-Diphtheria (Td): Every 10 years, 18 years and older.
- Varicella (VZV): Susceptibles only—two doses, 18 years and older.
- Measles, Mumps, Rubella (MMR): Women of childbearing age— one dose, 18–50 years.
- Pneumococcal: One dose, 65 years and older.
- Influenza: Yearly, 50 years and older.

Chemoprevention

- Discuss aspirin to prevent cardiovascular events:
    - Men—periodically, 40 years and older.
    - Women—periodically, 50 years and older.
- Discuss breast cancer chemoprevention with women at high risk.

Counseling

- Calcium intake: Women, periodically, 18 years and older.
- Folic acid: Women of childbearing age, 18–50 years.
- Tobacco cessation, drug and alcohol use, STDs and HIV, nutrition, physical activity, sun exposure, oral health, injury prevention, and polypharmacy: Periodically, 18 years and older.

Upper age limits should be individualized for each patient.

Personal Health Guide for Adults

If you don't understand something, be sure to ask your health care provider about it. This will help you get the answers you need to take care of your health.

After talking with your health care provider, keep written records of preventive screening recommendations. This will help you to know which services you need and how often you need them. Keeping health records can make it easier to keep accurate information about your health and will especially help you with details when you get treatments in the future.

Blood Pressure

Maintaining a good blood pressure will help protect you from heart disease, stroke, and kidney problems. Have your blood pressure checked regularly. Eating a healthy diet and getting regular physical activity are two ways you can help to keep your blood pressure under control. Some people will need to take medicine to help keep a healthy blood pressure.

If you have high blood pressure, talk with your health care provider about how to lower it by changing your diet, losing excess weight, exercising, or (if necessary) taking medicine. If you need to take medicine, be sure to take it every day, as prescribed. Ask your provider how often you need your blood pressure checked and what a healthy blood pressure is for you.

Immunizations

Adults need immunizations (shots) to prevent serious diseases. The following are common shots that most people need:

- Tetanus-diphtheria shot—Everyone needs this every 10 years.

- Rubella (German measles) shot—If you are a woman who is considering pregnancy and you have not had a shot for German measles, you should talk to your provider.

- Pneumococcal (pneumonia) shot—Everyone needs this one time at about age 65. People with health conditions such as asthma, emphysema, heart disease, diabetes, and certain other conditions should receive this at a younger age, and have it repeated at age 65.

- Influenza (flu) shots—Everyone over age 50 needs this every year. If you have lung, heart, or kidney disease, diabetes, HIV, or cancer you may need pneumococcal and flu shots before age 50. Health care workers may also benefit from annual flu shots.

- Hepatitis B—If you have contact with human blood or body fluids (such as semen or vaginal fluid), you may be at risk for hepatitis B. You may also be at risk if you have unprotected sex (vaginal, oral, or anal) or share needles during intravenous drug

71

use. Hepatitis B shots will protect you. Health care workers should also consider getting hepatitis B shots. Discuss this with your provider.

Cholesterol

Having your cholesterol checked is important, especially if you are a man age 45–65 or a woman age 45–65. Too much cholesterol can clog your blood vessels and cause heart disease and other serious problems. Your health care provider may check your levels of bad (LDL) and good (HDL) cholesterol.

You can lower your cholesterol level and keep a healthy level by changing your diet, losing excess weight, and getting regular exercise. If necessary, your provider may prescribe medication for you. Ask your provider what a healthy cholesterol level is for you and how often you need it checked. If you have high cholesterol, talk with your provider about a plan for lowering it.

Weight

Weighing too much or too little can lead to health problems. You should have your weight checked regularly by your health care provider. You can control/maintain your weight by eating a healthy diet and getting regular physical activity. Talk with your provider about what a healthy weight for you is and ways you can control your weight.

Colorectal Cancer

Colorectal cancer is the third leading cause of deaths from cancer. If it is caught early, it can be treated. If you are 50 years of age or older, you should have tests regularly to detect it. The tests you may have are:

- Fecal Occult Blood Test—to look for small amounts of blood in your stool. This test should be done yearly.

- Sigmoidoscopy—to look inside the rectum and colon using a small, lighted tube. Your health care provider will do this in the office or clinic. This test should be done every 5 to 10 years.

- Colonoscopy—similar to sigmoidoscopy, but uses a longer scope and examines the entire large intestine. It is usually done at a hospital as an outpatient procedure. If you have a family history of colon polyps or cancer, this may be a preferred test, and testing may need to begin younger than age 50.

Tell your health care provider if you have had polyps or if you have a family member(s) with cancer of the intestine, breast, ovaries, or uterus, you may need testing before age 50 or more often. Ask your health care provider at what age you need to start and how often you need these tests:

Preventive Care for Women

Mammogram

Women ages 40–50 should discuss when to begin getting mammograms with their health care provider. All women should begin having mammograms regularly by age 50. Some women may need mammograms earlier. A mammogram is an x-ray test that can detect a breast cancer when it is so small that it cannot be felt and when it can be most easily cured.

Talk with your health care provider about when to begin and how often to have mammograms. Make sure to tell your provider if your mother or a sister has had breast cancer. You may need to have mammograms more often than other women.

Pap Smear

You need to have Pap smears regularly. This simple test has saved the lives of many women by detecting cancer of the cervix early—when it is most easily cured. Cervical cancer frequently affects young women, so this is one test that is critical even for young, healthy women.

Talk to your health care provider about how often you need Pap smears. Tell your health care provider if you have had genital warts, sexually transmitted diseases (STDs/VD), multiple sexual partners, or abnormal Pap smears. You may need Pap smears more often than other women.

Additional Preventive Care

Following is a list of other preventive care. If you answer yes to any of the statements, discuss whether you need screening with your health care provider. If you:

- Have diabetes, or if you are over age 40 and African-American, or if you are over are over age 60: You should have routine eye examinations.

- Have had sexual intercourse without condoms, have had multiple sexual partners, or have had a sexually transmitted disease:

You may need AIDS (HIV), syphilis, gonorrhea, chlamydia, or hepatitis tests.

- Have injected illegal drugs or had a blood transfusion between 1978 and 1985: You may need an AIDS (HIV) and/or hepatitis test.

- Have had a family member with diabetes, are overweight, or have had diabetes during pregnancy: You may need a diabetes (glucose) test.

- Are over age 65: You may need a hearing test.

- Now or in the past, have ever consumed a lot of alcohol or have smoked or chewed tobacco: You may need a mouth examination.

- Are a man 50 years of age or older: You may need a prostate examination.

- Are a man aged 15–35 years, particularly if you have a testicle that is abnormally small or not in the normal position: You may need a testicular examination.

- Have had skin cancer in your family or if you have had a lot of sun exposure: You may need a skin examination.

- Have had radiation treatments of your upper body: You may need a thyroid examination.

- Have been exposed to tuberculosis (TB), or if you have recently moved from Asia, Africa, Central or South America, or the Pacific Islands, or if you have kidney failure, diabetes, HIV, alcoholism, or use illegal drugs: You may need a tuberculosis test (PPD).

American Heart Association Updates Heart Attack, Stroke Prevention Guidelines

To avert a first heart attack or stroke, physicians should routinely assess patients' general risk of cardiovascular disease beginning at age 20, according to new American Heart Association recommendations published in the July 16, 2003 *Circulation: Journal of the American Heart Association.*

The "AHA Guidelines for Primary Prevention of Cardiovascular Disease and Stroke: 2002 Update" also recommends that physicians calculate the risk of developing cardiovascular disease in the next 10 years for people age 40 and older or for anyone who has multiple risk factors.

"The imperative to prevent the first episode of coronary disease or stroke remains strong because many first-ever heart attacks or strokes are fatal or disabling," says Thomas Pearson, M.D., Ph.D., who chaired the consensus panel that worked on the update.

The updated guidelines incorporate new findings and expert opinion that have emerged since the American Heart Association published the recommendations in 1997. They reflect recent data on the degree of risk imposed by specific risk factors and the new efforts to categorize people more specifically according to their number and types of risk factors.

"Risk factor screening" includes having blood pressure, body mass index, waist circumference, and pulse recorded at least every two years, and cholesterol profile and glucose testing at least every five years beginning at age 20.

"Global risk estimation" combines information from all existing risk factors to determine a person's percentage risk for developing cardio-vascular disease in the next 10 years. Multiple areas of slight risk can be more important than one area of very high risk. This estimation is recommended every five years for people age 40 or older or for any-one with two or more risk factors.

"The challenge for healthcare professionals is to begin comprehensive risk reduction for more patients at an earlier stage of their disease," says Pearson.

The update integrates recommendations from other clinical guide-lines and consensus statements developed over the past five years—for example, the American Diabetes Association recommendation for managing high blood pressure and high cholesterol levels in diabetic patients and the U.S. Preventive Services Task Force recommenda-tions for routine health care examinations. Consolidating these vari-ous guidelines means that health care providers and patients can use a single source of information to evaluate individual risk for heart disease and stroke and to obtain the latest information about disease prevention.

The panel carefully reviewed the recommendations in each of these statements or guidelines to ensure the consistency.

Notable updates to the guidelines include:

- low-dose aspirin for people who have an increased risk for coro-nary heart disease; and

- blood-thinning drugs to reduce stroke risk in people who have atrial fibrillation—an abnormal heart rhythm that can propel blood clots from the heart toward the brain and increase the risk of stroke.

"The U.S. Preventive Services Task Force has always recommended aspirin for secondary prevention in people who already have heart disease, but now recommends low-dose aspirin for primary prevention, as well," says Pearson. "Aspirin can cause gastrointestinal bleeding and may increase the risk of hemorrhagic stroke (bleeding into the brain). But if a person has a 10-year risk of heart disease that exceeds 10 percent, the benefits of aspirin therapy greatly outweigh the risks."

Similarly, Pearson says studies have clearly shown that using blood-thinners to prevent clot formation, or treatment to eliminate abnormal heartbeats, substantially reduces the risk of stroke associated with atrial fibrillation.

The panel challenges healthcare providers to make prevention a high priority for all patients.

"Health care providers should be asking about smoking and measuring blood pressure and cholesterol levels," says Pearson. "The public should be encouraged to ask their physicians and other health care providers about these important issues in disease prevention."

Other recommendations to prevent heart attack and stroke:

- No exposure to tobacco smoke
- Blood pressure maintained below 140/90 mm Hg; below 130/85 mm Hg for people with kidney damage or heart failure; or below 130/80 mm Hg for people with diabetes
- An overall healthy eating pattern
- Cholesterol lowered to appropriate level based on individual risk
- At least 30 minutes of moderate-intensity physical activity on most (preferably all) days of the week
- Achieve and maintain desirable weight (body mass index 18.5–24.9 kg/m2);
- Normal fasting blood glucose (below 110 mg/dL)

Co-authors of this report are Steven N. Blair, P.E.D.; Stephen R. Daniels, M.D., Ph.D.; Robert H. Eckel, M.D.; Joan M, Fair, R.N., Ph.D.; Stephen P. Fortmann, M.D.; Barry A. Franklin, Ph.D.; Larry B. Goldstein, M.D.; Philip Greenland, M.D.; Scott M. Grundy, M.D., Ph.D.; Yuling Hong, M.D., Ph.D.; Nancy Houston-Miller, R.N.; Ronald M. Lauer, M.D.; Ira S. Ockene, M.D.; Ralph Sacco, M.D.; James F. Sallis Jr., Ph.D.; Sidney C. Smith Jr., M.D.; Neil J. Stone, M.D.; and Kathryn A. Taubert, Ph.D.

Chapter 10

Preventive Screenings for Women

Chapter Contents

Section 10.1

Regular Preventive Checkups

This section includes "HHS Urges Women to Get Regular Preventive Checkups," Agency for Healthcare Research and Quality, HHS Press Release, May 7, 2003; and "Women: Stay Healthy at Any Age—Checklist for Your Next Checkup," Agency for Healthcare Research and Quality, AHRQ Publication No. APPIP03-0008, April 2003.

Preventive Screenings Urged Nationwide on Day Following Mother's Day

On Monday, May 12, 2003 more than 600 community health centers, hospitals, and other health care providers nationwide were encouraging women to visit a health care professional as part of the Department of Health and Human Services' first National Women's Check-Up Day. The effort, scheduled for the day after Mother's Day, was part of the National Women's Health Week. "National Women's Check-Up Day is a perfect opportunity for women to talk to a doctor or health care professional about their health and get the information and care that they need," HHS Secretary Tommy G. Thompson said. "For many women, a visit to the doctor is the first and critical step towards treating and preventing disease. In addition, simple steps like the ones outlined in President Bush's Healthier U.S. initiative, can really make a difference—regular physical activity for 30 minutes a day, eating a nutritious diet, and stopping smoking can all have tremendous health benefits."

National Women's Check-Up Day emphasizes that getting a regular checkup and asking a doctor about screening for heart disease, diabetes, cancer, and sexually transmitted diseases (STDs) are often keys to improving women's health.

The new campaign recognizes that many of the leading causes of death among women can be successfully prevented or treated if the warning signs are caught early enough. For example:

- Heart disease is the number one killer of American women. Often thought of as a man's disease, more women die of heart disease each year than do men.

- Cancer is the second leading cause of death of American women. Lung cancer is the top cancer killer among American women, with an estimated 65,000 deaths in 2002, followed by breast cancer and colorectal cancer.

- Stroke is the number three killer of American women. Each year, 30,000 more women than men have strokes.

- Diabetes is the fifth leading cause of death in women. An estimated 17 million Americans have diabetes (8.1 million women), of which an estimated 6 million are undiagnosed.

- HIV and sexually transmitted diseases also have a major effect on women's health. There are an estimated 40,000 new HIV infections each year in the United States, with about 30 percent of reported infections occurring in women.

"While medical research and treatment are enabling women to live longer and healthier lives than ever before, far too many women die each year of diseases that could be treated if detected early on," Surgeon General Richard Carmona said. "By getting regular checkups, women can get the care and medical advice that can help them enjoy more tomorrows with the people they love."

Checklist for Your Next Checkup

What can you do to stay healthy and prevent disease? You can get certain screening tests, take preventive medicine if you need it, and practice healthy behaviors. Top health experts from the U.S. Preventive Services Task Force suggest that when you go for your next checkup, talk to your doctor or nurse about how you can stay healthy no matter what your age.

Screening Tests: What You Need and When

Screening tests, such as mammograms and Pap smears, can find diseases early when they are easier to treat. Some women need certain screening tests earlier, or more often, than others. Talk to your doctor about which of the tests listed below are right for you, when you should have them, and how often. The Task Force has made the following recommendations, based on scientific evidence, about which screening tests you should have.

- **Mammograms:** Have a mammogram every 1 to 2 years starting at age 40.

- **Pap Smears:** Have a Pap smear every 1 to 3 years if you have been sexually active or are older than 21.

- **Cholesterol Checks:** Have your cholesterol checked regularly starting at age 45. If you smoke, have diabetes, or if heart disease runs in your family, start having your cholesterol checked at age 20.

- **Blood Pressure:** Have your blood pressure checked at least every 2 years.

- **Colorectal Cancer Tests:** Have a test for colorectal cancer starting at age 50. Your doctor can help you decide which test is right for you.

- **Diabetes Tests:** Have a test to screen for diabetes if you have high blood pressure or high cholesterol.

- **Depression:** If you've felt down, sad, or hopeless, and have felt little interest or pleasure in doing things for 2 weeks straight, talk to your doctor about whether he or she can screen you for depression.

- **Osteoporosis Tests:** Have a bone density test at age 65 to screen for osteoporosis (thinning of the bones). If you are between the ages of 60 and 64 and weigh 154 lbs. or less, talk to your doctor about whether you should be tested.

- **Chlamydia Tests and Tests for Other Sexually Transmitted Diseases:** Have a test for chlamydia if you are 25 or younger and sexually active. If you are older, talk to your doctor to see whether you should be tested. Also, talk to your doctor to see whether you should be tested for other sexually transmitted diseases.

- **Hormones:** According to recent studies, the risks of taking the combined hormones estrogen and progestin after menopause to prevent long-term illnesses outweigh the benefits. Talk to your doctor about whether starting or continuing to take hormones is right for you.

- **Breast Cancer Drugs:** If your mother, sister, or daughter has had breast cancer, talk to your doctor about the risks and benefits of taking medicines to prevent breast cancer.

- **Aspirin:** Talk to your doctor about taking aspirin to prevent heart disease if you are older than 45 and have high blood pressure, high cholesterol, diabetes, or if you smoke.

- **Immunizations:** Stay up-to-date with your immunizations: Have a flu shot every year starting at age 50. Have a tetanus-diphtheria shot every 10 years. Have a pneumonia shot once at age 65. Talk to your doctor to see whether you need hepatitis B shots.

What Else Can You Do to Stay Healthy?

Don't Smoke. But if you do smoke, talk to your doctor about quitting. You can take medicine and get counseling to help you quit. Make a plan and set a quit date. Tell your family, friends, and co-workers you are quitting. Ask for their support. If you are pregnant and smoke, quitting now will help you and your baby.

Eat a Healthy Diet. Eat a variety of foods, including fruit, vegetables, animal or vegetable protein (such as meat, fish, chicken, eggs, beans, lentils, tofu, or tempeh), and grains (such as rice). Limit the amount of saturated fat you eat.

Be Physically Active. Walk, dance, ride a bike, rake leaves, or do any other physical activity you enjoy. Start small and work up to a total of 20–30 minutes most days of the week.

Stay at a Healthy Weight. Balance the number of calories you eat with the number you burn off by your activities. Remember to watch portion sizes. Talk to your doctor if you have questions about what or how much to eat.

Drink Alcohol Only in Moderation. If you drink alcohol, one drink a day is safe for women, unless you are pregnant. If you are pregnant, you should avoid alcohol. Since researchers don't know how much alcohol will harm a fetus, it's best not to drink any alcohol while you are pregnant. A standard drink is one 12-ounce bottle of beer or wine cooler, one 5-ounce glass of wine, or 1.5 ounces of 80-proof distilled spirits.

Screening Test Checklist

Take a checklist like the sample shown in Table 10.1 with you to your doctor's office and fill it out when you have had any of the tests listed. Talk to your doctor about when you should have these tests next, and note the month and year in the right-hand column. Also, talk to your doctor about which of the other tests you should have in the future, and when you need them.

Table 10.1. Sample Screening Test Record Checklist

Screening Test	The last time I had the following screening test was: (mm/yy)	I should schedule my next test for: (mm/yy)
Mammogram		
Pap smear		
Cholesterol		
Blood pressure		
Colorectal cancer		
Osteoporosis		
Chlamydia		

Additional Reading

For more information on staying healthy, order the following free publications in the "Put Prevention Into Practice (PPIP)" program from the Agency for Healthcare Research and Quality (call the AHRQ Publications Clearinghouse at 800-358-9295), or find them at: http://www.ahrq.gov/clinic/ppipix.htm

- *Women: Stay Healthy at Any Age—Checklist for Your Next Checkup*, (in English and Spanish), Publication No. APPIP 03-0008, April 2003.

- *Pocket Guide to Good Health for Adults*, Publication No. APPIP 03-0001, May 2003.

- *Staying Healthy at 50+* (in English and Spanish), Publication No. AHRQ 00-0002, January 2000.

Additional Information

Agency for Healthcare Research and Quality
540 Gaither Road
Rockville, MD 20850
Toll-Free: 800-358-9295
Phone: 301-427-1364
Website: www.ahrq.gov
E-mail: info@ahrq.gov

National Women's Health Information Center
Office on Women's Health
200 Independence Ave. S.W., Room 730B
Washington, DC 20201
Toll-Free: 800-994-9662
Toll-Free TDD: 888-220-5446
Phone: 202-690-7650
Fax: 202-205-2631
Website: www.4woman.gov/whw

The information in this section is based on research from the U.S. Department of Health and Human Services (HHS) and the U.S. Preventive Services Task Force (USPSTF), the leading independent panel of private-sector experts in prevention and primary care. The Task Force conducts rigorous scientific assessments of the effectiveness of a broad range of clinical preventive services. Its recommendations are considered the gold standard for preventive services delivered in the clinical setting.

Section 10.2

Breast Cancer Screening

This section includes "Mammography" National Center for Health Statistics, 2002; "Screening Mammograms: Questions and Answers," Cancer Facts 5.28, National Cancer Institute, reviewed May 3, 2002; and "Improving Methods for Breast Cancer Detection and Diagnosis," Cancer Facts 5.14, National Cancer Institute, reviewed June 12, 2001.

Mammography in the U.S.

- Percent of women 40 and over having a mammogram within the past 2 years—70.3% (2002)

- Percent of white, non-Hispanic women 40 and over having a mammogram within the past 2 years—72.1% (2000)

- Percent of black, non-Hispanic women 40 and over having a mammogram within the past 2 years—67.9% (2000)

- Percent of Hispanic women 40 and over having a mammogram within the past 2 years—61.4% (2000)

- Percent of women 40 and over and below poverty level having a mammogram within the past 2 years—55.2% (2000)

- Percent of women 40 and over and at or above poverty level having a mammogram within the past 2 years—72.2% (2000)

Source: National Center for Health Statistics. *Health, United States: 2002*, Table 82.

Screening Mammograms: Questions and Answers

What Is a Screening Mammogram?

A screening mammogram is an x-ray of the breast used to detect breast changes in women who have no signs or symptoms of breast cancer. It usually involves two x-rays of each breast. With a mammogram, it is possible to detect microcalcifications (tiny deposits of calcium in the breast, which sometimes are a clue to the presence of breast cancer) or a tumor that cannot be felt.

What Is a Diagnostic Mammogram?

A diagnostic mammogram is an x-ray of the breast that is used to diagnose unusual breast changes, such as a lump, pain, thickening, nipple discharge, or a change in breast size or shape. A diagnostic mammogram is also used to evaluate changes detected on a screening mammogram. This type of mammogram may be necessary if it is difficult to obtain a clear x-ray with a screening mammogram because of special circumstances, such as the presence of breast implants. A diagnostic mammogram takes longer than a screening mammogram because it involves more x-rays to obtain views of the breast from several angles. The technician may magnify a suspicious area to produce a detailed picture that can help the doctor make an accurate diagnosis.

When Does the National Cancer Institute (NCI) Recommend That Women Have Screening Mammograms?

- Women in their 40s and older should have mammograms every 1 to 2 years.

- Women who are at higher than average risk of breast cancer should talk with their health care providers about whether to have mammograms before age 40 and how often to have them.

What Are the Factors That Place a Woman at Increased Risk of Breast Cancer?

The risk of breast cancer increases gradually as a woman gets older. However, the risk of developing breast cancer is not the same for all women. Research has shown that the following factors increase a woman's chance of developing this disease:

- **Personal history of breast cancer:** Women who have had breast cancer are more likely to develop a second breast cancer.

- **Family history:** A woman's chance of developing breast cancer increases if her mother, sister, and/or daughter have a history of breast cancer (especially if they were diagnosed before age 50).

- **Certain breast changes on biopsy:** Having a diagnosis of atypical hyperplasia (a noncancerous condition in which cells have abnormal features and are increased in number) or lobular carcinoma in situ (LCIS) (abnormal cells found in the lobules of the breast) increases a woman's risk of breast cancer. Women who have had two or more breast biopsies for other benign conditions also have an increased chance of developing breast cancer. This increase is due to the condition that led to the biopsy, and not to the biopsy itself.

- **Genetic alterations:** Specific alterations in certain genes (BRCA1, BRCA2, and others) increase the risk of breast cancer. These alterations are rare; they are estimated to account for no more than 10 percent of all breast cancers.

- **Reproductive and menstrual history:** Evidence indicates that:
  - The older a woman is when she has her first child, the greater her chance of developing breast cancer.
  - Women who started menstruating at an early age (age 11 or younger), experienced menopause late (after age 55), or never had children are also at an increased risk of developing breast cancer.
  - Women who take hormone replacement therapy for a long time also appear to have an increased chance of developing breast cancer.

- **Breast density:** Breasts appear dense on a mammogram if they contain many glands and ligaments (called dense tissue), and do not have much fatty tissue. Because breast cancers nearly always develop in the dense tissue of the breast (not in the fatty tissue), older women who have mostly dense tissue on a mammogram are at an increased risk of breast cancer. Abnormalities in dense breasts can be more difficult to detect on a mammogram.

- **Radiation therapy (x-ray therapy):** Women who had radiation therapy to the chest (including the breasts) before age 30 are at an increased risk of developing breast cancer throughout their lives. This includes women treated for Hodgkin's disease. Studies show that the younger a woman was when she received her treatment, the higher her risk of developing breast cancer later in life.

- **Diet and lifestyle factors:** Diet is thought to play a role in breast cancer risk, although researchers have not yet identified specific dietary factors that affect risk. Differences in diet may explain the lower risk of breast cancer among Asian women compared with American women. Studies have found that obesity and weight gain in postmenopausal women increase breast cancer risk. A number of studies suggest that moderate alcohol consumption may also increase a woman's chance of developing breast cancer.

What Are the Chances That a Woman in the United States Might Get Breast Cancer?

Age is the most important risk factor for breast cancer. The older a woman is, the greater her chance of developing breast cancer. According to the National Cancer Institute Surveillance, Epidemiology, and End Results Program, 1973–1998, a woman's chance of being diagnosed with breast cancer is:

- from age 20 to age 30—1 out of 2,000
- from age 30 to age 40—1 out of 250
- from age 40 to age 50—1 out of 67
- from age 50 to age 60—1 out of 35
- from age 60 to age 70—1 out of 28
- Ever—1 out of 8

Most breast cancers occur in women over the age of 50; the number of cases is especially high for women over age 60. Breast cancer is relatively uncommon in women under age 40.

What Is the Best Method of Detecting Breast Cancer as Early as Possible?

A high-quality mammogram with a clinical breast exam (an exam done by a health care provider) is the most effective way to detect breast cancer early. Like any test, mammograms have both benefits and limitations. For example, some cancers cannot be detected by mammogram, but may be detectable by breast examination.

Checking one's own breasts for lumps or other unusual changes is called breast self-exam (BSE). Studies so far have not shown that BSE alone reduces the numbers of deaths from breast cancer. BSE should not take the place of clinical breast exam and mammography. Mammograms can detect breast cancer that cannot be felt.

What Are the Benefits of Screening Mammograms?

Several large studies conducted around the world show that breast cancer screening with mammograms reduces the number of deaths from breast cancer for women ages 40 to 69, especially those over age 50. Studies conducted to date have not shown a benefit for regular screening mammograms, or for a baseline screening mammogram, in women under age 40.

What Are Some of the Limitations of Screening Mammograms?

- **Finding cancer does not always mean saving lives**—Even though mammography can detect tumors that cannot be felt, finding a small tumor does not always mean that a woman's life will be saved. Mammography may not help a woman with a fast-growing or aggressive cancer that has already spread to other parts of her body before being detected.

- **False negatives**—False negatives occur when mammograms appear normal even though breast cancer is present. Overall, mammograms miss up to 20 percent of the breast cancers that are present at the time of screening. False negatives occur more often in younger women than in older women because the dense breasts of younger women make breast cancers more difficult to spot in mammograms. As women age, their breasts usually become more fatty (and therefore less dense), and breast cancers become easier to detect with screening mammograms.

- **False positives**—False positives occur when mammograms are read by a radiologist as abnormal, but no cancer is actually present. Although all abnormal mammograms should be followed up with additional testing (a diagnostic mammogram, ultrasound, and/or biopsy), most abnormalities turn out not to be cancer. False positives are more common in younger women, women who have had previous breast biopsies, women with a family history of breast cancer, and women who are taking estrogen (for example, hormone replacement therapy).

What Happens if Mammography Leads to the Detection of Ductal Carcinoma In Situ (DCIS)?

Over the past 30 years, improvements in mammography have resulted in an ability to detect a higher number of tissue abnormalities called DCIS. DCIS contains abnormal cells that are confined to the milk ducts of the breast. The cells have not invaded the surrounding breast tissue. Eighty percent of cases of DCIS are found by mammography because DCIS usually does not cause a lump that can be felt. Some of these cases later become invasive cancers. Today, it is not possible to predict which cases of DCIS will progress to invasive cancer. Therefore, DCIS is usually removed surgically. Until recently, DCIS was often treated with mastectomy, but breast-conserving surgery is now an option for many women with DCIS. Radiation therapy, with or without tamoxifen, also may be used. Women who have been diagnosed with DCIS should talk with their doctor to make an informed decision about treatment.

How Much Does a Mammogram Cost?

Screening mammograms generally cost between $100 and $150. Most states now have laws requiring health insurance companies to reimburse all or part of the cost of screening mammograms. Details can be provided by insurance companies and health care providers.

Medicare pays 80 percent of the cost of a screening mammogram each year for beneficiaries age 40 and older and one baseline mammogram for beneficiaries age 35 to 39. There is no deductible requirement for this benefit, but Medicare beneficiaries are responsible for a 20 percent copayment of the Medicare-approved amount.

Some state and local health programs and employers provide mammograms free or at low cost. For example, the Centers for Disease Control and Prevention (CDC) coordinates the National Breast and Cervical Cancer Early Detection Program. This program provides screening services, including clinical breast exams and mammograms, to low-income women throughout the United States and in several U.S. territories. Contact information for local programs is available on the CDC's Web site at http://www.cdc.gov/cancer/nbccedp/contacts.htm on the Internet, or by calling the CDC at 1-888-842-6355 (select option 7). Information on low-cost or free mammography screening programs is also available through the NCI's Cancer Information Service (CIS).

Where Can Women Get High-Quality Mammograms?

Women can get high-quality mammograms in breast clinics, radiology departments of hospitals, mobile vans, private radiology offices, and doctors' offices. The Mammography Quality Standards Act (MQSA) is a Federal law designed to ensure that mammograms are safe and reliable. Through the MQSA, all mammography facilities in the United States must meet stringent quality standards, be accredited by the Food and Drug Administration (FDA), and be inspected annually. The FDA ensures that facilities across the country meet MQSA standards. These standards apply to the following people at the facility:

- the technologist who takes the mammogram,
- the radiologist who interprets the mammogram, and
- the medical physicist who tests the mammography equipment.

All mammography facilities are required to display their FDA certificate. Women should look for the MQSA certificate at the mammography facility and check its expiration date. Women can ask their doctors or staff at the mammography facility about FDA certification before making an appointment. MQSA regulations also require mammography facilities to give patients an easy-to-read report on the results of their mammogram.

Information about local FDA-certified mammography facilities is available through the CIS at 800-422-6237. Also, a list of these facilities is on the FDA's Web site at http://www.fda.gov/cdrh/mammography/certified.html on the Internet.

What Should Women with Breast Implants Do about Screening Mammograms?

Women with breast implants should continue to have mammograms. (A woman who had an implant following breast cancer surgery should ask her doctor whether a mammogram of the reconstructed breast is necessary.) It is important to inform the facility about breast implants

89

when scheduling a mammogram. The technician and radiologist must be experienced in x-raying patients with breast implants. Implants can hide some breast tissue, making it more difficult for the radiologist to detect an abnormality on the mammogram. If the technologist performing the procedure is aware a woman has breast implants, steps can be taken to make sure that as much breast tissue as possible can be seen on the mammogram.

What Is Digital Mammography? How Is It Different from Conventional Mammography?

Digital mammography records x-ray images in computer code instead of on x-ray film, as with conventional mammography. In January 2000, the FDA approved a digital mammography system that may offer potential advantages over the use of standard x-ray film. Research studies so far have not shown that digital images are more effective in finding cancer than x-ray film images. However, NCI is directing additional studies to learn whether digital mammography is as good as or better than conventional mammography. Digital mammography may offer the following advantages over conventional mammography:

- The images can be stored and retrieved electronically, which makes long-distance consultations with other mammography specialists easier;

- Because the images can be adjusted by the radiologist, subtle differences between tissues may be noted;

- Digital mammography may reduce the number of follow-up procedures that are necessary; and

- The need for fewer exposures with digital mammography can reduce the already low levels of radiation.

Currently, digital mammography can be done only in facilities that are certified to practice conventional mammography and have received FDA approval to offer digital mammography. The procedure for having a mammogram with a digital system is the same as with conventional mammography.

Improving Methods for Breast Cancer Detection and Diagnosis

The National Cancer Institute (NCI) is funding numerous research projects to improve conventional mammography (an x-ray technique to visualize the internal structure of the breast) and develop other imaging technologies to detect, diagnose, and characterize breast tumors.

High-quality mammography is the most effective technology presently available for breast cancer screening. Efforts to improve mammography focus on refining the technology and improving how it is administered and x-ray films are interpreted. NCI is funding research to reduce the already low radiation dosage of mammography; enhance mammogram image quality; develop statistical techniques for computer-assisted interpretation of images; enable long-distance, electronic image transmission technology (telemammography/teleradiology) for clinical consultations; and improve image-guided techniques to assist with breast biopsies. (A breast biopsy is the removal of cells or tissues to look at under a microscope to check for signs of disease). NCI also supports research on technologies that do not use x-rays, such as magnetic resonance imaging (MRI), ultrasound, and breast-specific positron emission tomography (PET) to detect breast cancer. The following information describes the latest imaging techniques that are in use or being studied.

Ultrasound

Ultrasound, also called sonography, is an imaging technique in which high-frequency sound waves that cannot be heard by humans are bounced off tissues and internal organs. Their echoes produce a picture called a sonogram. Ultrasound imaging of the breast is used to distinguish between solid tumors and fluid-filled cysts. Ultrasound can also be used to evaluate lumps that are hard to see on a mammogram. Sometimes, ultrasound is used as part of other diagnostic procedures, such as fine needle aspiration (also called needle biopsy). Fine needle aspiration is the removal of tissue or fluid with a needle for examination under a microscope to check for signs of disease.

During an ultrasound examination, the clinician spreads a thin coating of lubricating jelly over the area to be imaged to improve conduction of the sound waves. A hand-held device called a transducer directs the sound waves through the skin toward specific tissues. As the sound waves are reflected back from the tissues within the breast, the patterns formed by the waves create a two-dimensional image of the breast on a computer.

Ultrasound is not used for routine breast cancer screening because it does not consistently detect certain early signs of cancer such as microcalcifications (tiny deposits of calcium in the breast that cannot be felt but can be seen on a conventional mammogram). A cluster of microcalcifications may indicate that cancer is present.

Digital Mammography

Digital mammography is a technique for recording x-ray images in computer code instead of on x-ray film, as with conventional mammography. The images are displayed on a computer monitor and can be enhanced (lightened or darkened) before they are printed on film. Images can also be manipulated; the radiologist (a doctor who specializes in creating and interpreting pictures of areas inside the body) can magnify or zoom in on an area. From the patient's perspective, the procedure for a mammogram with a digital system is the same as for conventional mammography.

Digital mammography may have some advantages over conventional mammography. The images can be stored and retrieved electronically, which makes long-distance consultations with other mammography specialists easier. Because the images can be adjusted by the radiologist, subtle differences between tissues may be noted. The improved accuracy of digital mammography may reduce the number of follow-up procedures. Despite these benefits, studies have not yet shown that digital mammography is more effective in finding cancer than conventional mammography.

The first digital mammography system received U.S. Food and Drug Administration (FDA) approval in 2000. An example of a digital mammography system is the Senographe® 2000D. Women considering digital mammography should talk with their doctor or contact a local FDA-certified mammography center to find out if this technique is available at that location. Only facilities that have been certified to practice conventional mammography and have FDA approval for digital mammography may offer the digital system.

Computer-Aided Detection

Computer-aided detection (CAD) involves the use of computers to bring suspicious areas on a mammogram to the radiologist's attention. It is used after the radiologist has done the initial review of the mammogram. In 1998, the FDA approved a breast imaging device that uses CAD technology. Others are in development. An example of a breast imaging device that uses CAD technology is the ImageChecker®. This device scans the mammogram with a laser beam and converts it into a digital signal that is processed by a computer. The image is then displayed on a video monitor, with suspicious areas highlighted for the radiologist to review. The radiologist can compare the digital image with the conventional mammogram to see if any of the highlighted areas were missed on the initial review and require further evaluation. CAD technology may improve the accuracy of screening mammography. The incorporation of CAD technology to digital mammography is under evaluation.

Magnetic Resonance Imaging

In magnetic resonance imaging (MRI), a magnet linked to a computer creates detailed pictures of areas inside the body without the use of radiation. Each MRI produces hundreds of images of the breast from side-to-side, top-to-bottom, and front-to-back. The images are then interpreted by a radiologist.

During an MRI of the breast, the patient lies on her stomach on the scanning table. The breast hangs into a depression or hollow in the table, which contains coils that detect the magnetic signal. The table is moved into a tube-like machine that contains the magnet. After an initial series of images has been taken, the patient may be given a contrast agent intravenously (by injection into a vein). The contrast agent is not radioactive; it is sometimes used to improve the visibility of a tumor. Additional images are then taken. The entire imaging session takes about 1 hour.

Breast MRI is not used for routine breast cancer screening, but clinical trials (research studies with people) are being performed to determine if MRI is valuable for screening certain women, such as young women at high risk for breast cancer. MRI cannot always accurately distinguish between cancer and benign (noncancerous) breast conditions. Like ultrasound, MRI cannot detect microcalcifications.

MRI is used primarily to evaluate breast implants for leaks or ruptures, and to assess abnormal areas that are seen on a mammogram or are felt after breast surgery or radiation therapy. It can be used after breast cancer is diagnosed to determine the extent of the tumor in the breast. MRI is also sometimes useful in imaging dense breast tissue, which is often found in younger women, and in viewing breast abnormalities that can be felt but are not visible with conventional mammography or ultrasound.

PET Scan

The positron emission tomography (PET) scan creates computerized images of chemical changes that take place in tissue. The patient is given an injection of a substance that consists of a combination of a sugar and a small amount of radioactive material. The radioactive sugar can help in locating a tumor because cancer cells take up or absorb sugar faster than other tissues in the body.

After receiving the radioactive drug, the patient lies still for about 45 minutes while the drug circulates throughout the body. If a tumor is present, the radioactive sugar will accumulate in the tumor. The patient then lies on a table, which gradually moves through the PET scanner 6 to 7 times during a 45-minute period. The PET scanner is used to detect the radiation. A computer translates this information into the images that are interpreted by a radiologist.

PET scans may play a role in determining whether a breast mass is cancerous. However, PET scans are more accurate in detecting larger and more aggressive tumors than they are in locating tumors that are smaller than 8 mm and/or less aggressive. They may also detect cancer when other imaging techniques show normal results. PET scans may be helpful in evaluating and staging recurrent disease (cancer that has come back).

An NCI-sponsored clinical trial is evaluating the usefulness of PET scan results in women who have breast cancer compared with the findings from other imaging and diagnostic techniques. This trial is also studying the effectiveness of PET scans in tracking the response of a tumor to treatment.

Electrical Impedance Scanning

Different types of tissue have different electrical impedance levels (electrical impedance is a measurement of how fast electricity travels through a given material). Some types of tissue have high electrical impedance, while others have low electrical impedance. Breast tissue that is cancerous has a much lower electrical impedance (conducts electricity much better) than normal breast tissue. Electrical impedance scanning devices are used along with conventional mammography to detect breast cancer. The T-Scan 2000, also known as the T-Scan, is an example of such a device. The FDA approved the T-Scan 2000 in 1999.

The electrical impedance scanning device, which does not emit any radiation, consists of a hand-held scanning probe and a computer screen that displays two-dimensional images of the breast. An electrode patch, similar to that used for an electrocardiogram, is placed on the patient's arm. A very small amount of electric current, about the same amount used by a small penlight battery, is transmitted through the patch and into the body. The current travels through the breast, where it is measured by the scanning probe placed over the breast. An image is generated from the measurements of electrical impedance. Because breast cancer cells conduct electricity better than normal breast cells and tend to have lower electrical impedance, breast tumors may appear as bright white spots on the computer screen.

This device can confirm the location of abnormal areas that were detected by a conventional mammogram. The scanner sends the image directly to a computer, allowing the radiologist to move the probe around the breast to get the best view of the area being examined. The device may reduce the number of biopsies needed to determine whether a mass is cancerous. It may also improve the identification of women who should have a biopsy.

The scanner is not approved as a screening device for breast cancer, and is not used when mammography or other findings clearly indicate the need for a biopsy. This device has not been studied with patients who have implanted electronic devices, such as pacemakers. It is not recommended for use on such patients.

Image-Guided Breast Biopsy Techniques

Imaging techniques play an important role in helping doctors perform breast biopsies, especially of abnormal areas that cannot be felt but can be seen on a conventional mammogram or with ultrasound. One type of needle biopsy, the stereotactic-guided biopsy, involves the precise location of the abnormal area in three dimensions using conventional mammography. (Stereotactic refers to the use of a computer and scanning devices to create three-dimensional images.) A needle is then inserted into the breast and a tissue sample is obtained. Additional samples can be obtained by moving the needle within the abnormal area.

Another type of needle biopsy uses a different system, known as the Mammotome® breast biopsy system. The FDA approved Mammotome in 1996; the hand-held version of the Mammotome received FDA clearance in September 1999. A large needle is inserted into the suspicious area using ultrasound or stereotactic guidance. The Mammotome is then used to gently vacuum tissue from the suspicious area. Additional tissue samples can be obtained by rotating the needle. This procedure can be performed with the patient lying on her stomach on a table. If the hand-held device is used, the patient may lie on her back or in a seated position.

There have been no reports of serious complications resulting from the Mammotome breast biopsy system. Women interested in this procedure should talk with their doctor.

Ductal Lavage

Ductal lavage is an investigational technique for collecting samples of cells from breast ducts for analysis under a microscope. A saline (salt water) solution is introduced into a milk duct through a catheter (a thin, flexible tube) that is inserted into the opening of the duct on the surface of the nipple. Fluid, which contains cells from the duct, is withdrawn through the catheter. The cells are checked under a microscope to identify changes that may indicate cancer or changes that may increase the risk for breast cancer. The usefulness of ductal lavage is still under study.

Imaging Clinical Trials

In March 1999, the NCI began funding the American College of Radiology Imaging Network (ACRIN) as part of the NCI's Clinical Trials Cooperative Group Program. (A cooperative group is a group of physicians, hospitals, or both that works with the NCI to identify important questions in cancer research and design clinical trials to answer these questions.) The Cooperative Group program is designed to promote and support clinical trials of new cancer treatments, explore methods of cancer prevention and early detection, and study quality of life issues and rehabilitation during and after treatment. ACRIN is dedicated to increasing the number and quality of clinical trials that involve imaging technologies to detect and diagnose cancer. The NCI actively participates in the planning, review, and monitoring of clinical trials that are organized by ACRIN.

People interested in taking part in a clinical trial should talk with their doctor. Information about clinical trials is available from the Cancer Information Service (CIS).

Additional Information

Cancer Information Service
National Cancer Institute (NCI)
Suite 3036A, MSC8322
6116 Executive Blvd.
Bethesda, MD 20892-8322
Toll-Free: 800-422-6237
Toll-Free TTY: 800-332-8615
Website: www.nci.nih.gov
E-mail: cancermail@icicc.nci.nih.gov

Section 10.3

Cervical Cancer/Pap Test

This section includes "Screening for Cervical Cancer: What's New From the USPSTF?" Agency for Healthcare Research and Quality (AHRQ), AHRQ Publication No. APPIP03-0004, January 2003; and "The Pap Test: Questions and Answers," Fact Sheet 5.16, National Cancer Institute (NCI), reviewed February 12, 2003.

Screening for Cervical Cancer

This information is based on the work of the U.S. Preventive Services Task Force (USPSTF). The USPSTF systematically reviews the evidence of effectiveness of a wide range of clinical preventive services—including screening, counseling, and chemoprevention (the use of medication to prevent diseases)—to develop recommendations for preventive care in the primary care setting.

This section presents highlights of USPSTF recommendations on this topic and should not be used to make treatment or policy decisions.

What Screening Is Recommended by the USPSTF?

- The U.S. Preventive Services Task Force (USPSTF) strongly recommends screening women for cervical cancer if they are sexually active and have a cervix.

- The USPSTF recommends against routinely screening women older than age 65 if they have had adequate recent screening with normal Pap smears and are not otherwise at increased risk for cervical cancer.

- The USPSTF recommends against routine Pap screening for women who have had a total hysterectomy for benign disease.

- The USPSTF concludes that the evidence is insufficient to recommend for or against new technologies (such as ThinPrep®) in place of conventional Pap tests.

- The USPSTF concludes that the evidence is insufficient to recommend for or against human papillomavirus (HPV) testing as a primary screening test for cervical cancer.

The Task Force concludes that screening should begin within 3 years of the start of sexual activity or age 21, whichever comes first, and should be done at least every 3 years. The risk for cervical cancer and the yield of screening decline through middle age.

For women older than 65 who have had normal Pap smears, the benefits of continued screening may not outweigh the potential harms, such as false-positive test results and invasive procedures. The Task Force also concludes that the yield of detecting vaginal neoplasms is too low to justify continuing screening after a total hysterectomy.

Most cases of cervical cancer occur in women who are not screened adequately. Clinicians, hospitals, and health plans should develop systems to identify and screen women, including older women, who have had no screening or who have been screened inadequately in the past.

Why Aren't Annual Pap Tests or Newer Technologies Recommended?

The USPSTF found no direct evidence that annual screening is more effective than less frequent screening in preventing cases of cervical cancer or death from cervical cancer. Cervical cancer usually progresses from precancerous lesions to invasive cancer over many years. Unless women are at increased risk for cervical cancer, screening less frequently is likely to be effective while reducing the number of false-positive results.

The available data are insufficient to determine whether newer, more expensive forms of Pap tests are better than conventional Pap tests. Although some data suggest new tests like ThinPrep® may detect more high-grade lesions, they may also increase false-positive results. HPV tests are not yet approved for use as primary screening tests for cervical cancer, but research is underway to determine whether HPV tests can identify women who need more or less frequent screening with Pap tests.

How Do These Recommendations Differ from Previous Task Force Recommendations?

These recommendations reinforce earlier recommendations that sexually active women get regular Pap testing at least every 3 years. The revised recommendations, however, raise the age at which routine

98

screening should begin, as a result of data suggesting that the risk for cervical cancer in adolescents is low and the risk for false-positive results is high. The recommendation against continuing routine screening in women after age 65, or after a total hysterectomy, are stronger than in 1996, reflecting new data on the low yield and potential harms of such screening.

The Pap Test: Questions and Answers

Key Points

- A Pap test and pelvic exam are important parts of a woman's routine health care because they can detect cancer or abnormalities that may lead to cancer of the cervix.
- Women should have a Pap test at least once every 3 years, beginning about 3 years after they begin to have sexual intercourse, but no later than age 21.
- If the Pap test shows abnormalities, further tests and/or treatment may be necessary.
- Human papillomavirus (HPV) infection is the primary risk factor for cervical cancer.

What is a Pap test?

The Pap test (sometimes called a Pap smear) is a way to examine cells collected from the cervix (the lower, narrow end of the uterus). The main purpose of the Pap test is to find abnormal cell changes that may arise from cervical cancer or before cancer develops.

What is a pelvic exam?

In a pelvic exam, the uterus, vagina, ovaries, fallopian tubes, bladder, and rectum are felt to find any abnormality in their shape or size. During a pelvic exam, an instrument called a speculum is used to widen the vagina so that the upper portion of the vagina and the cervix can be seen.

Why are a Pap test and pelvic exam important?

A Pap test and pelvic exam are important parts of a woman's routine health care because they can detect abnormalities that may lead to invasive cancer of the cervix. These abnormalities can be treated before cancer develops. Most invasive cancers of the cervix can be prevented if women have Pap tests regularly. Also, as with many types of cancer, cancer of the cervix is more likely to be treated successfully if it is detected early.

Who performs a Pap test?

Doctors and other specially trained health care professionals, such as physician assistants, nurse midwives, and nurse practitioners, may perform Pap tests and pelvic exams. These individuals are often called clinicians.

How is a Pap test done?

A Pap test is simple, quick, and painless; it can be done in a doctor's office, a clinic, or a hospital. While a woman lies on an exam table, the clinician inserts a speculum into her vagina to widen it. A sample of cells is taken from the cervix with a wooden scraper and/or a small cervical brush. The specimen (or smear) is placed on a glass slide and preserved with a fixative, or is rinsed in a vial of fixative, and is sent to a laboratory for examination.

How often should a woman have a Pap test?

Women should talk with their clinician about when and how often they should have a Pap test. Current general guidelines recommend that women have a Pap test at least once every 3 years, beginning about 3 years after they begin to have sexual intercourse, but no later than age 21. Experts recommend waiting about 3 years after the start of sexual activity to avoid overtreatment for common, temporary, abnormal changes. It is safe to wait 3 years, because cervical cancer usually develops slowly. Cervical cancer is extremely rare in women under age 25.

Women ages 65 to 70 who have had at least three normal Pap tests and no abnormal Pap tests in the last 10 years may decide, after talking with their clinician, to stop having Pap tests. Women who have had a hysterectomy (surgery to remove the uterus and cervix) do not need to have a Pap test, unless the surgery was done as a treatment for precancer or cancer.

When should the Pap test be done?

A woman should have this test when she is not menstruating; the best time is between 10 and 20 days after the first day of the last menstrual period. For about 2 days before a Pap test, she should avoid douching or using vaginal medicines or spermicidal foams, creams, or jellies (except as directed by a physician). These may wash away or hide abnormal cells.

How are the results of a Pap test reported?

Most laboratories in the United States use a standard set of terms called the Bethesda System to report test results. Under the Bethesda System, Pap test samples that have no cell abnormalities are reported as negative for intraepithelial lesion or malignancy. Samples with cell abnormalities are divided into the following categories:

- *ASC—atypical squamous cells.* Squamous cells are the thin flat cells that form the surface of the cervix. The Bethesda System divides this category into two groups:

   ASCUS—atypical squamous cells of undetermined significance. The squamous cells do not appear completely normal, but doctors are uncertain about what the cell changes mean. Sometimes the changes are related to HPV infection. ACSUS are considered mild abnormalities.

   ASC-H—atypical squamous cells cannot exclude a high-grade squamous intraepithelial lesion. The cells do not appear normal, but doctors are uncertain about what the cell changes mean. ASC-H may be at higher risk of being precancerous.

- *AGC—atypical glandular cells.* Glandular cells are mucus-producing cells found in the endocervical canal (opening in the center of the cervix) or in the lining of the uterus. The glandular cells do not appear normal, but doctors are uncertain about what the cell changes mean.

- *AIS—endocervical adenocarcinoma in situ.* Precancerous cells are found in the glandular tissue.

- *LSIL—low-grade squamous intraepithelial lesion.* Low-grade means there are early changes in the size and shape of cells. The word lesion refers to an area of abnormal tissue. Intraepithelial refers to the layer of cells that forms the surface of the cervix. LSILs are considered mild abnormalities caused by HPV infection.

- *HSIL—high-grade squamous intraepithelial lesion.* High-grade means that there are more marked changes in the size and shape of the abnormal (precancerous) cells, meaning that the cells look very different from normal cells. HSILs are more severe abnormalities and have a higher likelihood of progressing to invasive cancer.

How common are Pap test abnormalities?

About 55 million Pap tests are performed each year in the United States. Of these, approximately 3.5 million (6 percent) are abnormal and require medical follow-up.

What do abnormal results mean?

A physician may simply describe Pap test results to a patient as abnormal. Cells on the surface of the cervix sometimes appear abnormal but are very rarely cancerous. It is important to remember that abnormal conditions do not always become cancerous, and some conditions are more likely to lead to cancer than others. A woman may want to ask her doctor for specific information about her Pap test result and what the result means. There are several terms that may be used to describe abnormal results.

- **Dysplasia** is a term used to describe abnormal cells. Dysplasia is not cancer, although it may develop into very early cancer of the cervix. The cells look abnormal under the microscope, but they do not invade nearby healthy tissue. There are four degrees of dysplasia, classified as mild, moderate, severe, or carcinoma in situ, depending on how abnormal the cells appear under the microscope. Carcinoma in situ means that cancer is present only in the layer of cells on the surface of the cervix, and has not spread to nearby tissues.

- **Squamous intraepithelial lesion (SIL)** is another term that is used to describe abnormal changes in the cells on the surface of the cervix. The word squamous describes thin, flat cells that form the outer surface of the cervix. The word lesion refers to abnormal tissue. An intraepithelial lesion means that the abnormal cells are present only in the layer of cells on the surface of the cervix. A doctor may describe SIL as being low-grade (early changes in the size, shape, and number of cells) or high-grade (precancerous cells that look very different from normal cells).

- **Cervical intraepithelial neoplasia (CIN)** is another term that is sometimes used to describe abnormal tissue findings.

Neoplasia means an abnormal growth of cells. Intraepithelial refers to the layer of cells that form the surface of the cervix. The term CIN, along with a number (1 to 3), describes how much of the thickness of the lining of the cervix contains abnormal cells.

- **Atypical squamous cells** are findings that are unclear, and not a definite abnormality.

Cervical cancer, or invasive cervical cancer, occurs when abnormal cells spread deeper into the cervix or to other tissues or organs.

What if Pap test results are abnormal?

If the Pap test shows an ambiguous or minor abnormality, the physician may repeat the test to determine whether further follow-up is needed. Many times, cell changes in the cervix go away without treatment. In some cases, doctors may prescribe estrogen cream for women who have ASCUS and are near or past menopause. Because these cell changes are often caused by low hormone levels, applying an estrogen cream to the cervix for a few weeks can usually help to clarify the cause of the cell changes.

If the Pap test shows a finding of ASC-H, LSIL, or HSIL, the physician may perform a colposcopy using an instrument much like a microscope (called a colposcope) to examine the vagina and the cervix. The colposcope does not enter the body. During a colposcopy, the physician may coat the cervix with a dilute vinegar solution that causes abnormal areas to turn white. The physician may also perform a biopsy (a biopsy is the removal of a small piece of tissue for study in a lab).

The physician may also perform endocervical curettage. This test involves scraping cells from inside the endocervical canal with a small spoon-shaped tool called a curette. The doctor may also remove a small piece of cervical tissue for examination. This procedure is called a biopsy. The cells or tissue are sent to a lab for study under a microscope.

If the lab finds abnormal cells that have a high chance of becoming cancer, further treatment is needed. Without treatment, these cells may turn into invasive cancer. Treatment options include the following:

- **LEEP (loop electrosurgical excision procedure)** is surgery that uses an electrical current which is passed through a thin wire loop to act as a knife.

- **Cryotherapy** destroys abnormal tissue by freezing it.

- **Laser therapy** is the use of a narrow beam of intense light to destroy or remove abnormal cells.

- **Conization** removes a cone-shaped piece of tissue using a knife, a laser, or the LEEP technique.

For information about how Pap test abnormalities compare, and which tests and treatment options may be appropriate see Table 10.2.

Table 10.2. Pap Test Abnormalities Comparison

Pap Test Result	Abbreviation	Also Known As	Tests and Treatments May Include
Atypical squamous cells—undetermined significance	ASCUS		HPV testing; Repeat Pap test; Colposcopy and biopsy; Estrogen cream
Atypical squamous cells—cannot exclude HSIL	ASC-H		Colposcopy and biopsy
Atypical glandular cells	AGC		Colposcopy and biopsy and/or endocervical curettage
Endocervical adenocarcinoma in situ	AIS		Colposcopy and biopsy and/or endocervical curettage
Low-grade squamous intra-epithelial lesion	LSIL	Mild dysplasia or Cervical intraepithelial neoplasia 1 (CIN 1)	Colposcopy and biopsy
High-grade squamous intra-epithelial lesion	HSIL	Moderate dysplasia, Severe dysplasia, CIN 2, CIN 3, or Carcinoma in situ (CIS)	Colposcopy and biopsy and/or endocervical curettage; Further treatment with LEEP, cryotherapy, laser therapy, conization, or hysterectomy

How are human papillomaviruses (HPVs) associated with the development of cervical cancer?

Human papillomaviruses (HPVs) are a group of more than 100 viruses. Some types of HPV cause the common warts that grow on hands and feet. Some HPVs are sexually transmitted and cause wart-like growths on the genitals, but these types do not lead to cancer. More than a dozen other sexually transmitted HPVs have been linked to cervical cancer.

HPV infection is the primary risk factor for cervical cancer. However, although HPV infection is very common, only a very small percentage of women with untreated HPV infections develop cervical cancer.

Who is at risk for HPV infection?

HPV infection is more common in younger age groups, particularly among women in their late teens and twenties. Because HPVs are spread mainly through sexual contact, risk increases with number of sexual partners. Women who become sexually active at a young age, who have multiple sexual partners, and whose sexual partners have other partners are at increased risk. Women who are infected with the human immunodeficiency virus (HIV) are also at higher risk for being infected with HPVs and for developing cervical abnormalities. Nonsexual transmission of HPVs is rare. The virus often disappears but sometimes remains detectable for years after infection.

Does infection with a cancer-associated type of HPV always lead to a precancerous condition or cancer?

No. Most HPV infections appear to go away on their own without causing any kind of abnormality. However, persistent infection with cancer-associated HPV types increases the risk that mild abnormalities will progress to more severe abnormalities or cervical cancer. With regular follow-up care by trained clinicians, women with precancerous cervical abnormalities can be treated before cancer develops.

Have any studies been done to examine HPV testing and treatment options for mild Pap test abnormalities?

Findings of the ASCUS/LSIL Triage Study (ALTS), a major clinical trial (research study with people) funded and organized by the National Cancer Institute (NCI), suggest that HPV testing in women with ASCUS may help identify underlying abnormalities that need a doctor's attention. The study results suggest that testing cervical samples for HPVs can identify which ASCUS abnormalities need treatment. A negative HPV test can provide reassurance that cancer or a precancerous condition is not present.

What are false positive and false negative results?

The Pap test is a screening test and, like any such test, it is not 100-percent accurate. Although false positive and false negative results do not occur very often, they can cause anxiety and can affect a woman's health. A false positive Pap test means that a patient is told she has abnormal cells, but the cells are actually normal.

A false negative Pap test occurs when a specimen is called normal, but the woman has a significant abnormality that was missed. A false negative Pap test may delay the diagnosis and treatment of a precancerous condition. However, regular screening helps to compensate for the false negative result. If abnormal cells are missed at one time, chances are good that the cells will be detected the next time.

What methods are being developed to improve the accuracy of Pap tests?

In April 1996, the Consensus Development Conference on Cervical Cancer, which was convened by the National Institutes of Health (NIH), concluded that about half of false negative Pap tests are due to inadequate specimen collection. The other half are due to a failure to identify or interpret the specimens correctly. Although the conventional Pap test is effective in the majority of cases, the conference made it clear that new methods of collecting and reading specimens are needed to reduce the number of false negatives.

The Bethesda System requires laboratories to determine whether there are enough cervical cells in the specimen to make a proper evaluation. This requirement helps improve the quality of samples and sample collection. The Bethesda System requires a sample to be categorized as *satisfactory for evaluation* or *unsatisfactory for evaluation*.

One new method of collecting and analyzing samples is called liquid-based thin-layer slide preparation. This method may make it easier to screen for abnormal cells. Cervical cells are collected with a brush or other collection instrument. The instrument is rinsed in a vial of liquid preservative. The vial is sent to a laboratory, where an automated thin-layer slide device prepares the slide for viewing. Results of this method suggest that it is comparable to, or more sensitive than, standard Pap tests for the detection of significant abnormalities.

Computer automated readers are also being used to improve the reading of Pap tests. This technology uses a microscope that conveys a cellular image to a computer, which analyzes the image for the presence of abnormal cells

Section 10.4

Routine Tests during Pregnancy

This information was provided by KidsHealth, one of the largest resources online for medically reviewed health information written for parents, kids, and teens. For more articles like this one, visit www.KidsHealth.org or www.TeensHealth.org. © 2003 The Nemours Center for Children's Health Media, a division of The Nemours Foundation.

Prenatal Tests

Every parent-to-be spends happy hours envisioning a healthy baby. But these daydreams are often accompanied by moments of worry— what if the baby has a serious or untreatable health problem? What would I do? Would it be my fault?

Concerns like these are completely natural, and some may be exaggerated by news stories about genetics and genetic testing, which promises that someday parents may be able to pick only "desirable" traits in their unborn children. With all the medical information available, you may feel as though you have to undergo a battery of prenatal tests to make sure your baby is healthy.

Prenatal tests can serve a useful function in terms of identifying, and sometimes treating, health problems that could endanger both you and your unborn child. However, they have limitations. As an expecting parent, you should take the time to educate yourself about these tests and to think about what you would do if a health problem is detected.

Why Are Prenatal Tests Performed?

Prenatal tests do several different things. They can identify:

- treatable health problems in the mother that can affect the baby's health

- characteristics of the fetus, including size, sex, age, and placement in the uterus

- the chance that a baby has certain congenital, genetic, or chromosomal problems

- certain types of fetal abnormalities, including heart problems

The last two items on this list may seem the same, but there's a key difference. Some prenatal tests are screening tests and only reveal the possibility of a problem existing—they don't provide a definitive diagnosis. Other prenatal tests are diagnostic in nature, which means they can determine with a fair degree of certainty whether a fetus has a specific problem. Many women whose screening tests reveal the possibility of an abnormality have healthy babies, but in the interest of making the more specific determination, the screening test may be followed by a more invasive—and riskier—diagnostic test.

The issue of prenatal testing is further complicated by the fact that approximately 250 birth defects can be diagnosed in an unborn fetus—many more than can be treated or cured. This raises the question of what a parent will do once a defect or problem is detected.

What Do Prenatal Tests Find?

Among other things, routine prenatal tests can determine key things about the mother's health including her blood type, whether she suffers from gestational diabetes, her immunity to certain diseases, and whether she has a sexually transmitted disease (STD) or cervical cancer. All of these conditions can affect the health of the fetus. Prenatal tests also can determine things about the fetus' health, including whether it's one of the 2% to 3% of babies in the United States that the American College of Obstetricians and Gynecologists (ACOG) says have major congenital birth defects. There are different categories of defects screened by prenatal tests, including:

Dominant gene disorders: In dominant gene disorders, there's a 50-50 chance a child will inherit the gene from the affected parent and have the disorder. Dominant gene disorders include:

- **achondroplasia,** a rare abnormality of the skeleton causing shorter-than-normal arms and legs

- **Huntington disease,** a disease of the nervous system that causes neurologic deterioration affecting people in their 30s and 40s

Recessive gene disorders: Because there are so many genes in each cell, everyone carries some abnormal recessive genes, but most people don't have a defect because the normal gene overrules the abnormal one. But if a fetus has a pair of abnormal recessive genes (one from each parent), the child will have the disorder. It's more likely for this to happen in children born to certain ethnic groups or to parents who are blood relatives. Recessive gene disorders include:

- **cystic fibrosis** (most common among people of northern European descent), a disease that causes the respiratory system to produce thick mucus that clogs the lungs

- **sickle cell disease** (most common among people of African descent), a disease where red blood cells form a "sickle" shape, rather than the typical donut shape, get caught in blood vessels, and cut off oxygen to tissues

- **Tay-Sachs disease** (most common among people of European [Ashkenazi] Jewish descent), a disorder causing mental retardation, blindness, seizures, and death

- **beta thalassemia** (most common among people of Mediterranean descent), a disorder causing anemia

X-linked disorders: These disorders are determined by genes on the X-chromosome of the pair of chromosomes that determine sex. These disorders are much more common in boys because the pair of sex chromosomes in males contains only one X-chromosome (the other is a Y-chromosome). If the disease gene is present on the one X-chromosome, the X-linked disease shows up because there's no other paired gene to 'overrule' the disease gene. Hemophilia is one such X-linked disorder; people who have it lack a crucial clotting agent in their blood.

Chromosomal disorders: Some chromosomal disorders are inherited, but most are caused by a sporadic error in the genetics of the egg or sperm. The chance of a child having these disorders increases with the age of the mother. For example, according to the ACOG, one in 1,667 live babies born to 20-year-olds have Down syndrome; that number changes to one in 378 for 35-year-olds and one in 106 for 40-year-olds. Down syndrome causes mental retardation and physical defects.

Multifactorial disorders: This final category includes disorders that are caused by a mix of genetic and environmental factors. The frequency of these disorders varies from country to country; some can be detected during pregnancy. Multifactorial disorders include neural tube defects, which occur when the tube enclosing the spinal cord doesn't form properly. Neural tube defects include spina bifida and anencephaly. Spina bifida is also called "open spine" and occurs when the lower part of the neural tube doesn't close during embryo development, leaving the spinal cord and nerve bundles exposed. Anencephaly occurs when the brain and head don't develop properly, with the top half of the brain being completely absent. Neural tube defects have been associated with inadequate intake of folic acid during the early part of pregnancy, among other factors.

Other multifactorial disorders include:

- congenital heart defects
- club foot
- cleft lip and palate
- hip dislocations

Who Has Prenatal Tests?

Certain prenatal tests are considered routine—that is, almost all pregnant women receiving prenatal care get these tests. Others are recommended only for certain women, especially those who have what are known as high-risk pregnancies. George Macones, MD, the director of maternal/fetal medicine and director of obstetrics for the University of Pennsylvania Health System in Philadelphia, typically recommends non-routine tests to women who:

- are age 35 or older
- have had a premature baby
- have had a baby with a birth defect—especially heart or genetic problems
- have high blood pressure, diabetes, lupus, asthma, or a seizure disorder
- have or whose partner has an ethnic background where genetic disorders are common
- have or whose partner has a family history of mental retardation

Dr. Macones is also careful to point out that although he recommends these tests, ultimately it's up to the mother if she wants to have them. "I spend a lot of time talking to parents before the mother undergoes, for example, amniocentesis," he says. "Patients need to be educated before they make decisions."

In addition to talking to their obstetricians, women who have a family history of genetic problems in their families (or whose partners do) may want to consult with a genetic counselor who can help them construct a family tree going back as far as three generations.

To decide which tests are right for you, it's important to carefully discuss with your doctor what these tests are supposed to measure, how reliable they are, the potential risks, and your options and plans if the results indicate a disorder or defect.

Routine Prenatal Tests

On your first visit to the doctor for prenatal care, you'll undergo certain tests regardless of your age or genetic background.

Blood tests determine your blood type and Rh factor. If your blood is Rh positive and your partner's is Rh negative, you may develop antibodies that prove dangerous to your fetus. This can be treated through a course of injections. Blood tests also measure the level of iron in your blood and check for hepatitis B, syphilis, and HIV. You'll also be tested to see whether you're immune to rubella (German measles).

Urine tests check for kidney infections and signs of gestational diabetes and pregnancy-induced high blood pressure (which can cause a specific protein to show in the urine).

Cervical tests check for STDs (such as chlamydia and gonorrhea), cervical cancer, and Group B streptococcus infection. Group B streptococcus, which are bacteria that are not transmitted sexually, can cause serious infections in newborns.

Around the 16th to 18th week of pregnancy, most women will have a maternal blood screening test performed. Also known as a "triple-marker" test, it measures the levels of a protein produced by the fetus and two pregnancy-produced hormones in the mother's blood. This test can reveal the chances that a mother is carrying a fetus with neural tube defects or Down syndrome.

It's at this point that most women will also have their first ultrasound test, which helps the doctor identify the position of the baby and its gender as well as helping to detect Down syndrome, other chromosome abnormalities, structural defects such as spina bifida and anencephaly, and inherited metabolic disorders.

111

Around the 24th week of pregnancy, an additional screening for gestational diabetes may be performed.

Chart of Prenatal Tests

This chart includes some tests that are now performed almost routinely in the United States and those that are performed only in high-risk pregnancies or if the doctor suspects an abnormality in the fetus.

Chorionic Villus Sampling (CVS)

- **Why Is This Test Performed?** Chorionic villi are microscopic finger-like projections that make up the placenta. They develop from the same fertilized egg as the fetus and reflect the fetal genetic makeup. This newer alternative to amniocentesis removes some of the chorionic villi and tests them for chromosomal abnormalities, such as Down syndrome. Its advantage over amniocentesis is that it can be performed earlier, allowing more time for expectant parents to receive counseling and make decisions.

- **Should I Have This Test?** If you are older than age 35, have a family history of genetic disorders (or a partner who does), or have a previous child with a birth defect, your doctor may recommend this test for you. ACOG says this test carries between a 0.5% and 1% risk of miscarriage. It may cause intrauterine growth retardation, prematurity, or early labor. Other risks include infection and spotting or bleeding (this is more common in the transcervical test).

- **When Should I Have This Test?** 10 to 12 weeks.

- **How Is the Test Performed?** This test is performed in one of two ways:

  - **Transcervical:** Using ultrasound as a guide, a thin tube is passed from the vagina into the cervix. Gentle suction removes a sample of tissue from the chorionic villi. No anesthetic is used, although some women do experience a pinch and cramping.

  - **Transabdominal:** A needle is inserted through the abdominal wall—this minimizes chances of intrauterine infection, and in women whose uterus is tipped, reduces the chance of miscarriage. After the sample is taken, the doctor will check the fetal heart rate. You should rest for a couple hours afterward.

- **When Are the Results Available?** Less than 1 week for Down syndrome or about 2 weeks for a thorough analysis.

Maternal Blood Screening

- **Why Is This Test Performed?** Doctors use this to test the mother's blood only for alpha-fetoprotein (AFP). AFP is the protein produced by the fetus, and it appears in varying amounts in the mother's blood and the amniotic fluid at different times during pregnancy. A certain level in the mother's blood is considered normal, but higher or lower levels may indicate a problem. This test has been expanded, however, to include two pregnancy hormones called estriol and human chorionic gonadotropin (HCG), which is why it's now sometimes referred to as a "triple screen." This test calculates a woman's individual risk of birth defects based on the levels of the three (or more) substances plus her age, weight, race, and whether she has diabetes requiring insulin treatment. It's important to note that this screening test determines risk only—it doesn't diagnose a condition.

- **Should I Have This Test?** All women are offered this test. Remember that this is a screening, not a definite test—it indicates whether a woman is likely to be carrying an affected fetus. It's also not foolproof—spina bifida may go undetected, and some women with high levels have been found to be carrying a healthy baby. Further testing is recommended to confirm a positive result.

- **When Should I Have This Test?** 16 to 18 weeks.

- **How Is the Test Performed?** Blood is drawn from the mother.

- **When Are the Results Available?** 3 to 5 days, although it may take up to a week or two.

Amniocentesis

- **Why Is This Test Performed?** This test is used most often to detect Down syndrome and other chromosome abnormalities, structural defects such as spina bifida and anencephaly, and inherited metabolic disorders. Other common birth defects, such as heart disorders and cleft lip and palate, can't be determined using this test. Late in the pregnancy, this test can reveal if a baby's lungs are strong enough to allow the baby to breathe normally after birth, which can help the doctor make decisions about inducing labor.

- **Should I Have This Test?** If you are older than age 35, have a family history of genetic disorders (or a partner who does), or have a previous child with a birth defect, your doctor may recommend this test for you. This test can be very accurate—close to 100%—but only certain disorders can be detected. According to the Centers for Disease Control and Prevention (CDC), the rate of miscarriage with this procedure is between one in 400 and one in 200. The procedure also carries a lower risk of uterine infection (less than one in 1,000), which can cause miscarriage.

- **When Should I Have This Test?** 16 to 18 weeks.

- **How Is the Test Performed?** A needle is inserted through the abdominal wall into the uterus, removing some of the amniotic fluid. A local anesthetic may be used. Some women report they experience cramping when the needle enters the uterus or pressure while the doctor retrieves the sample. The doctor will check the fetus' heartbeat after the procedure to make sure it's normal. Most doctors recommend rest for a couple hours after the procedure. One ounce of fluid is withdrawn and sent to a lab for testing. The cells in the fluid are grown in a special culture and then analyzed. The specific tests conducted depend on personal and family medical history.

- **When Are the Results Available?** Up to 1 month (with the possibility that the lab will ask for a repeat), but tests of lung maturity are available immediately.

Ultrasound

- **Why Is This Test Performed?** In this test, sound waves are bounced off the baby's bones and tissues to construct an image showing the baby's shape and position in the uterus. Ultrasounds were once used only in high-risk pregnancies but have become so common that they are often part of routine prenatal care. In addition to showing the fetus' age, rate of growth, position, movement, breathing, and heart rate, it shows the number of fetuses and the amount of amniotic fluid in the uterus. The test is used most often to detect Down syndrome and other chromosome abnormalities, structural defects such as spina bifida and anencephaly, and inherited metabolic disorders. Congenital heart defects, gastrointestinal and kidney malformations, and cleft lip or palate may also be determined. Ultrasound can indicate the position of the placenta in late pregnancy (which may be blocking the baby's way out of the uterus). They can be used to detect pregnancies outside the uterus and they can guide other tests by showing placement of the fetus.

- **Should I Have This Test?** Most women have this test. You may want to ask your doctor about ultrasound. Find out if it's the most appropriate test for you and discuss the risks and benefits. There are no proven side effects of ultrasound to the mother or fetus, although it's still being studied.

- **When Should I Have This Test?** 16 to 18 weeks (it can be done earlier and later if necessary, especially if your doctor wants to monitor fetal growth).

- **How Is the Test Performed?** Women need to have a full bladder for a transabdominal ultrasound to be performed in the early months—you may be asked to drink a lot of water and not urinate. You'll lie on an examining table, and your abdomen will be coated with a special ultrasound gel. A technician will pass a transducer back and forth over your abdomen, while a computer translates the waves into an image called a sonogram. You may want to ask to have the picture interpreted for you, even in late pregnancy—it often doesn't look like a baby to the untrained eye. Sometimes, if the radiologist isn't getting a good enough image from the ultrasound, he or she will determine that a transvaginal ultrasound is necessary. This is especially common in early pregnancy. For this procedure, your bladder should be empty. Instead of a transducer being moved over your abdomen, the high-frequency waves will be emitted by a probe called an endovaginal transducer, which is placed in your vagina. This technique often provides improved images of the uterus and ovaries. A radiologist, who is a physician experienced in obstetric ultrasound, will analyze the images and send a signed report with his or her interpretation to your doctor.

- **When Are the Results Available?** Immediately (but a full evaluation may take up to 1 week).

Glucose Screening

- **Why Is This Test Performed?** Glucose screening checks for gestational diabetes, a short-term form of diabetes that develops in some women during pregnancy. Gestational diabetes occurs in 1% to 3% of pregnancies and can cause health problems for the baby.

- **Should I Have This Test?** Most women have this test at 24 weeks, but if you've had high sugar in two routine urine tests, your doctor may order it earlier.

- **When Should I Have This Test?** 24 weeks.

- **How Is the Test Performed?** Blood is drawn after you've consumed a sugary drink. If the reading is high, you'll have a glucose-tolerance test, which means you'll drink a glucose solution on an empty stomach and have your blood drawn once every hour for 3 hours.

- **When Are the Results Available?** Immediately.

Nonstress Test

- **Why Is This Test Performed?** If you've gone beyond your due date, this test uses external fetal monitoring to determine fetal movement. This test is used mostly in high-risk pregnancies or when the doctor is uncertain of fetal movement. The nonstress test can help a doctor make sure that the baby is receiving enough oxygen and that the nervous system is responding. A nonresponsive baby doesn't necessarily mean that the baby is in danger.

- **Should I Have This Test?** Your doctor may recommend this if you have a high-risk pregnancy or if you have a low-risk pregnancy and you're past your due date.

- **When Should I Have This Test?** 1 week after due date.

- **How Is the Test Performed?** The doctor will measure the response of the fetus' heart rate to each movement the fetus makes as reported by the mother or observed by the doctor on an ultrasound screen. If the fetus doesn't move during the test, he may be asleep and the doctor may use a buzzer to wake him.

- **When Are the Results Available?** Immediately.

Contraction Stress Test

- **Why Is This Test Performed?** This test stimulates the uterus with Pitocin, a synthetic form of oxytocin (a hormone secreted during childbirth), and determines the effect of contractions on fetal heart rate. It's usually recommended when a nonstress test indicates a problem and can determine whether the baby's heart rate remains stable during contractions.

- **Should I Have This Test?** This test is usually ordered if the nonstress test indicates a problem. It does have a high false-positive rate, though, and can cause labor to be induced prematurely.

- **When Should I Have This Test?** After 40 weeks.
- **How Is the Test Performed?** Mild contractions are brought on either by injections of Pitocin or by squeezing the mother's nipples (which causes oxytocin to be secreted). The fetus' heart rate is then monitored.
- **When Are the Results Available?** Immediately.

Percutaneous Umbilical Vein Sampling (PUVS)

- **Why Is This Test Performed?** This test obtains fetal blood by guiding a needle into the umbilical vein. It's primarily used in addition to ultrasound and amniocentesis if your doctor needs to quickly check your baby's chromosomes for defects or disorders or if your doctor is concerned that your baby may be anemic. The advantage to this test is its speed. There are situations (such as when a fetus shows signs of distress) in which it's helpful to know whether the fetus has a fatal chromosomal defect. If the fetus is suspected to be anemic, this test is the only way to confirm this, and it also allows transfusion while the needle is in place.
- **Should I Have This Test?** This test is used late in a pregnancy after an abnormality has been noted on an ultrasound, when amniocentesis results are not conclusive, if the fetus may have Rh disease, or if you've been exposed to an infectious disease that could potentially affect fetal development.
- **When Should I Have This Test?** Between 18 and 36 weeks.
- **How Is the Test Performed?** A fine needle is passed through your abdomen and uterus into the fetal vein in the umbilical cord and blood is withdrawn for testing.
- **When Are the Results Available?** 3 days.

Talking to Your Doctor about Prenatal Tests

Prenatal tests can be stressful, and because many aren't definitive, even a negative result may not ease any anxiety you may be experiencing. Because many women who have abnormal tests end up having healthy babies and because many of the problems that are detected cannot be treated, some women decide to forgo some of the testing.

One important thing to consider is what you will do in the event that a birth defect is discovered. Implicit in much of this testing is that you can make a decision to terminate the pregnancy based on the results. Your obstetrician or a genetic counselor can help you establish priorities, give you facts, and discuss your options.

It's important to remember that tests are offered to women—they are not mandatory. You should feel free to ask your doctor why he or she is ordering a certain test, what the risks and benefits of the test are, and most importantly, what the results will—and won't—tell you.

"The women who are most stressed about tests are the women who don't understand what the results are going to be like," Dr. Macones says. "It's important that doctors educate the patient—if not right in the office, then by giving her literature about each type of test."

If you think that your doctor isn't answering your questions adequately, you should say so. You don't have to accept the answer "I do this test on all of my patients." Questions to ask include:

- How much will the test cost? Will it be covered by insurance?
- What do I need to do to prepare?
- How long before I get the results? How accurate is this test?
- What are you looking to get from these test results? What do you hope to learn?
- Is the procedure painful? Is it dangerous to me or the fetus? Do the potential benefits outweigh the risks?
- What could happen if I don't undergo this test?

Preventing Birth Defects

The best thing that mothers-to-be can do to avoid birth defects is to make sure they take care of their bodies during pregnancy by:

- not smoking (and avoiding second-hand smoke)
- avoiding alcohol
- eating a healthy diet and taking prenatal vitamins
- getting exercise and plenty of rest
- getting prenatal care

Dr. Macones also points out that there are women who should talk to their doctor before becoming pregnant (including women with diabetes and seizure disorders) to obtain genetic counseling.

Chapter 11

Preventive Screenings for Men

Chapter Contents

Section 11.1

Medical Tests for Prostate Problems

"Medical Tests for Prostate Problems," National Kidney and Urologic Diseases Information Clearinghouse, NIH Publication No. 02-5105, July 2002.

The prostate is a walnut-sized gland in men that produces fluid that is a component of semen. The gland has two or more lobes—or sections—enclosed by an outer layer of tissue. Located in front of the rectum and just below the bladder, where urine is stored, the prostate surrounds the urethra, which is the canal through which urine passes out of the body.

The most common prostate problem in men under 50 is inflammation or infection, which is called prostatitis. Prostate enlargement is another common problem. Since the prostate normally continues to grow as a man matures, prostate enlargement, also called benign prostatic hyperplasia or BPH, is the most common prostate problem for men over 50. Older men are at risk for prostate cancer as well, but it is much less common than BPH.

Sometimes, different prostate problems have similar symptoms. For example, one man with prostatitis and another with BPH may both have a frequent, urgent need to urinate. Other men with BPH may have different symptoms. For example, one man may have trouble beginning a stream of urine, while another may have to get up to go to the bathroom frequently at night. A man in the early stages of prostate cancer may have no symptoms at all. This confusing array of symptoms makes a thorough medical examination and testing very important. Diagnosing the problem may require a series of tests.

Talking to Your Doctor or Nurse

Letting your doctor or nurse know you have a problem is the first step. Try to give as many details about the problem as you can, including when it began and how often it occurs. Tell the doctor or nurse whether you have had recurrent urinary tract infections or symptoms such as pain after ejaculation or during urination, sudden strong urges, or hesitancy and weak urine stream. You should talk about the medicines you take, both prescription medicines and those you can buy over the counter, because they might be part of the problem. You should also talk about how much fluid you typically drink each day, whether you use caffeine or alcohol, and whether your urine has an unusual color or odor. In turn, the doctor or nurse will ask you about your general medical history, including any major illnesses or surgeries. Other typical questions are as follows:

- Over the past month or so, how often have you had to urinate again in less than two hours?

- Over the past month, from the time you went to bed at night until the time you got up in the morning, how many times a night did you typically get up to urinate?

- Over the past month or so, how often have you had a sensation of not emptying your bladder completely after you finished urinating?

- Over the past month or so, how often have you had a weak urinary stream?

- Over the past month or so, how often have you had to push or strain to begin urinating?

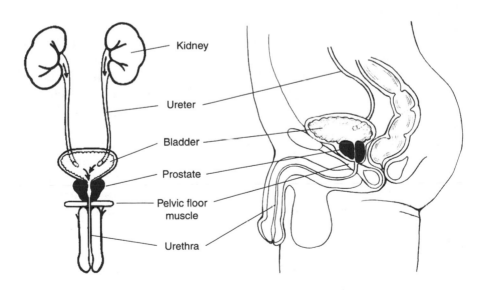

Figure 11.1. *Male Urinary Tract, Front and Side Views*

Your answers to these questions may help your doctor or nurse identify the problem or determine what tests are needed. You may also receive a symptom score evaluation that can be used as a baseline to see how effective later treatments are at relieving those symptoms.

Preparing for the Exam

The common tests your doctor or nurse will perform first require no special preparation. Digital rectal exams (DRE) and blood tests for prostate-specific antigen (PSA) are often included in routine physical examinations for men over 50. For African-American men and men with a family history of prostate cancer, it is recommended that tests be given starting at age 40. Some organizations even recommend that these tests be given to all men starting at age 40.

If you have urination problems or if the DRE or PSA test indicates that you might have a problem, you will probably be given additional tests that may require some preparation. Ask your doctor or nurse whether you should change your diet or fluid intake or stop taking any medications. If the tests involve inserting instruments into the urethra or rectum, you may be given antibiotics before and after the test to prevent infection.

Procedures

Digital Rectal Exam (DRE)

This exam is usually done first. Many doctors perform a DRE as part of a routine physical exam for any man over 50, some even at 40, whether the man has urinary problems or not. You may be asked to bend over a table or to lie on your side holding your knees close to your chest. The doctor slides a gloved, lubricated finger into the rectum and feels the part of the prostate that lies next to it. You may find the DRE slightly uncomfortable, but it is very brief. This exam tells the doctor whether the gland has any bumps, irregularities, soft spots, or hard spots that require additional tests. If a prostate infection is suspected, the doctor might massage the prostate during the DRE to obtain fluid for examination under a microscope.

PSA Blood Test

To rule out cancer, your doctor may recommend a PSA blood test. The amount of PSA, a protein produced by prostate cells, is often higher in the blood of men who have prostate cancer. However, an elevated level of PSA does not necessarily mean you have cancer. The Food and Drug Administration has approved a PSA test for use in conjunction with a DRE to help detect prostate cancer in men age 50 or older and for monitoring men with prostate cancer after treatment. However, much remains unknown about how to interpret the PSA test, its ability to discriminate between cancer and benign prostate conditions, and the best course of action if the PSA is high.

Because so many questions are unanswered, the relative magnitude of the test's potential risks and benefits is unknown. When added to DRE screening, PSA enhances detection, but PSA tests are known to have relatively high false-positive rates, and they also may identify a greater number of medically insignificant tumors.

The PSA test first became available in the 1980s, and its use led to an increase in the detection of prostate cancer between 1986 and 1991. In the mid-1990s, deaths from prostate cancer began to decrease, and some observers credit PSA testing for this trend. Others, however, point out that statistical trends do not necessarily prove a cause-and-effect relationship, and the benefits of screening for prostate cancer are still being studied. The National Cancer Institute is conducting the Prostate, Lung, Colorectal, and Ovarian Cancer Screening Trial, or PLCO Trial, to determine whether certain screening tests reduce the number of deaths from these cancers. DRE and PSA exams are being studied to see whether yearly screening will decrease the risk of dying from prostate cancer.

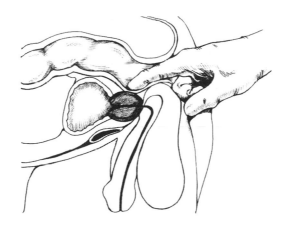

Figure 11.2. *Digital Rectal Exam (DRE)*

Until a definitive answer is found, doctors and patients should weigh the benefits of PSA testing against the risks of follow-up diagnostic tests and cancer treatments. The procedures used to diagnose prostate cancer may cause significant side effects, including bleeding and infection. Treatment for prostate cancer often causes erectile dysfunction, or impotence, and may cause urinary incontinence.

Urinalysis

Your doctor or nurse may ask for a urine sample to test with a dipstick or to examine under a microscope. A chemically treated dipstick will change color if the urine contains nitrite, a byproduct of bacterial infection. Traces of blood in the urine may indicate that a kidney stone or infection is present, or the sample might reveal bacteria or infection-fighting white blood cells. You might be asked to urinate into two or three containers to help locate the infection site. If signs of infection appear in the first container but not in the others, the infection is likely to be in the urethra. Your doctor or nurse might ask you to urinate into the first container, then stop the stream for a prostate

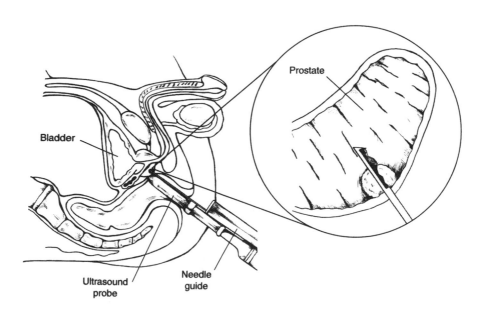

Figure 11.3. *Transrectal Ultrasound and Prostate Biopsy*

massage before completing the test. If urine taken after prostate massage or the prostate fluid itself contains significantly more bacteria, it is a strong sign that you have bacterial prostatitis.

Transrectal Ultrasound and Prostate Biopsy

If prostate cancer is suspected, your doctor may recommend transrectal ultrasound. In this procedure, the doctor or technician inserts a probe slightly larger than a pen into the rectum. The probe directs high-frequency sound waves at the prostate, and the echo patterns form an image of the gland on a television monitor. The image shows how big the prostate is and whether there are any irregularities, but cannot unequivocally identify tumors.

To determine whether an abnormal-looking area is indeed a tumor, the doctor can use the probe and the ultrasound images to guide a biopsy needle to the suspected tumor. The needle collects a few pieces of prostate tissue for examination under a microscope.

Magnetic Resonance Imaging (MRI) and Computed Axial Tomography (CAT) Scans

MRI and CAT scans both use computers to create three-dimensional or cross-sectional images of internal organs. These tests can help identify abnormal structures, but they cannot distinguish between cancerous tumors and noncancerous prostate enlargement. Once a biopsy has confirmed cancer, a doctor might use these imaging techniques to determine how far the cancer has spread. Experts caution, however, that MRI and CAT scans are very expensive and rarely add useful information. They recommend using these techniques only when the PSA score is very high or the DRE suggests an extensive cancer, or both.

Urodynamic Tests

If your problem appears to be related to blockage, your doctor or nurse may recommend tests that measure bladder pressure and urine flow rate. You may be asked to urinate into a special device that measures how quickly the urine is flowing and records how many seconds it takes for the peak flow rate to be reached. Another test measures postvoid residual, the amount of urine left in your bladder when you have finished urinating. A weak stream and difficulty emptying the bladder completely may be signs of urine blockage caused by an enlarged prostate that is squeezing the urethra.

Intravenous Pyelogram (IVP)

IVP is an x-ray of the urinary tract. In this test, dye is injected into a vein, and x-ray pictures are taken at 0, 5, 10, and 15 minutes to see the progression of contrast through the kidney and ureter. The dye makes the urine visible on the x-ray and shows any narrowing or blockage in the urinary tract. This procedure can help identify problems in the kidneys, ureters, or bladder that may have resulted from urine retention or backup.

Abdominal Ultrasound

For an abdominal ultrasound exam, a technician will apply gel to your lower abdomen and sweep a handheld transducer across the area to receive a picture of your entire urinary tract. Like the IVP, an abdominal ultrasound can show damage in the upper urinary tract that results from urine blockage at the prostate.

Cystoscopy

After a solution numbs the inside of the penis, the doctor inserts a small tube through the urethral opening at the tip of the penis. The tube, called a cystoscope, contains a lens and a light system, which allow the doctor to see the inside of the urethra and the bladder. The doctor can then determine the location and degree of the obstruction.

After the Test

You may have mild discomfort for a few hours after urodynamics and cystoscopy. Drinking two 8-ounce glasses of water each hour for 2 hours should help. Ask your doctor whether you can take a warm bath. If not, you may be able to hold a warm, damp washcloth over the urethral opening to relieve the discomfort. A prostate biopsy may also produce pain in the area of the rectum and the perineum (between the rectum and the scrotum).

Your doctor may give you an antibiotic to take for 1 or 2 days to prevent an infection, but not always. If you have signs of infection—including pain, chills, or fever—call your doctor at once.

Getting the Results

Results for simple tests can be discussed with your doctor or nurse immediately after the test. Other tests may take a few days. You will have the chance to ask questions about the results and possible treatments for your problem.

Additional Information

American Foundation for Urologic Disease
1128 North Charles St.
Baltimore, MD 21201
Toll-Free: 800-828-7866
Phone: 410-468-1800
Website: www.afud.org
E-mail: admin@afud.org

The Prostatitis Foundation
1063 30th Street, Box 8
Smithshire, IL 61478
Toll-Free: 888-891-4200
Fax: 309-325-7184
Website: www.prostate.org

Cancer Information Service
National Cancer Institute (NCI)
Suite 3036A, MSC8322
6116 Executive Blvd.
Bethesda, MD 20892-8322
Toll-Free: 800-4 CANCER (800-422-6237)
Toll-Free TTY: 800-332-8615
Website: www.nci.nih.gov (NCI's primary website) or http://cancernet.nci.nih.gov (material for professionals, patients, and the public)
E-mail: cancermail@icicc.nci.nih.gov

National Kidney and Urologic Diseases Information Clearinghouse
3 Information Way
Bethesda, MD 20892-3580
Toll-Free: 800-891-5390
Phone: 301-654-4415
Website: http://kidney.niddk.nih.gov/index.htm
E-mail: nkudic@info.niddk.nih.gov

Section 11.2

Testicular Cancer Screen

PDQ® Cancer Information Summary, National Cancer Institute, Bethesda, MD, "Testicular Cancer (PDQ®) Screening–Patient." Updated 06/2003. Available at: http://cancer.gov. Accessed 11/06/2003.

What Is Screening?

Screening for cancer is examination (or testing) of people for early signs of a certain type of cancer even though they have no symptoms. Scientists have studied patterns of cancer in the population to learn which people are more likely to get certain types of cancer. They have also studied what things around us and what things we do in our lives may cause cancer. This information helps doctors recommend who should be screened for certain types of cancer, what types of screening tests people should have, and how often these tests should be done. Not all screening tests are helpful, and most have risks such as bleeding, infection, or pain of the testicle or groin due to a biopsy for an abnormal screening test. For this reason, scientists at the National Cancer Institute are studying many screening tests to find out how useful they are.

If your doctor suggests certain cancer screening tests as part of your health care plan, this does not mean he or she thinks you have cancer. Screening tests are done when you have no symptoms. Since decisions about screening can be difficult, you may want to discuss them with your doctor and ask questions about the potential benefits and risks of screening tests and whether they have been proven to decrease the risk of dying from cancer.

If you have signs or symptoms of cancer, your doctor will order certain tests to see whether you have cancer. These are called diagnostic tests.

The purposes of this summary on testicular cancer screening are to:

- Give information on testicular cancer and what makes it more likely to occur (risk factors).

- Describe testicular cancer screening methods.

- Give current evidence about the effectiveness of screening tests.

You can talk to your doctor or health care professional about cancer screening and whether it would be likely to help you.

Testicular Cancer Screening

The testicles are male sex glands involved in the production of sperm. They are located behind the penis in a pouch of skin called the scrotum. The testicles are the body's main source of male hormones.

Risk of Testicular Cancer

Testicular cancer is rare. Despite a slow increase in the number of new cases, the number of deaths due to testicular cancer has decreased dramatically since the 1960s as a result of treatment improvements. Anything that increases a person's chance of developing a disease is called a risk factor. Some risk factors for testicular cancer are as follows:

Age: Young men have a higher risk of testicular cancer. In men, testicular cancer is the most common cancer between the ages of 20 to 34, the second most common cancer between the ages of 35 to 39, and the third most common cancer between the ages of 15 to 19.

Family History: Men with a family history of testicular cancer may have an increased risk of developing testicular cancer.

Hereditary Conditions: Men born with gonadal dysgenesis or Klinefelter's syndrome have a greater risk of developing testicular cancer.

Personal History: Men with undescended testicles have a higher-than-average risk of developing testicular cancer. Men who have already had testicular cancer have a higher risk of developing a tumor in the other testicle.

Race: Testicular cancer is more common among white men than black men. Hispanic, American Indian, and Asian men develop testicular cancer at a higher rate than black men, but less than white men.

Screening Tests for Testicular Cancer

Most testicular cancers are first detected by the patient, either unintentionally or by self-examination. Some are discovered by routine physical examination. However, no studies have been done to determine whether self-examination or examination during routine physicals can help reduce the number of deaths caused by testicular cancer.

Additional Information

National Cancer Institute
NCI Public Inquiries Office
Suite 3036A, MSC8322
6116 Executive Blvd.
Bethesda, MD 20892-8322
Toll-Free: 800-422-6237
Toll-Free TTY: 800-332-8615
Website: www.nci.nih.gov

Part Three

Screenings and Diagnostic Tests for Specific Concerns

Chapter 12

Cardiovascular Disease Diagnosis

Chapter Contents

Section 12.1

Heart Attack and Stroke

This section includes "Tests to Diagnose Heart Disease," and "Heart Attack, Stroke, and Cardiac Arrest Warning Signs." Reproduced with permission from the American Heart Association World Wide Web Site, www.americanheart.org. © 2003. Copyright American Heart Association.

Tests to Diagnose Heart Disease

Several tests diagnose possible heart disease. The choice of which (and how many) tests to perform depends on several things including, a patient's risk factors, history of heart problems, current symptoms, and the doctor's interpretation of these factors.

People being evaluated for possible heart disease are usually given simple tests first. Then more complicated ones may be used, if needed. Specific tests depend on the patient's particular problem(s) and the physician's assessment.

Some of these tests are noninvasive. That means they don't involve inserting needles, instruments, or fluids into the body. Those that do are called invasive tests.

Most of these tests are described in other sections of this *Sourcebook*.

What are some examples of noninvasive tests?

- Resting electrocardiogram (ECG or EKG)
- Signal-averaged electrocardiogram (SAECG)
- Chest x-ray
- Holter monitor (ambulatory electrocardiogram)
- Echocardiogram
- Exercise stress test
- Computed tomography (CT) scan
- Magnetic resonance imaging (MRI)
- Magnetic resonance angiography (MRA)

What are nuclear imaging tests?

These are invasive; each requires a needle puncture in an arm vein.

- MUGA scan
- Thallium stress test
- Technetium stress test
- Pharmacologic stress test
- PET test
- Stress echocardiography

What are some other imaging tests?

- Transesophageal echocardiogram (TEE)
- Cardiac catheterization (cath)—also known as coronary angiography

Heart Attack, Stroke, and Cardiac Arrest Warning Signs

Act in Time

The American Heart Association and the National Heart, Lung, and Blood Institute have launched a new *Act in Time* campaign to increase people's awareness of heart attack and the importance of calling 9-1-1 immediately at the onset of heart attack symptoms.

Dial 9-1-1 Fast

Heart attack and stroke are life-and-death emergencies—every second counts. If you see or have any of the listed symptoms, immediately call 9-1-1. Not all these signs occur in every heart attack or stroke. Sometimes they go away and return. If some occur, get help fast! Today heart attack and stroke victims can benefit from new medications and treatments unavailable to patients in years past. For example, clot-busting drugs can stop some heart attacks and strokes in progress, reducing disability, and saving lives. But to be effective, these drugs must be given relatively quickly after heart attack or stroke symptoms first appear. So again, don't delay—get help right away!

Statistics

Coronary heart disease is America's No. 1 killer. Stroke is No. 3 and a leading cause of serious disability. That's why it's so important to reduce your risk factors, know the warning signs, and know how to respond quickly and properly if warning signs occur.

Heart Attack Warning Signs

Some heart attacks are sudden and intense—the movie heart attack, where no one doubts what's happening. But most heart attacks start slowly, with mild pain or discomfort. Often people affected aren't sure what's wrong and wait too long before getting help. Here are signs that can mean a heart attack is happening:

- **Chest discomfort.** Most heart attacks involve discomfort in the center of the chest that lasts more than a few minutes, or that goes away and comes back. It can feel like uncomfortable pressure, squeezing, fullness, or pain.

- **Discomfort in other areas of the upper body.** Symptoms can include pain or discomfort in one or both arms, the back, neck, jaw, or stomach.

- **Shortness of breath.** This feeling often comes along with chest discomfort. But it can occur before the chest discomfort.

- **Other signs.** These may include breaking out in a cold sweat, nausea, or lightheadedness.

If you or someone you're with has chest discomfort, especially with one or more of the other signs, don't wait longer than a few minutes (no more than 5) before calling for help. Call 9-1-1. Get to a hospital right away.

Calling 9-1-1 is almost always the fastest way to get lifesaving treatment. Emergency medical services staff can begin treatment when they arrive—up to an hour sooner than if someone gets to the hospital by car. The staff is also trained to revive someone whose heart has stopped. You'll get treated faster in the hospital if you come by ambulance, too.

If you can't access the emergency medical services (EMS), have someone drive you to the hospital right away. If you're the one having symptoms, don't drive yourself, unless you have absolutely no other option.

Stroke Warning Signs

The American Stroke Association says these are the warning signs of stroke:

- Sudden numbness or weakness of the face, arm, or leg, especially on one side of the body
- Sudden confusion, trouble speaking, or understanding
- Sudden trouble seeing in one or both eyes
- Sudden trouble walking, dizziness, loss of balance, or coordination
- Sudden, severe headache with no known cause

If you or someone with you has one or more of these signs, don't delay! Immediately call 9-1-1 or the emergency medical services (EMS) number so an ambulance (ideally with advanced life support) can be sent for you. Also, check the time so you'll know when the first symptoms appeared. It's very important to take immediate action. If given within three hours of the start of symptoms, a clot-busting drug can reduce long-term disability for the most common type of stroke.

Cardiac arrest strikes immediately and without warning. Here are the signs:

- Sudden loss of responsiveness. No response to gentle shaking.
- No normal breathing. The victim does not take a normal breath when you check for several seconds.
- No signs of circulation. No movement or coughing.

If cardiac arrest occurs, call 9-1-1 and begin CPR immediately. If an automated external defibrillator (AED) is available and someone trained to use it is nearby, involve them.

Additional Information

American Heart Association
7272 Greenville Ave.
Dallas, TX 75231
Toll-Free: 800-242-8721
Website: www.americanheart.org

American Stroke Association
7272 Greenville Ave.
Dallas, TX 75231
Toll-Free: 888-478-7653
Website: www.strokeassociation.org

Section 12.2

Detecting High Blood Pressure

This section includes "Your Guide to Lowering High Blood Pressure," National Heart, Lung, and Blood Institute, updated May 2003; and "NHLBI Issues New High Blood Pressure Clinical Practice Guidelines," Press Release, National Heart, Lung, and Blood Institute (NHLBI), May 14, 2003.

High Blood Pressure Detection

You can find out if you have high blood pressure by having your blood pressure checked regularly. Most doctors will diagnose a person with high blood pressure on the basis of two or more readings, taken on several occasions. A consistent blood pressure reading of 140/90 mmHg or higher is considered high blood pressure, another term for hypertension.

Some people experience high blood pressure only when they visit the doctor's office. This condition is called "white-coat hypertension." If your doctor suspects this, you may be asked to monitor your blood pressure at home or asked to wear a device called an ambulatory blood pressure monitor. This device is usually worn for 24 hours and can take blood pressure every 30 minutes. In this section you will learn more about diagnosing high blood pressure.

How Do I Know if I Have High Blood Pressure?

High blood pressure often has no signs or symptoms. The only way to find out if you have high blood pressure is to be tested for it. Using the familiar blood pressure cuff, your doctor or nurse can easily tell if your blood pressure is high.

How Is Blood Pressure Tested?

Having your blood pressure tested is quick and easy. Blood pressure is measured in millimeters of mercury (mmHg) and recorded as two numbers, systolic pressure over diastolic pressure. For example, the doctor or nurse might say "130 over 80" as a blood pressure reading.

Both numbers in a blood pressure reading are important. As we grow older, systolic blood pressure is especially important.

To test your blood pressure, your doctor will use a familiar device with a long name. It is called a sphygmomanometer (pronounced sfig'-mo-ma-nom-e-ter).

Tips for Having Your Blood Pressure Taken

- Don't drink coffee or smoke cigarettes 30 minutes before having your blood pressure measured.

- Before the test, sit for five minutes with your back supported and your feet flat on the ground. Rest your arm on a table at the level or your heart.

- Wear short sleeves so your arm is exposed.

- Go to the bathroom prior to the reading. A full bladder can change your blood pressure reading.

- Get two readings, taken at least two minutes apart, and average the results.

- Ask the doctor or nurse to tell you the blood pressure reading in numbers.

When systolic and diastolic blood pressures fall into different categories, the higher category should be used to classify blood pressure level. For example, 160/80 mmHg would be stage 2 hypertension (high blood pressure).

Table 12.1. Categories for Blood Pressure Levels in Adults Ages 18 and Older

Category	Blood Pressure Level (mmHg)		
	Systolic		*Diastolic*
Normal	< 120	and	< 80
Prehypertension	120-139	or	80-89
High Blood Pressure			
Stage 1 Hypertension	140-159	or	90-99
Stage 2 Hypertension	≥160	or	≥100

< means less than
≥ means greater than or equal to

What Device Can I Use to Take My Own Blood Pressure?

Tests at home can be done with the familiar blood pressure cuff and a stethoscope, or with an electronic monitor, such as a digital read-out monitor. Also, be sure that the person who will use the device reads the instructions before taking blood pressure readings. Your doctor, nurse, or pharmacist can help you check the device and teach you how to use it. You also may ask for their help in choosing the right one for you. Blood pressure devices can be bought at various places, such as discount chain stores and pharmacies.

National Heart, Lung and Blood Institute Issues New High Blood Pressure Clinical Practice Guidelines

On May 14, 2003, the National Heart, Lung, and Blood Institute (NHLBI) released new clinical practice guidelines for the prevention, detection, and treatment of high blood pressure. The guidelines, which were approved by the Coordinating Committee of the NHLBI's National High Blood Pressure Education Program (NHBPEP), feature altered blood pressure categories, including a new prehypertension level—which covers about 22 percent of American adults or about 45 million persons.

The new guidelines also streamline the steps by which doctors diagnose and treat patients, and recommend the use of diuretics as part of the drug treatment plan for high blood pressure in most patients. The guidelines were prepared by a special committee of the NHBPEP, which represents 46 professional, voluntary, and Federal organizations, and reviewed by 33 national hypertension experts and policy leaders. The NHBPEP issues new guidelines when warranted by scientific advances. The last guidelines were issued in November 1997.

"Since 1997, much more has been learned about the risk of high blood pressure and the course of the disease," said NHLBI Director Dr. Claude Lenfant. "Americans' lifetime risk of developing hypertension is much greater than we'd thought. For instance, those who do not have hypertension at age 55 have a 90 percent risk of going on to develop the condition. We also now know that damage to arteries begins at fairly low blood pressure levels—those formerly considered normal and optimal," he continued. "In fact, studies show that the risk of death from heart disease and stroke begins to rise at blood pressures as low as 115 over 75, and that it doubles for each 20 over 10 millimeters of mercury (mmHg) increase. So the harm starts long before people get treatment. Unless prevention steps are taken, stiffness and other damage to arteries worsen with age and make high blood pressure more and more difficult to treat. The new prehypertension category reflects this risk and, we hope, will prompt people to take preventive action early."

"The past six years have brought results from more than 30 clinical studies worldwide, many of which were funded by the NHLBI," said Dr. Aram V. Chobanian, Dean of Boston University School of Medicine in MA and Chair of the Joint National Committee that produced the new guidelines. "These findings have been remarkably consistent in demonstrating the critical importance of lowering blood pressure, irrespective of age, gender, race, or socio-economic status. The data allow us to create a set of recommendations that are easier to use than past guidelines, which should in turn make it easier for clinicians to treat their patients' hypertension."

High blood pressure is a major risk factor for heart disease and the chief risk factor for stroke and heart failure, and also can lead to kidney damage. It affects about 50 million Americans—one in four adults. Treatment seeks to lower blood pressure to less than 140 mm Hg systolic and less than 90 mmHg diastolic for most persons with hypertension (less than 130 systolic and less than 80 diastolic for those with diabetes and chronic kidney disease).

The guidelines include new data on U.S. control, awareness, and treatment rates for high blood pressure. According to a national survey, 70 percent of Americans are aware of their high blood pressure, 59 percent are being treated for it, and 34 percent of those with hypertension have it under control. Those percentages represent a slight improvement over rates for 10 years ago, when 68 percent of Americans were aware of their high blood pressure, 54 percent were being treated for it, and 27 percent of those with hypertension had it under control. By contrast, about 25 years ago, 51 percent were aware of their high blood pressure, 31 percent were being treated, and 10 percent of those with hypertension had it under control.

"Though improved, the treatment and control rates are still too low," said Chobanian. "The new guidelines zero in on this problem, recommending factors that often lead to inadequate control such as not prescribing sufficient medication. The guidelines stress that most patients will need more than one drug to control their hypertension and that lifestyle measures are a crucial part of treatment. Another key factor is the need for clinicians to pay more attention to systolic blood pressure in those ages 50 and older," he continued. "From mid-life on, systolic hypertension is a more important cardiovascular risk factor than diastolic. It's also much more common and harder to control."

Key aspects of the new guidelines include:

- A new prehypertension level and merging of other categories. The new report changes the former blood pressure definitions to: normal, less than 120/less than 80 mmHg; prehypertension, 120–139/80—89 mmHg; stage 1 hypertension, 140–159/90–99 mm Hg; stage 2 hypertension, at or greater than 160/at or greater than 100 mmHg. The 1997 categories were optimal, normal, high-normal, and hypertension stages 1, 2, and 3.

"Stages 2 and 3 were combined because their treatment is essentially the same," said Chobanian. "The new prehypertension category should alert people to their real risk from high blood pressure."

The guidelines do not recommend drug therapy for those with prehypertension unless it is required by another condition, such as diabetes or chronic kidney disease. But the report advises them—and encourages those with normal blood pressures—to make any needed lifestyle changes. These include losing excess weight, becoming physically active, limiting alcoholic beverages, and following a heart-healthy eating plan, including cutting back on salt and other forms of sodium. The report also recommends that, for overall cardiovascular health, persons quit smoking.

As in the 1997 guidelines, the new report recommends Americans follow the DASH—Dietary Approaches to Stop Hypertension—eating plan, which is rich in vegetables, fruit, and nonfat dairy products. Clinical studies have shown that DASH significantly lowers blood pressure. The decreases are often comparable to those achieved with blood pressure-lowering medication.

- Simplified and strengthened drug treatment recommendations. The guidelines recommend use of a diuretic, either alone or in combination with another drug class, as part of the treatment plan in most patients. The report notes that even though many studies have found diuretics to be effective in preventing hypertension's cardiovascular complications, they are currently not being sufficiently used.

The guidelines also list other drug classes that have been shown to be effective in reducing hypertension's cardiovascular complications and that may be considered to begin therapy: angiotensin converting enzyme (ACE) inhibitors, angiotensin receptor blockers, beta-blockers, and calcium channel blockers. The report also gives the compelling indications—or high-risk conditions—for which such drugs are recommended as initial therapy.

- Use of additional drugs for severe hypertension or to lower blood pressure to the desired level. According to the new report, most persons will need two, and at times three or more, medications to lower blood pressure to the desired level.

- The guidelines also recommend clinicians work with patients to agree on blood pressure goals and develop a treatment plan.

"No treatment will work unless patients stay on it, no matter how careful the clinician," said NHBPEP Coordinator Dr. Ed Roccella. "The guidelines incorporate information from behavioral studies and offer advice to clinicians on how to motivate patients to stick with their treatment. It's crucial to build trust and make sure patients understand their treatment and feel able to voice their concerns."

The bottom line is that Americans must change how they think about blood pressure," said Roccella. "The sooner they take action, the better. It's vital that they adopt a heart-healthy lifestyle early, even if their blood pressure is normal."

Section 12.3

Screening Adults for Lipid Disorders

This section includes "Screening Adults for Lipid Disorders: What's New from the USPSTF," Agency for Healthcare Research and Quality (AHRQ), AHRQ Publication No. APPIP 01-0011, March 2001; "Another Reason to Test Your Cholesterol," © 2003 American Association for Clinical Chemistry. Reprinted with permission. For additional information on clinical lab testing, visit the Lab Tests Online website at www.labtestsonline.org; and "New Palm Test for Cholesterol," FDA Updates, *FDA Consumer*, September-October 2002, U.S. Food and Drug Administration.

What Are Lipid Disorders?

- Lipid disorders are abnormal levels of cholesterol in the blood that put men and women at risk for heart disease.

- Some cholesterol is necessary to maintain cell membranes and other aspects of health. However, too much cholesterol can lead to heart disease.

- Heart disease is the leading cause of death in the United States. Heart attacks kill nearly 500,000 men and women each year.

- Cholesterol is carried through the blood bound to two types of lipoproteins. Low-density lipoprotein (LDL) carries most of the cholesterol in the blood. High levels of LDL can cause cholesterol to deposit in blood vessels, clogging the arteries.

- High-density lipoprotein (HDL) helps remove cholesterol from the blood and helps prevent cholesterol from building up.

- The risk for heart disease increases as levels of LDL increase and as levels of HDL decrease. Lipid disorders are risk factors for heart disease, the leading cause of death in the United States.

Who Should Be Screened for Lipid Disorders?

The third U.S. Preventive Services Task Force (USPSTF) recommends that:

- All men aged 35 and older and all women aged 45 and older should be screened routinely for lipid disorders. This extends the recommendations of the second USPSTF, which recommended that adults be screened until age 65.

- Younger adults—men aged 20–35 and women aged 20–45—should be screened if they have other risk factors for heart disease. These risk factors include tobacco use, diabetes, a family history of heart disease or high cholesterol, or high blood pressure. This recommendation expands on the recommendations of the second USPSTF, which focused on screening middle-aged men and women.

- Clinicians should measure HDL in addition to measuring total cholesterol or LDL. There is insufficient evidence to recommend for or against measuring triglycerides.

The third USPSTF makes no recommendation for or against routine cholesterol screening in young adult men and women who are not at risk for heart disease.

Why Screen for Lipid Disorders?

Heart disease may be the first sign of abnormal cholesterol levels. Screening can detect cholesterol abnormalities and lead to treatment before heart disease develops or worsens.

Does Treatment Work?

Several large studies have shown that patients who took cholesterol-lowering drugs for 5–7 years and had either high total cholesterol or low HDL cholesterol decreased their risk of heart disease by about 30 percent. In the one study that included women, the treatment appeared to be as effective in postmenopausal women as in men.

Reducing dietary saturated fat and losing weight can lower total and LDL cholesterol as much as 10–20 percent in some men and women. On average, however, most patients achieve reductions in total cholesterol of about 2–6 percent after modifying their lifestyles.

The Take-Home Message

All men aged 35 and older and all women aged 45 and older should be screened routinely for lipid disorders to find out whether their cholesterol levels increase their risk for heart disease. Younger adults should be screened for lipid disorders if they are otherwise at risk for heart disease.

Clinicians should consider overall risk of heart disease in making treatment decisions. Clinicians should counsel all patients about changing their lifestyles (reducing dietary saturated fat, exercising, and losing weight) to improve their lipid levels. Many men and women, especially those at highest risk, may need medications to best control their lipid abnormalities. Drug treatment is usually more effective than dietary changes alone for reducing total cholesterol.

Another Reason to Test Your Cholesterol

On July 1, 2002, the American Heart Association reported that a recent study in the Netherlands found an association between low levels of high-density lipoprotein (HDL or good cholesterol) and cognitive impairment, including dementia. Although additional research is needed to confirm these findings, they seem to suggest yet another reason to have your cholesterol, especially HDL, checked regularly.

The study measured the levels of HDL as well as total cholesterol, low-density lipoprotein (LDL or bad cholesterol), and triglycerides in 561 patients 85 years of age and older. Statistically significant differences were found in mental ability such that patients with lower concentrations of HDL in their blood had poorer scores on the Mini-Mental State Examination than did those with higher levels of HDL. This association was strongest among those patients who did not have evidence of heart disease or stroke. Patients with the lowest levels of HDL were four times as likely to have dementia as those with the highest levels of HDL. There did not appear to be a difference in mental ability based on LDL or triglycerides levels, however.

The American Heart Association recommends that adults maintain HDL cholesterol levels between 40 and 50 (men) or between 50 and 60 (women) milligrams per deciliter. In the new study, patients in the group with the lowest levels of HDL had concentrations around 35.9 milligrams per deciliter while those in the group with the highest levels had values around 63.7 milligrams per deciliter. The AHA recommends three steps to maintaining a healthy concentration of HDL: not smoking, keeping at a healthy weight, and exercising.

New Palm Test for Cholesterol

The Food and Drug Administration has cleared a new laboratory test to measure cholesterol levels in the skin of adults with severe coronary artery disease. *Cholesterol 1,2,3*, manufactured by International Medical Innovations Inc., of Toronto, can help determine the amount of cholesterol in skin using the palm of the hand. Other tests currently used by laboratories measure cholesterol from blood samples.

To do the palm cholesterol test, an applicator pad, much like an adhesive bandage, is placed on the palm of the hand. Drops of solution are added to the pad for three minutes. A hand-held reader attached to a computer reads the amount of blue color in the pad. The results are displayed on the computer screen. The deeper the blue, the more cholesterol is present.

Specifically, the new test is for people suspected of having severe coronary artery disease, defined as 50 percent closure of two or more arteries, and those with a history of heart attack. *Cholesterol 1,2,3* is not intended to be used as a substitute for the standard blood tests, nor can it substitute for an evaluation of other risk factors used to identify coronary artery disease.

Skin contains about 11 percent by weight of all body cholesterol. When severe coronary artery disease is present, the numeric values obtained with the skin cholesterol test increase. The test was not shown to be useful in identifying people with less severe coronary artery disease, and should not be used as a screening tool to determine coronary artery disease risk in the general population.

The test cannot be used on people with skin diseases on the hand or on those who recently applied skin lotions or topical medications.

Additional Information

American Academy of Family Physicians
11400 Tomahawk Creek Parkway
Leawood, KS 66211-2672
Toll-Free: 800-274-2237; Phone: 913-906-6000
Website: www.aafp.org
E-mail: fp@aafp.org

American College of Cardiology
Heart House
9111 Old Georgetown Road
Bethesda, MD 20814
Toll-Free: 800-253-4636; Phone: 301-897-5400
Fax: 301-897-9745
Website: www.acc.org
E-mail: resource@aac.org

American College of Physicians/American Society of Internal Medicine
190 N. Independence Mall West
Philadelphia, PA 19106-1572
Toll-Free (customer service): 800-523-1546, ext. 2600
Phone: 215-351-2600
Website: www.acponline.org

American Heart Association
National Center
7272 Greenville Avenue
Dallas, TX 75231
Toll-Free: 800-242-8721
Website: www.americanheart.org

Healthfinder®
P.O. Box 1133
Washington, DC 20013-1133
Website: www.healthfinder.gov
E-mail: healthfinder@nhic.org

National Heart, Lung, and Blood Institute (NHLBI) /National Cholesterol Education Program
NHLBI Information Center
P.O. Box 30105
Bethesda, MD 20824-0105
Phone: 301-592-8573
Fax: 301-592-8563
Website: www.nhlbi.nih.gov/about/ncep/index.htm
E-mail: nhlbiinfo@rover.nhlbi.nih.gov

Section 12.4

High Levels of C-Reactive Protein Linked to Heart Disease

"Inflammation, Heart Disease and Stroke: The Role of C-Reactive Protein," August 21, 2003. Reproduced with permission from the American Heart Association World Wide Web Site, www.americanheart.org. © 2003. Copyright American Heart Association.

Inflammation, Heart Disease, and Stroke: The Role of C-Reactive Protein

How Does Inflammation Relate to Heart Disease and Stroke Risk?

Inflammation is the process by which the body responds to injury. Laboratory evidence and findings from clinical and population studies suggest that inflammation is important in atherosclerosis (athero-skleh-RO'sis). This is the process in which fatty deposits build up in the lining of arteries.

C-reactive protein (CRP) is one of the acute phase proteins that increase during systemic inflammation. It's been suggested that testing CRP levels in the blood may be a new way to assess cardiovascular disease risk. A high sensitivity assay for CRP test (hs-CRP) is now widely available.

The American Association and the Centers for Disease Control and Prevention recently published a joint scientific statement about using inflammatory markers in clinical and public health practice. This statement was developed after systematically reviewing the evidence of association between inflammatory markers (mainly CRP) and coronary heart disease and stroke.

What Is the Role of CRP in Predicting Recurrent Cardiovascular and Stroke Events?

A growing number of studies have examined whether hs-CRP can predict recurrent cardiovascular disease and stroke and death in different settings. High levels of hs-CRP consistently predict new coronary events in patients with unstable angina and acute myocardial infarction (heart attack). Higher hs-CRP levels also are associated with lower survival rate of these people. Many studies suggested that after adjusting for other prognostic factors, hs-CRP was still useful as a risk predictor.

Recent studies also suggest that higher levels of hs-CRP may increase the risk that an artery will reclose after it's been opened by balloon angioplasty. High levels of hs-CRP in the blood seem to predict prognosis and recurrent events in patients with stroke and peripheral arterial disease.

What Is the Role of hs-CRP in Predicting New Cardiovascular Events?

Most studies show that the higher the hs-CRP levels, the higher the risk of developing heart attack. In fact, scientific studies have found that the risk for heart attack in people in the upper third of hs-CRP levels is twice that of those whose hs-CRP is in the lower third. These prospective studies include men, women, and the elderly. Recent studies also found an association between sudden cardiac death, peripheral arterial disease, and hs-CRP. However, not all of the established cardiovascular risk factors were controlled for when the association was examined. The true independent association between hs-CRP and new cardiovascular events hasn't yet been established.

What Causes Low-Grade Inflammation?

No one knows for sure what causes the low-grade inflammation that seems to put otherwise healthy people at risk. However, the new findings are consistent with the hypothesis that an infection—possibly one caused by a bacteria or a virus—might contribute to or even cause atherosclerosis.

Possible infectious bacteria include *Chlamydia pneumoniae* (klah-MID'e-ah nu-MO'ne-i) and *Helicobacter pylori* (HEL'ih-ko-bak ter pi-LO'ri). Possible viral agents include herpes simplex virus and cytomegalovirus (si to-meg ah-lo-VI'rus). Thus, it may be that antimicrobial or antiviral therapies will someday join other therapies used to prevent heart attacks.

This idea clearly needs to be tested in clinical trials. However, the notion that chronic infection can lead to unsuspected disease isn't foreign to most doctors. For example, bacterial infection with *Helicobacter pylori* is now known to be the major cause of stomach ulcers. The treatment for this condition now routinely includes antibiotic therapy. Patients with autoimmune diseases and cancer also often have elevated CRP levels.

Should I Have My CRP Level Measured?

If a person's cardiovascular risk score—judged by global risk assessment—is low (the possibility of developing cardiovascular disease is less than 10 percent in 10 years, no test is immediately warranted. If the risk score is in the intermediate range (10–20 percent in 10 years), such a test can help predict a cardiovascular and stroke event and help direct further evaluation and therapy. However, the benefits of such therapy based on this strategy remain uncertain. A person with a high risk score (greater than 20 percent in 10 years) or established heart disease or stroke should be treated intensively regardless of hs-CRP levels.

What Is the Normal Range of hs-CRP Level?

- If hs-CRP level is lower than 1.0 mg/L, a person has a low risk of developing cardiovascular disease.
- If hs-CRP is between 1.0 and 3.0 mg/L, a person has an average risk.
- If hs-CRP is higher than 3.0 mg/L, a person is at high risk.
- If, after repeated testing, patients have persistently unexplained, markedly elevated hs-CRP (greater than 10.0 mg/L), other evaluation should be considered to exclude noncardiovascular causes.

Chapter 13

Peripheral Vascular Disease (PVD) Diagnosis

Peripheral vascular disease (PVD) is a common circulation problem in which the arteries that carry blood to the legs or arms become narrowed or clogged. PVD is sometimes called peripheral arterial disease, or PAD. Many people also refer to the condition as hardening of the arteries. The following information was prepared by the Society of Cardiovascular and Interventional Radiology (SIR) to provide general information for consumers on PVD.

Peripheral Vascular Disease: An Overview

What Is Peripheral Vascular Disease?

Peripheral vascular disease, or PVD, is a condition in which the arteries that carry blood to the arms or legs become narrowed or clogged. This interferes with the normal flow of blood, sometimes causing pain, but often causing no symptoms at all. The most common cause of PVD is atherosclerosis (often called hardening of the arteries). Atherosclerosis is a gradual process in which cholesterol and scar tissue build up, forming a substance called plaque that clogs the blood vessels. In some cases, PVD may be caused by blood clots that lodge in the arteries and restrict blood flow.

"Peripheral Vascular Disease." The information in this chapter is reprinted with permission from the Society of Interventional Radiology (SIR). © 2003 Society of Interventional Radiology. All Rights Reserved. For additional information, visit the SIR website at www.sirweb.org.

How Common Is PVD?

PVD affects about 1 in 20 people over the age of 50, or 10 million people in the United States. More than half the people with PVD experience leg pain, numbness, or other symptoms—but many people dismiss these signs as "a normal part of aging" and don't seek medical help. Only about half of those with symptoms have been diagnosed with PVD and are seeing a doctor for treatment.

Incidence of Peripheral Vascular Disease (PVD)

- PVD affects 10 million people in the United States including 5% of the over 50 population
- Only a quarter of PVD sufferers are receiving treatment
- Symptomatic constitutes 50% of cases (5 million)
- Of these, 2.5 million go undiagnosed
- Of the 2.5 million diagnosed cases, 2.1 million are medically managed (e.g., exercise)

What Are the Symptoms of PVD?

The most common symptom of PVD is painful cramping in the leg or hip, particularly when walking. This symptom, also known as claudication, occurs when there is not enough blood flowing to the leg muscles during exercise. The pain typically goes away when the muscles are given a rest.

Other symptoms may include numbness, tingling, or weakness in the leg. In severe cases, you may experience a burning or aching pain in your foot or toes while resting, or develop a sore on your leg or foot that does not heal. People with PVD also may experience a cooling or color change in the skin of the legs or feet, or loss of hair on the legs. In extreme cases, untreated PVD can lead to gangrene, a serious condition that may require amputation of a leg, foot, or toes. If you have PVD, you are also at higher risk for heart disease and stroke. Unfortunately, the disease often goes undiagnosed because many people do not experience symptoms in the early stages of PVD or they mistakenly think the symptoms are a normal part of aging.

PVD Symptoms

- Leg or hip pain during walking
- The pain stops when you rest

- Numbness, tingling, or weakness in the legs
- Burning or aching pain in feet or toes when resting
- Sore on leg or foot that won't heal
- Cold legs or feet
- Color change in skin of legs or feet
- Loss of hair on legs

Who Is at Risk for PVD?

As many as 8 million people in the U.S. may have PVD. The disease affects everyone, although men are somewhat more likely than women to have PVD. Those who are at highest risk are:

- over the age of 50,
- smokers,
- diabetic,
- overweight,
- people who do not exercise, or
- people who have high blood pressure or high cholesterol.

A family history of heart or vascular disease may also put you at higher risk for PVD.

How Is PVD Diagnosed?

The most common test for PVD is the ankle-brachial index (ABI), a painless exam in which a special stethoscope is used to compare the blood pressure in your feet and arms. Based on the results of your ABI, as well as your symptoms and risk factors for PVD, the physician can decide if further tests are needed. When the ABI indicates that an individual may have PVD, other imaging techniques may be used to confirm the diagnosis, including duplex ultrasound, magnetic resonance angiography (MRA), and computed tomography (CT) angiography.

The Ankle-Brachial Index (ABI) Test for PVD

The ABI is a simple, painless test to help your physician determine if you have PVD. The blood pressure in your arms and ankles is checked using a regular blood pressure cuff and a special ultrasound stethoscope called a Doppler. The pressure in your ankle is compared to the pressure in your arm to determine how well your blood is flowing and whether further tests are needed.

How Can I Find Out If I Have PVD?

If you suspect that you may have PVD, it is important that you see your personal physician for an evaluation. If you are concerned about PVD, you can take the following self-test to determine if you are at risk. You also may want to participate in Legs For Life™—National Screening for PVD Leg Pain.

Peripheral Vascular Disease (PVD) Self-Test

Your answers to these questions will help you know if you are at risk.

- Do you have cardiovascular (heart) problems such as high blood pressure, heart attack, stroke?
- Do you have diabetes?
- Do you have a family history of diabetes or cardiovascular problems (immediate family such as parent, sister, brother)?
- Do you have aching, cramping, or pain in your legs when you walk or exercise, but then the pain goes away when you rest?
- Do you have pain in your toes or feet at night?
- Do you have any ulcers or sores on your feet or legs that are slow in healing?
- Do you smoke?
- Have you ever smoked?
- Are you more than 25 pounds overweight?
- Do you eat fried or fatty foods three times a week or more?
- Do you have an inactive lifestyle?

The more yes answers you have, the more important it is for you to see your doctor.

Chapter 14

Colorectal Cancer Screening

On July 15, 2002, the U.S. Preventive Services Task Force, in its strongest ever recommendation for colorectal cancer screening, urged that all adults age 50 and over get screened for the disease, the nation's second leading cause of cancer deaths. Various screening tests are available, making it possible for patients and their clinicians to decide which test is most appropriate for each individual.

"When it comes to colon cancer, screening saves lives," Health and Human Services Secretary Tommy G. Thompson said. "Less than half of all Americans over the age of 50 are currently being screened for colorectal cancer. This new recommendation—based on the best medical evidence available—should encourage more Americans to get one of the key screening tests to identify colon cancer early when people are more likely to recover."

An estimated 143,300 U.S. adults will be diagnosed with colorectal cancer in 2002, and nearly 57,000 will die from it. Of cancer deaths, only lung cancer kills more Americans.

This recommendation strengthens the Task Force's previous position in 1996, when it "simply recommended" screening. It now "strongly recommends" screening for colorectal cancer because new studies show even more clearly that various screening methods are effective

This chapter includes "U.S. Preventive Services Task Force Urges Colorectal Cancer Screening for All Americans 50 and Over," Press Release, Agency for Healthcare Research and Quality (AHRQ), 7/15/2002; and "Colorectal Cancer Screening: Questions and Answers," Fact Sheet 5.31, National Cancer Institute (NCI), reviewed: 4/03/2002.

in diagnosing cancer and preventing deaths. The Task Force is an independent panel of experts that is sponsored by the Agency for Healthcare Research and Quality (AHRQ). Its recommendation was published in the July 16, 2002 *Annals of Internal Medicine*.

Although several screening tests are effective in diagnosing colorectal cancer at an early stage when it is treatable, the Task Force noted that current information is insufficient to recommend one method over another. Options include at-home fecal occult blood test (FOBT); flexible sigmoidoscopy; a combination of home FOBT and flexible sigmoidoscopy; colonoscopy; and double-contrast barium enema. Screening can also lead to early detection of adenomatous polyps— pre-cancerous growths that can be removed to prevent them from progressing to cancer.

The Task Force found good evidence that annual FOBT reduces deaths from colorectal cancer and fair evidence that sigmoidoscopy alone, or in combination with FOBT, reduces deaths. It noted that colonoscopy or barium enema were also likely to be effective screening tools, although the Task Force did not find direct evidence that colonoscopy or barium enema are effective in reducing colorectal cancer deaths. The Task Force could not determine whether the increased accuracy of colonoscopy, which allows doctors to examine the entire colon, offsets the procedure's inconvenience, costs, and potential complications, such as a small risk for bleeding and perforation of the colon.

"There is no single best test for all patients and clinical practice settings—each test has advantages and disadvantages," said Alfred O. Berg, M.D., M.P.H., Chair of the Task Force. "Clinicians should talk to patients about the benefits and potential harms with each option. The decision to screen should be based on patient preferences and available resources for testing and follow-up."

Most cases of colorectal cancer occur in people at average risk for the disease, a category that includes people 50 and over. About 20 percent of colorectal cancers occur in those at high risk for the disease, including people with a personal history of ulcerative colitis or a family history of colorectal cancer in a first-degree relative; that is, a mother, father, sister, or brother who received a diagnosis before age 60. For those at high risk, the Task Force indicated that screening could begin at a younger age but didn't recommend a specific time schedule.

The Task Force, the leading independent panel of private-sector experts in prevention and primary care, conducts rigorous, impartial assessments of all the scientific evidence for a broad range of preventive services. Its recommendations are considered the gold standard for clinical preventive services. The Task Force based its conclusion on a report published in the July 16 *Annals of Internal Medicine* from a research team led by Michael Pignone, M.D., M.P.H., at AHRQ's Evidence-based Practice Center at RTI International-University of North Carolina. The Task Force grades the strength of evidence from "A" (strongly recommends) to "D" (recommends against). The Task Force recommendation for colorectal cancer screening is an "A" recommendation.

Colorectal Cancer Screening: Questions and Answers

What Is Colorectal Cancer?

Colorectal cancer is a disease in which cells in the colon or rectum become abnormal and divide without control or order, forming a mass called a tumor. (The colon and rectum are parts of the body's digestive system that remove nutrients from food and water and store solid waste until it passes out of the body.) Cancer cells invade and destroy the tissue around them. They can also break away from the tumor and spread to form new tumors in other parts of the body.

What Methods Are Used to Screen People for Colorectal Cancer?

Health care providers may suggest one or more of the tests listed below for colorectal cancer screening.

- A fecal occult blood test (FOBT) checks for hidden blood in the stool. Studies have proven that this test, when performed every 1 to 2 years in people age 50 to 80, reduces the number of deaths due to colorectal cancer.

- A sigmoidoscopy is an examination of the rectum and lower colon using a lighted instrument called a sigmoidoscope. Sigmoidoscopy can find precancerous or cancerous growths in the rectum and lower colon. Studies suggest that regular screening with sigmoidoscopy after age 50 can reduce the number of deaths from colorectal cancer.

- A colonoscopy is an examination of the rectum and entire colon using a lighted instrument called a colonoscope. Colonoscopy can find precancerous or cancerous growths throughout the colon, including the upper part of the colon, where they would be missed by sigmoidoscopy. However, it is not known whether this benefit outweighs the increased risks of colonoscopy, which include bleeding and puncturing of the lining of the colon. More research is needed to address these issues.

- A double contrast barium enema (DCBE) is a series of x-rays of the entire colon and rectum. The x-rays are taken after the patient is given an enema with a barium solution and air is introduced into the colon. The barium and air help to outline the colon and rectum on the x-rays. Research shows that DCBE is more effective at detecting larger growths than smaller ones.

A digital rectal exam (DRE) is often part of a routine physical examination. In a DRE, the health care provider inserts a lubricated, gloved finger into the rectum to feel for abnormal areas. The test is often used to examine nearby structures, such as the prostate in men. Unlike the colorectal cancer screening tests described above, DRE allows for examination of only the lowest part of the rectum.

Scientists are still studying colorectal cancer screening methods, both alone and in combination, to determine how effective they are. Studies are also under way to clarify the risks of each test.

How Can People and Their Health Care Providers Decide Which Colorectal Cancer Screening Test to Use and How Often to Be Screened?

Several major organizations, including the U.S. Preventive Services Task Force (a group of experts convened by the U.S. Public Health Service) and the American Cancer Society, have developed guidelines for colorectal cancer screening. Although their recommendations vary regarding which screening tests to use and how often to be screened, all of these organizations support screening for colorectal cancer. People should talk with their health care provider about when to begin screening for colorectal cancer, what tests to have, the benefits and risks of each test, and how often to schedule appointments.

The decision to have a certain test will take into account several factors:

- Person's age, medical history, family history, and general health;
- Accuracy of the test;
- Risks associated with the test;
- Preparation required before the test;
- Sedation necessary during the test;

- Follow-up care after the test;
- Convenience of the test; and
- Cost and insurance coverage of the test.

Table14.1 outlines some of the advantages and disadvantages of the colorectal cancer screening tests described in this chapter.

Do Insurance Companies Pay for Colorectal Cancer Screening?

Insurance coverage varies. People should check with their health insurance provider to determine their colorectal cancer screening benefits. Medicare covers several colorectal cancer screening tests for its beneficiaries.

What Happens If a Colorectal Cancer Screening Test Shows an Abnormality?

If screening tests find an abnormality, the health care provider will perform a physical exam and evaluate the person's personal and family medical history. Additional diagnostic tests may be ordered. These may include x-rays of the gastrointestinal tract, sigmoidoscopy, or colonoscopy. The health care provider may also order a blood test called a CEA assay to measure carcinoembryonic antigen, a protein that is sometimes present in higher levels in patients with colorectal cancer.

If an abnormal area is found during a sigmoidoscopy or colonoscopy, a biopsy is performed to determine if cancer is present.

Are New Tests under Study for Colorectal Cancer Screening?

Several new tests for colorectal cancer screening and diagnosis are under study. For example, virtual colonoscopy (also called computed tomographic colonography) is a procedure that uses special x-ray equipment to produce pictures of the colon. A computer then assembles these pictures into detailed images that can show polyps and other abnormalities. Because it is less invasive and does not require sedation, virtual colonoscopy may cause less discomfort and take less time than conventional colonoscopy. However, unlike conventional colonoscopy, it is not possible to remove polyps or perform a biopsy during this test. An additional procedure, such as conventional colonoscopy, is needed if the virtual procedure finds a potential problem. Clinical

Table 14.1. Advantages and Disadvantages of Colorectal Cancer Screening Tests (continued on next page)

Fecal Occult Blood Test (FOBT)

Advantages

No preparation of the colon is necessary. Samples can be collected at home. Cost is low compared to other colorectal screening tests. There is no risk of infection or tears in the lining of the colon.

Disadvantages

This test fails to detect most polyps and some cancers. False positive results are possible. (False positive means the test suggests an abnormality when none is present.) Dietary and other limitations, such as increasing fiber intake and avoiding meat, certain vegetables, vitamin C, iron, and aspirin, are necessary for several days before the test. Additional procedures, such as colonoscopy, may be necessary if the test indicates an abnormality.

Sigmoidoscopy

Advantages

The test is usually quick, with few complications. Discomfort is minimal. The doctor can perform a biopsy (the removal of tissue for examination under a microscope by a pathologist) and remove polyps during the test, if necessary. Less extensive preparation of the colon is necessary with this test than for a colonoscopy.

Disadvantages

This test allows the doctor to view only the rectum and the lower part of the colon. Any polyps in the upper part of the colon will be missed. There is a very small risk of infection or tears in the lining of the colon. Additional procedures, such as colonoscopy, may be necessary if the test indicates an abnormality.

Colonoscopy

Advantages

This test allows the doctor to view the rectum and the entire colon. The doctor can perform a biopsy and remove polyps during the test, if necessary.

Disadvantages

The test may not detect some small polyps and cancers. Thorough preparation of the colon is necessary before the test. Sedation is usually needed. Complications, such as infection and/or tears in the lining of the colon, can occur.

Table 14.1. Advantages and Disadvantages of Colorectal Cancer Screening Tests (continued from previous page)

Double Contrast Barium Enema (DCBE)

Advantages

This test usually allows the doctor to view the rectum and the entire colon. Complications are rare. No sedation is necessary. Discomfort is minimal.

Disadvantages

The test may not detect some small polyps and cancers. Thorough preparation of the colon is necessary before the test. False positive results are possible. The doctor cannot perform a biopsy or remove polyps during the test. Additional procedures are necessary if the test indicates an abnormality.

trials (research studies with people) are under way to compare the advantages and disadvantages of virtual colonoscopy with those of other colorectal cancer screening tests.

Genetic testing of stool samples is also under study as a possible way to screen for colorectal cancer. The lining of the colon is constantly shedding cells into the stool. Testing stool samples for genetic alterations that occur in colorectal cancer cells may help doctors find evidence of cancer. Research conducted thus far has shown that this test can detect colorectal cancer in people already diagnosed with this disease by other means. However, more studies are needed to determine whether the test can detect colorectal cancer in people who do not have symptoms.

References

Dong SM, Traverso G, Johnson C, et al. Detecting colorectal cancer in stool with the use of multiple genetic targets. *Journal of the National Cancer Institute* 2001; 93(11):858–865.

Fenlon HM, Nunes DP, Schroy III PC, et al. A comparison of virtual and conventional colonoscopy for the detection of colorectal polyps. *The New England Journal of Medicine* 1999; 341(20):1496–1503.

Levin B. Overview of colorectal cancer screening in the United States. *Journal of Psychological Oncology* 2001; 19(3/4):9–19.

Lieberman DA, Harford WV, Ahnen DJ, et al. One-time screening for colorectal cancer with combined fecal occult-blood testing and examination of the distal colon. *New England Journal of Medicine* 2001; 345(8):555–560.

Lieberman DA, Weiss DG, Bond JH, et al. Use of colonoscopy to screen asymptomatic adults for colorectal cancer. *New England Journal of Medicine* 2000; 343(3):162–168.

Mandel JS, Church TR, Ederer F, Bond JH. Colorectal cancer mortality: Effectiveness of biennial screening for fecal occult blood. *Journal of the National Cancer Institute* 1999; 91(5):434–437.

Ransohoff DF, Sandler RS. Screening for colorectal cancer. *New England Journal of Medicine* 2002; 346(1):40–44.

Winawer SJ, Stewart ET, Zauber AG, et al. A comparison of colonoscopy and double-contrast barium enema for surveillance after polypectomy. *New England Journal of Medicine* 2000; 342(24):1766–1772.

Additional Information

National Cancer Institute
NCI Public Inquiries Office
Suite 3036A, MSC8322
6116 Executive Blvd.
Bethesda, MD 20892-8322
Toll-Free: 800-422-6237
Toll-Free TTY: 800-332-8615
Website: www.nci.nih.gov

The NCI booklet "What You Need To Know About™ Cancer of the Colon and Rectum," provides more information about the diagnosis and treatment of colorectal cancer. This publication and other cancer resources are available from the National Cancer Institute.

Chapter 15

Diabetes Diagnosis

Diabetes Overview

Almost everyone knows someone who has diabetes. An estimated 17 million people, 6.2 percent of the population, in the United States have diabetes mellitus—a serious, lifelong condition. About 5.9 million people have not yet been diagnosed. Each year, about 1 million people age 20 or older are diagnosed with diabetes.

What Is Diabetes?

Diabetes is a disorder of metabolism—the way our bodies use digested food for growth and energy. Most of the food we eat is broken down into glucose, the form of sugar in the blood. Glucose is the main source of fuel for the body.

After digestion, glucose passes into the bloodstream, where it is used by cells for growth and energy. For glucose to get into cells, insulin must be present. Insulin is a hormone produced by the pancreas, a large gland behind the stomach.

When we eat, the pancreas is supposed to automatically produce the right amount of insulin to move glucose from blood into our cells.

This chapter includes excerpts from "Diabetes Overview," National Institute of Diabetes and Digestive and Kidney Diseases (NIDDK), NIH Publication No. 02-3873, May 2003; and "Diabetes Grows at Alarming Rate," National Institute of Diabetes and Digestive and Kidney Diseases (NIDDK), October 2001.

In people with diabetes, however, the pancreas either produces little or no insulin, or the cells do not respond appropriately to the insulin that is produced. Glucose builds up in the blood, overflows into the urine, and passes out of the body. Thus, the body loses its main source of fuel even though the blood contains large amounts of glucose.

What Are the Types of Diabetes?

The three main types of diabetes are

- Type 1 diabetes
- Type 2 diabetes
- Gestational diabetes

Type 1 Diabetes

Type 1 diabetes is an autoimmune disease. An autoimmune disease results when the body's system for fighting infection (the immune system) turns against a part of the body. In diabetes, the immune system attacks the insulin-producing beta cells in the pancreas and destroys them. The pancreas then produces little or no insulin. Someone with type 1 diabetes needs to take insulin daily to live.

At present, scientists do not know exactly what causes the body's immune system to attack the beta cells, but they believe that autoimmune, genetic, and environmental factors, possibly viruses, are involved. Type 1 diabetes accounts for about 5 to 10 percent of diagnosed diabetes in the United States.

Type 1 diabetes develops most often in children and young adults, but the disorder can appear at any age. Symptoms of type 1 diabetes usually develop over a short period, although beta cell destruction can begin years earlier.

Symptoms include increased thirst and urination, constant hunger, weight loss, blurred vision, and extreme fatigue. If not diagnosed and treated with insulin, a person can lapse into a life-threatening diabetic coma, also known as diabetic ketoacidosis.

Type 2 Diabetes

The most common form of diabetes is type 2 diabetes. About 90 to 95 percent of people with diabetes have type 2. This form of diabetes usually develops in adults age 40 and older and is most common in adults over age 55. About 80 percent of people with type 2 diabetes are overweight. Type 2 diabetes is often part of a metabolic syndrome that includes obesity, elevated blood pressure, and high levels of blood lipids. Unfortunately, as more children and adolescents become overweight, type 2 diabetes is becoming more common in young people.

When type 2 diabetes is diagnosed, the pancreas is usually producing enough insulin, but, for unknown reasons, the body cannot use the insulin effectively, a condition called insulin resistance. After several years, insulin production decreases. The result is the same as for type 1 diabetes—glucose builds up in the blood and the body cannot make efficient use of its main source of fuel.

The symptoms of type 2 diabetes develop gradually. They are not as sudden in onset as in type 1 diabetes. Some people have no symptoms. Symptoms may include fatigue or nausea, frequent urination, unusual thirst, weight loss, blurred vision, frequent infections, and slow healing of wounds or sores.

Gestational Diabetes

Gestational diabetes develops only during pregnancy. Like type 2 diabetes, it occurs more often in African Americans, American Indians, Hispanic Americans, and people with a family history of diabetes. Though it usually disappears after delivery, the mother is at increased risk of getting type 2 diabetes later in life.

What Tests Are Recommended for Diagnosing Diabetes?

The fasting plasma glucose test is the preferred test for diagnosing type 1 or type 2 diabetes. However, a diagnosis of diabetes is made for any one of three positive tests, with a second positive test on a different day:

- A random plasma glucose value (taken any time of day) of 200 mg/dL or more, along with the presence of diabetes symptoms.

- A plasma glucose value of 126 mg/dL or more, after a person has fasted for 8 hours.

- An oral glucose tolerance test (OGTT) plasma glucose value of 200 mg/dL or more in the blood sample, taken 2 hours after a person has consumed a drink containing 75 grams of glucose dissolved in water. This test, taken in a laboratory or the

Table 15.1. Diabetes Grows at Alarming Rate. Diagnosed Diabetes in U.S. Adults Aged 18 Years or Older (continued on next page)

	Total Number of People with Diagnosed Diabetes in 2000	Percent of People with Diagnosed Diabetes in 2000	Rate of Increase in Percent of People with Diagnosed Diabetes from 1990 to 2000
United States	15 million	7.3	49
State	(*in thousands*)		
Alabama	241	8.0	43
Alaska	16	4.4	42*
Arizona	180	7.4	90
Arkansas	122	6.9	35*
California	1569	8.4	105
Colorado	135	6.0	94
Connecticut	123	6.3	19
Delaware	35	6.9	17
Dist of Columbia	28	7.3	49*
Florida	812	7.9	39
Georgia	357	7.7	57
Hawaii	47	6.4	23
Idaho	43	5.7	78
Illinois	567	7.3	83
Indiana	279	6.9	21
Iowa	121	6.7	43
Kansas	110	6.9	68*
Kentucky	191	6.9	21
Louisiana	200	7.4	40
Maine	53	6.9	47
Maryland	258	8.0	86
Massachusetts	257	7.3	92
Michigan	455	7.6	55
Minnesota	170	6.1	91
Mississippi	154	8.8	28
Missouri	261	7.2	13
Montana	35	5.5	96

Table 15.1. Diabetes Grows at Alarming Rate. Diagnosed Diabetes in U.S. Adults Aged 18 Years or Older (continued from previous page)

State	Total Number of People with Diagnosed Diabetes in 2000 (*in thousands*)	Percent of People with Diagnosed Diabetes in 2000	Rate of Increase in Percent of People with Diagnosed Diabetes from 1990 to 2000
Nebraska	57	5.4	17
Nevada	87	7.1	65*
New Hampshire	39	5.0	11
New Jersey	350	6.7	52*
New Mexico	74	7.1	37
New York	832	7.7	48
North Carolina	368	7.3	22
North Dakota	24	6.3	80
Ohio	521	7.5	60
Oklahoma	140	5.8	12
Oregon	133	6.9	86
Pennsylvania	620	7.6	29
Rhode Island	43	7.4	64*
South Carolina	195	8.5	35
South Dakota	28	6.3	66
Tennessee	275	7.6	31
Texas	902	7.1	48
Utah	66	6.7	81
Vermont	19	5.6	65
Virginia	320	6.6	53
Washington	229	6.1	39
West Virginia	103	7.9	5
Wisconsin	222	6.2	51
Wyoming	16	5.5	53*

Data source: Behavioral Risk Factor Surveillance System, Centers for Disease Control and Prevention. Estimates include people with gestational diabetes.

* 5-year rate of increase in percent of people with diabetes from 1995 to 2000

Prepared October, 2001

doctor's office, measures plasma glucose at timed intervals over a 3-hour period.

Gestational diabetes is diagnosed based on plasma glucose values measured during the OGTT. Glucose levels are normally lower during pregnancy, so the threshold values for diagnosis of diabetes in pregnancy are lower. If a woman has two plasma glucose values meeting or exceeding any of the following numbers, she has gestational diabetes: a fasting plasma glucose level of 95 mg/dL, a 1-hour level of 180 mg/dL, a 2-hour level of 155 mg/dL, or a 3-hour level of 140 mg/dL.

What Are the Other Forms of Impaired Glucose Metabolism, Also Called Prediabetes?

People with prediabetes, a state between normal and diabetes, are at risk for developing diabetes, heart attacks, and strokes. About 16 million people ages 40 to 74 in the United States have prediabetes. There are two forms of prediabetes.

Impaired Fasting Glucose: A person has impaired fasting glucose (IFG) when fasting plasma glucose is 110 to 125 mg/dL. This level is higher than normal but less than the level indicating a diagnosis of diabetes.

Impaired Glucose Tolerance: Impaired glucose tolerance (IGT) means that blood glucose during the oral glucose tolerance test is higher than normal but not high enough for a diagnosis of diabetes. IGT is diagnosed when the glucose level is 141 to 199 mg/dL 2 hours after a person is given a drink containing 75 grams of glucose.

Additional Information

National Diabetes Information Clearinghouse
1 Information Way
Bethesda, MD 20892-3560
Toll-Free: 800-860-8747
Phone: 301-654-3327
Fax: 301-907-8906
Website: http://diabetes.niddk.nih.gov
E-mail: ndic@info.niddk.nih.gov

American Diabetes Association National Service Center
1701 North Beauregard Street
Alexandria, VA 22311
Toll-Free: 800-342-2383
Phone: 703-549-1500
Website: www.diabetes.org
E-mail: AskADA@diabetes.org

Juvenile Diabetes Research Foundation International
120 Wall Street, 19th Floor
New York, NY 10005
Toll-Free: 800-533-2873
Phone: 212-785-9500
Website: www.jdrf.org
E-mail: info@jdrf.org

Chapter 16

Diagnosing Osteoporosis

"An accurate diagnosis, which is relatively simple, can save women from a lot of suffering, fractures, and emotional damage." Carmen Sanchez, Spain, osteoporosis patient.

People with osteoporosis suffer from a reduction in their bone mass and bone quality—put simply, their bones become fragile, leading to an increased risk of fractures. Bone density loss is usually gradual and without noticeable symptoms. The only reliable way to determine loss of bone mass is to have a bone mineral density (BMD) test.

Who Should Be Tested?

Strong risk factors for osteoporosis include:

- Estrogen deficiency:
    - Early menopause (age < 45 years)
    - Absence or cessation of menstrual periods (amenorrhea > 1 year)
    - Primary or secondary hypogonadism in both genders
- Prolonged corticosteroid therapy (prednisolone, or equivalent, 7.5 mg or more daily with an expected use of 3 months or more)

"Osteoporosis: What You Need to Know: Diagnosis," © 2003 International Osteoporosis Foundation. Reprinted with permission. For additional information, visit www.osteofound.org.

- Maternal family history of hip fracture
- Low body mass index (< 19 kg/m2)
- Chronic disorders associated with osteoporosis: anorexia nervosa, malabsorption syndromes including chronic liver disease and inflammatory bowel disease, primary hyperparathyroidism, post-transplantation, chronic renal failure, hyperthyroidism, prolonged immobilization, and Cushing's syndrome
- Previous fragility fracture, particularly of the hip, spine, or wrist
- Loss of height, thoracic kyphosis (widows hump)

Other risk factors:

- Female (women are more at risk than men)
- Asian or Caucasian
- Poor diet low in calcium
- Lack of exercise
- Smoking
- Regular and excessive alcohol consumption

People with a strong risk of osteoporosis are advised to consult their doctors for a bone mineral density test. In the USA, for example, guidelines recommend that all women aged 65 and up should have a BMD test and that postmenopausal women under age 65 who have one or more risk factors (in addition to being postmenopausal and female) should have a BMD test.

How Osteoporosis Is Diagnosed

The most common diagnostic tool is a bone mineral density (BMD) test. This is a painless and noninvasive scan which, depending on the technology, measures bone density in the hip, spine, wrist, heel, or hand.

According to World Health Organization (WHO) guidelines, a BMD score in a postmenopausal Caucasian woman that is more than 2.5 standard deviations below the average for the young healthy female population implies a diagnosis of osteoporosis. For every standard deviation (SD) below peak bone mineral density fracture risk increases by 50% to 100%. The same BMD values are being provisionally used for men because currently data on BMD and fracture in men is scarce.

Summary of WHO Definitions of Osteoporosis Based on Bone Density Levels Based on DXA Measurement at Hip or Spine

Normal: BMD is within +1 or -1 SD of the young adult mean.

Osteopenia (low bone mass): BMD is between -1 and -2.5 standard deviations below young adult mean.

Osteoporosis: BMD is -2.5 SD or more than the young adult mean.

Severe (established) osteoporosis: BMD is more than -2.5 SD and one or more osteoporotic fractures have occurred.

Methods of Diagnosis

A variety of methods is available to assess bone density. All are painless and noninvasive. The most common types of tests are listed below:

DXA (Dual Energy X-Ray Absorptiometry)

DXA is a special low radiation x-ray capable of detecting quite low percentages of bone loss. DXA scans are the most commonly used method of BMD measurement. They are used to measure spine and hip bone densities.

- **pDXA** (Peripheral Dual Energy X-Ray Absorptiometry): pDXA measures the forearm, finger, and heel

- **SXA** (Single-Energy X-Ray Absorptiometry): SXA measures the heel

QCT (Quantitative Computed Tomography)

QCT scans the trabecular bones of the lower spine—these are bones that change as you grow older. pQCT measures the forearm.

QUS (Quantitative Ultrasound)

QUS uses sound waves to measure density at the heel, shin and finger.

The Importance of Early Diagnosis

Through early detection, people with osteopenia (low bone mass) or osteoporosis, can take action to stop the progressive loss of bone mass. By making positive lifestyle changes and following appropriate treatment strategies in consultation with a doctor, osteoporosis can be prevented and treated.

Chapter 17

Tests That Evaluate
Asthma and Lung Disease

Tests to Diagnose Asthma

Sometimes, your doctor can be fairly certain whether or not you have asthma based on your symptoms and physical examination. Often, though, more information is needed to distinguish between asthma and other respiratory problems. After all, asthma is not the only medical problem that can lead to breathing difficulties. If there is doubt about your diagnosis, your physician may ask you to perform some tests that provide additional information regarding how well your lungs work or whether you have allergies. These are called *pulmonary function tests* (PFTs) or allergy tests.

Pulmonary Function Tests

Spirometry

The most commonly used pulmonary function test is called spirometry (from the Greek *spiro*—breathing, and *metry*—measurement). Patients are asked to breathe in to the tops of their lungs, then to blow out as fast and as completely as possible into a machine (the spirometer) which measures how much and how fast they can exhale. The

"Tests Done to Evaluate Asthma," reprinted with permission from the University of Chicago Asthma Center, © 2003 University of Chicago Asthma Center. For additional information on living with asthma, visit http://asthma.bsd.uchicago.edu.

exhalation speed is reported in two numbers—the forced expiratory volume in the first second of exhalation (or FEV1), and the fastest or peak instantaneous expiratory flow rate during exhalation (or peak flow, abbreviated as PF or PEF). The total volume of air exhaled is called the forced vital capacity, or FVC.

During an asthma attack, FEV1 and PF become reduced (indicating obstruction to airflow through the bronchial tubes caused by airway narrowing). FVC often falls, too. These numbers provide your health care provider with an objective measurement of how severely narrowed your airways are at the time. They are more accurate than your own impression of how severe your asthma is just then, and they are much more accurate than your doctor's impression. This is why asthmatics should measure their own peak flow rates at home, using a simple, portable peak flow meter, rather than simply relying on their own impressions of how they are doing.

Post-Bronchodilator Spirometry

Some other diseases besides asthma can also reduce FEV1, PF, and FVC, and for this reason doctors sometimes request additional tests. Commonly, an asthmatic patient will be asked to repeat spirometry after inhaling a quick-reliever medicine, like albuterol. Patients with asthma typically show substantial improvements in FEV1 and PF (over 20% or more) after inhaling such a medicine. Patients with other lung diseases (such as emphysema or chronic bronchitis from smoking) often do not exhibit such immediate benefit. So if the measurements are substantially better after the quick reliever medicine than they were before, it suggests that the person has asthma.

Lung Volume Determination, Diffusing Capacity Measurement, and Arterial Blood Gases

After forcibly exhaling from the top to the bottom of the lungs (as one does during spirometry), there is still some air remaining within the lungs, and this is normal. To determine how much air is left in the lungs after complete exhalation (this amount is called the residual volume), pulmonary function labs use two kinds of procedures. The preferred way is for the patient to perform some panting maneuvers while sitting inside a big plastic box (a body box, or body plethysmograph), but it is also possible to infer residual volume by measuring the dilution of inhaled, non-absorbed gases like helium. While sitting inside a plastic box may seem weird, neither of these procedures is painful or dangerous at all. From these measurements, your doctor can also calculate the biggest size your lungs can achieve at full inhalation (called total lung capacity, equal to residual volume plus FVC).

In one additional test called diffusing capacity measurement, the ability of your lung to absorb inhaled gas is measured. Finally, occasionally it may be necessary to measure how much oxygen and carbon dioxide are actually in your blood. This is usually done by sampling blood from an artery in your wrist. The information gained from all these auxiliary tests can usually provide fairly strong evidence for or against asthma.

Bronchial Provocation

Sometimes all the tests listed are normal, even in a person who actually has asthma. This is because airflow obstruction in asthma is very commonly episodic—that is, airflow obstruction occurs during asthma attacks, but at other times, lung function is normal. In this case, your doctor may ask you to perform bronchial provocation testing.

There are certain substances that when inhaled will narrow everyone's airways to some degree. These substances are called bronchoconstrictors, and include histamine and methacholine. However, a characteristic of asthmatics' airways is that they tend to narrow more than those of normal people, and at lower doses of bronchoconstrictor than are required to cause narrowing of normal airways.

To perform a bronchial provocation test, the patient inhales increasing doses of bronchoconstrictor (usually methacholine), starting with tiny doses. The patient has spirometry after each dose to see how much bronchoconstriction was induced. From this test, your doctor can infer whether the reactivity of your airways is normal or high. Very high airway reactivity to methacholine or histamine is almost exclusively seen in patients with asthma.

Exercise or Cold Air Bronchial Provocation

Many patients with asthma experience airway narrowing after exercise or after breathing cold air. For this reason, it is sometimes useful to measure spirometry after a patient performs exercise or breathes cold air from a special laboratory apparatus. These sorts of bronchial challenge tests can also reveal quite specific evidence for asthma, if there is substantial exercise—or cold air-induced bronchoconstriction.

Allergy Tests

Many, though certainly not all, patients with asthma have allergies to one or more substances in the environment (called allergens). An asthmatic patient can improve his/her asthma control, or at least reduce the likelihood of inducing an asthma attack, by limiting contact with substances to which he or she is allergic.

To determine whether allergies are present, and to which environmental allergens, your doctor may perform a series of skin prick tests, in which a drop of allergen is placed on the forearm, and a tiny prick into the very top of the skin is made with a needle. Surprisingly, this doesn't really hurt. When allergy to the substance is present, an itchy red reaction occurs.

Another kind of test for allergies is performed on a regular blood sample, and measures the quantity of a particular kind of antibody (immunoglobulin E, or IgE) that is often elevated in people with multiple allergies.

Chapter 18

Allergy Testing

What Is Allergy Testing?

If you are allergic, you are reacting to a particular substance. Any substance that can trigger an allergic reaction is called an allergen. To determine which specific substances are triggering your allergies, your allergist/immunologist will safely and effectively test your skin, or sometimes your blood, using tiny amounts of commonly troublesome allergens.

Allergy tests are designed to gather the most specific information possible so your doctor can determine what you are allergic to and provide the best treatment.

Who Should Be Tested for Allergies?

Adults and children of any age who have symptoms that suggest they have an allergic disease. Allergy symptoms can include:

- Respiratory symptoms: itchy eyes, nose, or throat; nasal congestion, runny nose, watery eyes, chest congestion, or wheezing.
- Skin symptoms: hives, generalized itchiness, or atopic dermatitis.
- Other symptoms: anaphylaxis (severe life-threatening allergic reactions), abdominal symptoms (cramping, diarrhea) consistently following particular foods, stinging insect reactions other than large local swelling at the sting site.

"Tips to Remember: What is Allergy Testing?" © 2003 American Academy of Allergy, Asthma, and Immunology (AAAAI), reprinted with permission. For further information about allergies, visit the AAAAI website at www.aaaai.org

Generally, inhaled allergens such as dust mites, tree, grass, or weed pollens will produce respiratory symptoms, and ingested (food) allergies will produce skin and/or gastrointestinal symptoms or anaphylaxis, but both types of allergens (ingested and inhaled) can produce the spectrum of allergy symptoms.

What Are the Reasons for Undergoing Allergy Skin Testing?

To help you manage your allergy symptoms most effectively, your allergist/immunologist must first determine what is causing your allergy. For instance, you don't have to get rid of your cat if you are allergic to dust mites but not cats.

Allergy tests provide concrete specific information about what you are and are not allergic to. Once you have identified the specific allergen(s) causing your symptoms, you and your physician can develop a treatment plan aimed at controlling or eliminating your allergy symptoms. With your allergy symptoms under control you should see a considerable improvement in the quality of your life. Improved sleep quality because of less congestion, days without constant sneezing and blowing your nose, improved ability to exercise, and better control of your atopic dermatitis (eczema) are some of improvements you may gain from your allergy treatment plans.

Which Allergens Will I Be Tested For?

Because your physician has made a diagnosis of allergies, you know that one or more allergens is causing your allergic reaction—itching, swelling, sneezing, wheezing, and other symptoms. Your symptoms are probably caused by one of these common allergens:

- Products from dust mites (tiny bugs you can't see) that live in your home;
- Proteins from furry pets, which are found in their skin secretions (dander), saliva, and urine (it's actually not their hair);
- Molds in your home or in the air outside;
- Tree, grass, and weed pollen; and/or cockroach droppings.

More serious allergic reactions can be caused by:

- Venoms from the stings of bees, wasps, yellow jackets, fire ants, and other stinging insects;
- Foods;
- Natural rubber latex, such as gloves or balloons; or

- Drugs, such as penicillin.

All of these allergens are typically made up of proteins. Allergy tests find which of these proteins you may be reacting to.

The allergen extracts or vaccines used in allergy tests are made commercially and are standardized according to U.S. Food and Drug Administration (FDA) requirements. Your allergist/immunologist is able to safely test you for allergies to substances listed using these allergen extracts.

Types of Allergy Tests

Prick Technique: The prick technique involves introducing a small amount of allergen into the skin by making a small puncture through a drop of the allergen extract. If you have an allergy, the specific allergens that you are allergic to will cause a chain reaction to begin in your body.

People with allergies have an allergic antibody called *IgE (immunoglobulin E)* in their body. This chemical, which is only found in people with allergies, activates special cells called mast cells. These mast cells release chemicals called mediators, such as histamine, the chemical that causes redness and swelling. With testing, this swelling occurs only in the spots where the tiny amount of allergen to which you are allergic has been introduced. So, if you are allergic to ragweed pollen but not to cats, the spot where the ragweed allergen touched your skin will swell and itch a bit, forming a small dime-sized hive. The spot where the cat allergen scratched your skin will remain normal. This reaction happens quickly within your body.

Test results are available within 15 minutes of testing, so you don't have to wait long to find out what is triggering your allergies. And you won't have any other symptoms besides the slightly swollen, small hives where the test was done; this goes away within 30 minutes.

Intradermal: Involves injecting a small amount of allergen under the skin with a syringe. This form of testing is more sensitive than the prick skin test method. This form of allergy testing may be used if the prick skin tests are negative.

Other Allergy Testing Techniques

Scratch tests: The term scratch test refers to a technique not commonly used at the present, which involves abrading the skin and then dropping the allergen on the abraded site.

Challenge testing: Involves introducing small amounts of the suspected allergen by oral, inhaled, or other routes. With the exception of food and medication, challenges are rarely performed. When they are performed, they must be closely supervised by an allergist/immunologist.

Blood (RAST) test: Sometimes your allergist/immunologist will do a blood test, called a RAST (radioallergosorbent) test. Since this test involves drawing blood, it costs more, and the results are not available as rapidly as skin tests. RAST tests are generally used only in cases in which skin tests cannot be performed, such as on patients taking certain medications, or those with skin conditions that may interfere with skin testing.

Other types of allergy testing methods the American Academy of Allergy, Asthma and Immunology considers to be unacceptable are: applied kinesiology (allergy testing through muscle relaxation), cytotoxicity testing, urine autoinjection, skin titration (Rinkel method), provocative and neutralization (subcutaneous) testing, or sublingual provocation. If your physician plans to conduct any of these tests on you, please see an AAAAI member allergist/immunologist for appropriate allergy testing.

Who Can Be Tested for Allergies?

Adults and children of any age can be tested for allergies. Because different allergens bother different people, your allergist/immunologist will take your medical history to determine which test is the best for you. Some medications can interfere with skin testing. Antihistamines, in particular, can inhibit some of the skin test reactions. Use of antihistamines should be stopped one to several days prior to skin testing.

Your allergist/immunologist can provide you with more information on allergy testing.

Additional Information

American Academy of Allergy, Asthma, and Immunology
611 East Wells Street
Milwaukee, WI 53202
Toll-Free: 800-822-2762
Website: www.aaaai.org
E-mail: info@aaaai.org

Chapter 19

Vision Exams

When to See an Eye M.D.

Eye M.D.

An eye M.D. is an ophthalmologist—a medical doctor (or DO) who specializes in eye and vision care. Eye M.D.s are specially trained to provide the full spectrum of eye care, from prescribing glasses and contact lenses to complex and delicate eye surgery.

Read to see when you and your family should visit an eye M.D. for a complete eye examination. Early detection and treatment of eye problems, along with protecting your eyes from accidental injury, are the best ways to take care of your vision throughout life.

If you have any of these risk factors for eye problems, you may need to see your eye M.D. more often than recommended:

- Family history of eye problems
- African American over age 40
- Diabetes
- History of eye injury

This chapter includes "When to See an Eye M.D.," updated 2003, © 2002 American Academy of Ophthalmology. Used by permission. All rights reserved. For more information, visit www.aao.org; and "Standard Ophthalmic Exam," © 2003 A.D.A.M., Inc. Reprinted with permission.

Before Age 3

Since it is possible for your child to have a serious vision problem without being aware of it, your child should have his or her eyes screened during regular pediatric appointments. Vision testing is recommended for all children starting around 3 years of age.

If there is a family history of vision problems or if your child appears to have any of the following conditions speak to your eye M.D. promptly about when and how often your child's eyes should be examined:

- Strabismus (crossed eyes)
- Amblyopia (lazy eye)
- Ptosis (drooping of the upper eyelid)

Age 3 to 19

To ensure your child's or teenager's eyes remain healthy, he or she should have his or her eyes screened every one to two years during regular checkup appointments.

Age 20 to 39

Most young adults have healthy eyes, but they still need to take care of their vision by wearing protective eyewear when playing sports, doing yard work, working with chemicals, or taking part in other activities that could cause an eye injury.

Have a complete eye exam at least once between the ages of 20 and 29 and at least twice between the ages of 30 and 39.

Also, be aware of symptoms that could indicate a problem. See an eye M.D. if you experience any eye conditions, such as:

- Visual changes or pain
- Flashes of light
- Seeing spots or ghost-like images
- Lines appear distorted or wavy
- Dry eyes with itching and burning

Age 40 to 64

The adult and middle-aged groups can be affected by eye problems. Preventive measures should be taken to protect eyes from injury and detect disease early. Schedule an eye exam with your eye M.D. every two to four years.

Age 65 and Over

Seniors age 65 and over should have complete eye exams by their eye M.D. every one to two years to check for cataracts, glaucoma, age-related macular degeneration, diabetic retinopathy, and other eye conditions.

Standard Ophthalmic Exam

Alternative names: Routine eye examination; Eye exam—standard

Definition

A series of tests performed by an ophthalmologist or optometrist (eye doctor) that measure the refraction and visual acuity of the eye and test for disease.

How the Test Is Performed

The eye doctor will start by asking a series of questions about your medical and ocular history and any noticeable eye problems.

Visual acuity (vision) is determined in each eye using the Snellen Chart. This chart consists of random letters of different sizes. The letters for normal vision (20/20) are 3/8-inch tall when viewed at 20 feet. People with normal vision can read these letters. A refraction test may also be performed where the doctor puts several lenses in front of the eyes to determine if glasses are needed.

Eye movement and peripheral vision are tested by moving a light or object through the field of vision. The eye's reaction to light (pupillary response) is also measured. Color blindness is tested using multicolored dots that form numbers. Color blind people are not able to detect certain numbers or may see a different number than people who are not color blind.

Glaucoma testing (tonometry) is performed with a puff of air directed at the eye or using a blue circle of light that comes very close to the eye. Evaluation of the cornea and the front part of the eye is performed while seated at a slit lamp, a device which magnifies the doctors view.

The retina, fundus (back of the eye), retinal vessels, and optic nerve head (optic disc) are viewed with an ophthalmoscope (a device made up of a light and magnifier). This procedure is known as an ophthalmoscopy. Drops that dilate the pupil are usually used to allow more of the fundus to be viewed.

How to Prepare for the Test

- Make an appointment with the eye doctor (some take walk-in patients).
- Avoid eye strain the day of the test.
- Arrange transportation, since your pupils will be dilated.

Infants and Children

The physical and psychological preparation you can provide for this or any test or procedure depends on your child's age, interests, previous experience, and level of trust.

How the Test Will Feel

The tests cause no pain or discomfort.

Why the Test Is Performed

This test should be performed on a regular basis to detect eye problems early and help determine the cause of noticeable changes in vision. Some professions (such as pilots, military, personnel, and professional drivers) require eye tests.

Various eye and medical problems can be found by a routine eye test. People with diabetes should have their eyes examined at least once a year.

Normal Values

- 20/20 (normal) vision
- able to differentiate colors
- no signs of glaucoma
- normal optic nerve, retinal vessels, and fundus

What Abnormal Results Mean

- glaucoma
- myopia

- hyperopia
- damaged optic nerves, vessels, or fundus
- astigmatism
- presbyopia
- corneal abrasion (or dystrophy)
- color blindness
- strabismus (motility disturbance between eyes)
- eye diseases
- cataracts
- trauma
- corneal ulcers and infections
- blocked tear duct
- amblyopia (lazy eye)
- age-related macular degeneration (ARMD)
- diabetic retinopathy

What the Risks Are

If your pupils are dilated during the ophthalmoscopy, vision will be blurred and sunlight can damage your eye. Wear dark glasses or shade your eyes to avoid discomfort.

Special Considerations

Many eye diseases, if detected early, are curable or can be treated.

The information provided herein should not be used during any medical emergency or for the diagnosis or treatment of any medical condition. A licensed physician should be consulted for diagnosis and treatment of any and all medical conditions. Call 911 for all medical emergencies.

Chapter 20

Hearing Screening

Hearing screening tests provide a quick and cost effective way to separate people into two groups: a pass group and a fail group. Those who pass hearing screening are presumed to have no hearing loss. Those who fail are in need of an in-depth evaluation by an audiologist and may also need follow-up care from other professionals.

Hearing screening occurs from birth throughout the adult years when requested, when conditions occur that increase risk for hearing loss, or when mandated by state and local laws or practices.

It is recommended that all hearing screening programs be conducted under the supervision of an audiologist holding the American Speech-Language-Hearing Association's (ASHA) Certificate of Clinical Competence (CCC).

Newborns and Infants

Hearing screening for newborns before they leave the hospital or maternity center is becoming a common practice. Without such programs, the average age of hearing loss identification will stay at 12–25 months.

When hearing loss is detected late, language development is already delayed. Children are more likely to perform below their grade level, and are more likely to be held back, drop out of school, and fail to earn a high school diploma. These consequences are in sharp contrast to those

---

This chapter includes "Hearing Screening," and "Hearing Assessment," 2003 American Speech-Language-Hearing Association. Copyright by the American Speech-Language-Hearing Association. Reprinted with permission.

for children who are identified early, receive early intervention, and then are found to function at the level of their peers by the time they enter school.

Screening Techniques

Screening procedures for newborns and infants can detect permanent bilateral or unilateral, sensory or conductive hearing loss, averaging 30 to 40 dB or more in the frequency region important for speech recognition (approximately 500–4000 Hz).

The screening of newborns and infants involves use of non-invasive, objective physiologic measures that include otoacoustic emissions (OAEs) and/or auditory brainstem response (ABR). Both procedures can be done painlessly while the infant is resting quietly.

Otoacoustic emissions are inaudible sounds from the cochlea when audible sound stimulates the cochlea. The outer hair cells of the cochlea vibrate, and the vibration produces an inaudible sound that echoes back into the middle ear. This sound can be measured with a small probe inserted into the ear canal. Persons with normal hearing produce emissions. Those with hearing loss greater than 25–30 dB do not. OAEs can detect blockage in the outer ear canal, middle ear fluid, and damage to the outer hair cells in the cochlea.

Auditory brainstem response is an auditory evoked potential that originates from the auditory nerve. It is often used with babies. Electrodes are placed on the head, and brain wave activity in response to sound is recorded. ABR can detect damage to the cochlea, the auditory nerve, and the auditory pathways in the stem of the brain.

ASHA-certified audiologists (and state licensed where applicable) should be designated as the manager of these screening programs.

What Happens If an Infant Does Not Pass the Screening?

Infants who do not pass a screening are often given a second screening to confirm findings and then referred for follow-up audiological and medical evaluations that should occur no later than 3 months of age. These evaluations confirm the presence of hearing loss; determine the type, nature, and (whenever possible) the cause of the hearing loss; and help identify options for treatment.

Even if the infant passes screening, certain conditions do not produce immediate hearing loss. Rather, the hearing loss occurs later in the child's development.

An infant with any of the following indicators for progressive or delayed-onset hearing loss should receive audiologic monitoring every six months until age 3 years:

1. Parental or caregiver concern regarding hearing, speech, language, and/or developmental delay.

2. Family history of permanent childhood hearing loss.

3. Characteristics or other findings associated with a syndrome known to include a sensorineural and/or conductive hearing loss.

4. Postnatal infections associated with sensorineural hearing loss including bacterial meningitis.

5. In utero infections such as cytomegalovirus, herpes, rubella, syphilis, and toxoplasmosis.

6. Neonatal indicators—specifically hyperbilirubinemia at a serum level requiring exchange transfusion, persistent pulmonary hypertension of the newborn associated with mechanical ventilation, and conditions requiring the use of extracorporeal membrane oxygenation (ECMO).

7. Syndromes associated with progressive hearing loss such as neurofibromatosis, osteopetrosis, and Usher's syndrome.

8. Neurodegenerative disorders, such as Hunter syndrome, or sensory motor neuropathies, such as Friedreich's ataxia and Charcot-Marie-Tooth syndrome.

9. Head trauma.

10. Recurrent or persistent otitis media with effusion for at least 3 months.

Legal Requirements

The Individuals with Disabilities Education Act (IDEA) in its regulations requires states to develop and implement a statewide system of early intervention services for infants and toddlers. It is required that infants and toddlers with disabilities be identified and evaluated using at-risk criteria and appropriate audiologic screening techniques. After a hearing loss is confirmed, coordination of services should be facilitated by the infant's medical manager and the IDEA coordinating agencies.

Contact your local school district or your state or local health department to find out how to obtain screenings/evaluations and intervention services through your state's Early Intervention program.

Older Infants and Toddlers

Infants and toddlers (7 months through 2 years) should be screened for hearing loss as needed, requested, mandated, or when conditions place them at risk for hearing disability.

Infants not tested as newborns should be screened before three months of age. Other infants should be screened who received neonatal intensive care or special care, or who display other indicators that place them at risk for hearing loss.

Older infants and toddlers who have a greater chance of hearing loss because of certain risk factors should also be screened. This screening should be done even if an initial hearing screening is passed because some causes of hearing loss do not take effect until later in the child's development. These children's hearing should be monitored at least every 6 months until 3 years of age, and at regular intervals thereafter dependent upon the risk factor.

Risk Factors

Parental, caregiver, and/or health care provider concerns regarding hearing, speech, language, and/or developmental delay based on observation and/or standardized developmental screening.

1. Family history of permanent childhood hearing loss.

2. Characteristics or other findings associated with a syndrome known to include a sensorineural and/or conductive hearing loss.

3. Infections associated with sensorineural hearing loss including bacterial meningitis, mumps.

4. In utero infections such as cytomegalovirus, herpes, rubella, syphilis, and toxoplasmosis.

5. Neonatal indicators—specifically hyperbilirubinemia at a serum level requiring exchange transfusion, persistent pulmonary hypertension of the newborn associated with mechanical ventilation, and conditions requiring the use of extracorporeal membrane oxygenation (ECMO).

6. Syndromes associated with progressive hearing loss such as neurofibromatosis, osteopetrosis, and Usher's syndrome.

7. Neurodegenerative disorders, such as Hunter syndrome, or sensory motor neuropathies, such as Friedreich's ataxia and Charcot-Marie-Tooth syndrome.

8. Head trauma.

9. Recurrent or persistent otitis media with effusion for at least 3 months.

10. Anatomic disorders that affect eustachian tube function.

11. Neurofibromatosis type II or neurodegenerative disorders.

Screening Techniques

Screening procedures to detect hearing impairment that exceeds 20–30 dB HL are applicable to this age group. Two screening methods are suggested as the most appropriate tools for children who are functioning at a development age of 7 months to 3 years, visual reinforcement audiometry (VRA) and conditioned play audiometry (CPA). Both of these methods are behavioral techniques that require involvement and cooperation of the child.

Visual reinforcement audiometry (VRA) is the method of choice for children between 6 months and 2 years of age. The child is trained to look toward (localize) a sound source. When the child gives a correct response, e.g., looking to a source of sound when it is presented, the child is rewarded through a visual reinforcement such as a toy that moves or a flashing light.

Conditioned play audiometry (CPA) can be used as the child matures. It is widely used between 2 and 3 years of age. The child is trained to perform an activity each time a sound is heard. The activity may be putting a block in a box, placing pegs in a hole, putting a ring on a cone, etc. The child is taught to wait, listen, and respond.

With both of these methods, sounds of different frequencies are presented at a sound level that children with normal hearing can hear.

It is ideal if the child will allow earphones to be placed on his or her head so that independent information can be obtained for each ear. If the child refuses earphone placement or earphone placement is otherwise not possible, sounds are presented through speakers inside a sound booth. Since sound field screening does not give ear specific information, a unilateral hearing loss (hearing loss in only one ear) may be missed.

Alternative procedures, such as otoacoustic emissions (OAEs) or auditory brainstem response (ABR) may be used if the child is unable to be conditioned.

ASHA certified audiologists are the professionals who have the knowledge, skill, and expertise to screen for hearing impairment in this age group.

What Happens If a Toddler Does Not Pass the Screening?

A toddler who does not pass the screening should be rescreened or referred for audiologic evaluation. Confirmation of hearing status should be obtained within 1 month, but no later than 3 months, after the initial screening.

Legislative requirements are the same as for younger children.

Preschoolers

The goal of screening for hearing loss in preschoolers (ages 3–5 years) is to identify children most likely to have hearing loss that may interfere with communication, development, health, or future school performance. In addition, because hearing loss in this age range is so often associated with middle ear disease, it is also recommended that children in this age group be screened for outer and middle ear disorders (acoustic immittance screening).

Some children may pass an initial hearing screening, but still be at risk for hearing loss that fluctuates, is progressive (gets worse over time), or is acquired later in development.

Risk Factors

1. Parental, caregiver, and/or health care provider concerns regarding hearing, speech, language, and/or developmental delay based on observation and/or standardized developmental screening.

2. Family history of permanent childhood hearing loss.

3. Characteristics or other findings associated with a syndrome known to include a sensorineural and/or conductive hearing loss.

4. Infections associated with sensorineural hearing loss including bacterial meningitis, mumps.

5. In utero infections such as cytomegalovirus, herpes, rubella, syphilis, and toxoplasmosis.

6. Neonatal indicators—specifically hyperbilirubinemia at a serum level requiring exchange transfusion, persistent pulmonary hypertension of the newborn associated with mechanical ventilation, and conditions requiring the use of extracorporeal membrane oxygenation (ECMO).

7. Syndromes associated with progressive hearing loss such as neurofibromatosis, osteopetrosis, and Usher's syndrome.

8. Neurodegenerative disorders, such as Hunter syndrome, or sensory motor neuropathies, such as Friedreich's ataxia and Charcot-Marie-Tooth syndrome.

9. Head trauma.

10. Recurrent or persistent otitis media with effusion for at least 3 months.

11. Ototoxic medications, including but not limited to chemotherapeutic agents or aminoglycosides used in multiple courses or in combination with loop diuretics.

12. Apgar scores of 0–4 at 1 minute or 0–6 at 5 minutes.

13. Neurofibromatosis type II or neurodegenerative disorders.

14. Anatomic disorders that affect eustachian tube function.

Screening procedures to detect unilateral or bilateral sensorineural and/or conductive hearing loss greater than 20 dB HL in the frequency region from 1000 through 4000 Hz are applicable to this age group.

Conditioned play audiometry (CPA) is the most commonly employed procedure.

Acoustic Immittance screening may include tympanometry, acoustic reflex, and static acoustic impedance.

Tympanometry introduces air pressure into the ear canal making the eardrum move back and forth. A special machine then measures the mobility of the eardrum. Tympanograms, or graphs, are produced which show stiffness, floppiness, or normal eardrum movement.

197

Acoustic reflex measures the response of a tiny ear muscle that contracts when a loud sound occurs. The loudness level at which the acoustic reflex occurs and/or the absence of the acoustic reflex give important diagnostic information.

Static acoustic measures estimate the physical volume of air in the ear canal. This test is useful in identifying a perforated eardrum or whether ear ventilation tubes are still open.

Screening should be limited to audiologists holding a Certificate of Clinical Competence (CCC-A) from the American Speech-Language Hearing Association and state licensure where applicable; speech-language pathologists holding a Certificate of Clinical Competence (CCC-SLP) from the American Speech-Language Hearing Association and state licensure where applicable; and other personnel under the supervision of an ASHA-certified audiologist.

What Happens If a Preschooler Does Not Pass the Screening?

If the child cannot be conditioned to the play audiometry, the child will be screened using infant-toddler procedures or will be recommended for a more in-depth audiologic assessment.

If the child did condition and did not pass the screening, then referral for audiological assessment by an ASHA-certified audiologist will be made.

Hearing status of children referred after screening should be confirmed within 1 month, but no later than 3 months, after the initial screening.

Legislative Requirements

The Individuals with Disabilities Education Act (IDEA) in its regulations for student ages 3–21 requires states to identify children with disabilities, including hearing loss, residing in the state. Contact your local school district or your state's education department to find out how to obtain screenings/evaluations for children with suspected disabilities.

School Age (5–18 years)

School-age children should be screened for hearing loss as needed, requested, mandated, or when conditions place them at risk for hearing disability. Screening for hearing loss identifies the school-age children most likely to have hearing impairment that may interfere with development, communication, health, and education. School age children with even minimal hearing loss are at risk for academic and communication difficulties.

Periodic screenings are recommended because of the increased potential for hearing loss due to overexposure to high levels of noise and the importance of identifying children at risk for hearing impairment that may affect their future educational, vocational, or social opportunities.

School age children should be screened at the following times:

1. On first entry into school.

2. Every year from kindergarten through 3ʳᵈ grade.

3. In 7ᵗʰ grade.

4. In 11ᵗʰ grade.

5. Upon entrance into special education.

6. Upon grade repetition.

7. Upon entering a new school system without evidence of having passed a previous hearing screening.

School age children who already receive regular audiologic management need not participate in a screening program.

Hearing screening should be done in other years when:

1. Parent/care provider, health care provider, teacher, or other school personnel have concerns regarding hearing, speech, language, or learning abilities.

2. There is family history of late or delayed onset hereditary hearing loss.

3. Otitis media with effusion (fluid in the middle ear) recurs or persists for at least 3 months.

4. There are skull or facial abnormalities, especially those that can cause changes to the structure of the pinna and ear canal.

5. Characteristics or other findings occur that are associated with a syndrome known to include hearing loss.

6. Head trauma occurs with loss of consciousness.

7. There is reported exposure to potentially damaging noise levels or to drugs that frequently cause hearing loss.

Screening Techniques Used for School-Age Students

Screening procedures to detect unilateral or bilateral sensorineural and/or conductive hearing loss greater than 20 dB HL in the frequency region from 1000 through 4000 Hz are applicable to this age group.

Conventional audiometry where students are instructed to raise their hand (or point to the appropriate ear) when they hear a tone is the commonly used procedure. Conditioned play audiometry (CPA) is also used.

Who Should Carry Out the Screening?

Screening practitioners should be limited to:

1. Audiologists holding a Certificate of Clinical Competence (CCC-A) from the American Speech-Language Hearing Association and state licensure where applicable.

2. Speech-Language Pathologists holding a Certificate of Clinical Competence (CCC-SLP) from the American Speech-Language Hearing Association and state licensure where applicable.

3. Support personnel under supervision of a certified audiologist.

What Happens If a School-Age Student Does Not Pass the Screening?

1. The student should be reinstructed, earphones repositioned, and rescreened in the same session.

2. If the student does not pass the rescreening, he or she should be referred for audiologic assessment.

3. Hearing status of referred students should be confirmed within one month, and no later than 3 months, after initial screening.

Legislative Mandates

The Individuals with Disabilities Education Act (IDEA) in its regulations for students aged 3–21 years requires states to identify children with disabilities residing in the state. "The identification of children with hearing loss" is included in the definition of audiology.

Contact your local school district or your state's education department to find out how to obtain screenings/evaluations for children with suspected disabilities.

Adults

Hearing loss is a prevalent chronic condition among adults of all ages. It is recognized that hearing loss increases as a function of age, especially for frequencies at 2000 Hz and above. However, adults tend to ignore its effects, delay their decision to seek audiologic services, and tend to put off recommended treatments.

While more than 30% of people over 65 have some type of hearing loss, 14% of those between 45 and 64 have hearing loss. Close to 8 million people between the ages of 18 and 44 have hearing loss.

Adult hearing screening programs are considered voluntary. It is recommended however, that adults be screened at least every decade through age 50 and at 3-year intervals thereafter.

Screening Techniques Used for Adults

Screening procedures to detect unilateral or bilateral sensorineural and/or conductive hearing loss greater than 25 dB HL in the frequency region from 1000 through 4000 Hz are applicable to this age group.

Techniques for hearing screening include case history [regarding history of hearing loss, unilateral hearing loss, sudden or rapid progression of hearing loss, unilateral tinnitus, acute or chronic dizziness, recent drainage from the ear(s), and/or pain of discomfort in the ear(s)], visual inspection of the ear, pure-tone screening, and screening by self-assessed judgment of hearing difficulty.

Conventional audiometry where individuals are instructed to raise their hand (or point to the appropriate ear) when they hear a tone is the commonly used procedure for the pure-tone screening.

Who Should Carry Out the Screening?

Screening practitioners should be limited to:

1. Audiologists holding a Certificate of Clinical Competence (CCC-A) from the American Speech-Language Hearing Association and state licensure where applicable.

2. Speech-Language Pathologists holding a Certificate of Clinical Competence (CCC-SLP) from the American Speech-Language Hearing Association and state licensure where applicable.

3. Support personnel under supervision of a certified audiologist.

What Happens If an Individual Does Not Pass the Screen?

The individual is counseled regarding hearing loss. Counseling may result in a recommendation for audiologic evaluation. However, the individual may decline audiologic evaluation or further medical follow-up.

1. The individual should be referred for audiologic assessment if case history discussion indicates a condition indicating a risk for hearing loss.

2. The individual should be referred for audiologic assessment and/or cerumen (wax) management if visual inspection indicates any physical abnormality of the outer ear, or if there is otoscopic identification of ear canal abnormality, or impacted cerumen.

Hearing Assessment

Individuals throughout their lives have their hearing assessed on the basis of self-referral, family/caregiver referral, failure of an audiologic screening, follow-up to previous audiologic assessment, case history for risk indicators, or referral from other professionals.

Purpose

The purpose of audiological assessment is to quantify and qualify hearing in terms of the degree of hearing loss, the type of hearing loss and the configuration of the hearing loss.

With regard to **degree of hearing loss**, the audiologist is looking for quantitative information. Hearing levels are expressed in decibels based on the pure tone average for the frequencies 500 to 4000 Hz and discussed using descriptors related to severity: normal hearing (-10 to +15 dB HL), slight/minimal hearing loss (16–25 dB HL), mild hearing loss (26–30 dB HL), moderate hearing loss (31–50 dB HL), moderate to severe hearing loss (51–70 dB HL), severe hearing loss (71–90 dB HL), and profound hearing loss (91 dB HL or greater).

With regard to the **type of hearing loss**, the audiologist is looking for information that suggests the point in the auditory system where the loss is occurring. The loss may be conductive (a temporary or permanent hearing loss typically due to abnormal conditions of the outer and/or middle ear), sensorineural (typically a permanent hearing loss due to disease, trauma, or inherited conditions affecting the nerve cells in the cochlea, the inner ear, or the eighth cranial nerve), mixed (a combination of conductive and sensorineural components), or a central auditory processing disorder (a condition where the brain has difficulty processing auditory signals that are heard).

With regard to the **configuration of the hearing loss**, the audiologist is looking at qualitative attributes such as bilateral versus unilateral hearing loss; symmetrical versus asymmetrical hearing loss; high-frequency versus low frequency hearing loss; flat versus sloping versus precipitous hearing loss; progressive versus. sudden hearing loss; and stable versus. fluctuating hearing loss.

Audiological evaluation is also carried out for purposes of monitoring an already identified hearing loss. Once a particular hearing loss has been identified, a treatment and management plan is put into place. The plan may include medical or surgical intervention, prescription of personal hearing aids, prescription/provision of assistive listening devices, skills development through aural (audiologic) habilitation/rehabilitation, or simply monitoring of the condition through periodic assessment.

Once a treatment and management plan is in place, it is still important for an individual's hearing loss to be checked periodically to determine its stability. Is it fluctuating? Has it improved as a result of medical intervention? Is it progressing? Have new conditions come into play that have affected the original condition?

It is also important that a person's ability to hear using amplification (i.e., personal hearing aids and any assistive listening devices that are used in place of, or in conjunction with, personal amplification) be monitored and documented. This monitoring would include functional gain assessment, real ear measurement, electroacoustic analysis, listening check, and even informal functional assessment in the person's typical listening environment (i.e., the classroom, the workplace, the home).

The Assessment Itself

An audiologic evaluation is sometimes thought of as just a hearing test, but more than just the ability to hear sounds is involved. The audiologic evaluation consists of a battery of tests each providing specific stand alone information. Yet, the tests are complementary to one another. The audiologic evaluation consists of several different components.

Case History

The audiologist will ask several questions during the case history. For example:

- What brought you here today?

- Have you noticed difficulty with your hearing? What have you noticed? For how long? When do you think the hearing loss began?

- Does your hearing problem affect both ears or just one ear?

- Has your difficulty with hearing been gradual or sudden?

- Do you have ringing (tinnitus) in your ears?

- Do you have a history of ear infection?

- Have you noticed any pain in your ears or any discharge from your ears?

- Do you experience dizziness?

- Is there a family history of hearing loss? Do you have greater difficulty hearing women's, men's, or children's voices?

- Do people comment on the volume setting of your television?

- Has someone said that you speak too loudly in conversation?

- Do you frequently have to ask people to repeat?

- Do you hear people speaking, but can't understand what is being said?

- Do you have any history of exposure to noise in recreational activities, at work, or in the military?

- Are there situations where it is particularly difficult for you to follow conversation? Noisy restaurant? Theater? Car? Large groups?

For children, questions will also be asked regarding:

- speech and language development
- health history

- recognition of and response to familiar sounds
- the startle response to loud, unexpected sounds
- the presence of other disabilities
- any previous hearing screening or testing results

Physical Examination

The audiologist will look at the outer ear (the pinna) checking for any misformation. The audiologist will use an otoscope, an instrument that contains a light and a magnifying lens, to examine the ear canal and eardrum. The ear canal is examined for the presence of excessive wax (cerumen), or foreign objects (food, toys, pieces of cotton swabs, etc.). The eardrum (tympanic membrane) is examined for any perforation and signs of fluid or infection. The audiologist will look for any indicators suggesting the need for referral for a medical evaluation and/or treatment.

Tests of Hearing and Listening

The audiologist will conduct tests of hearing tones. This is called pure-tone audiometry. The results are recorded on a graph called an audiogram. The audiologist will also determine speech reception threshold or the faintest speech that can be heard half the time. Then the audiologist will determine word recognition or ability to recognize words at a comfortable loudness level.

Tests of Middle Ear Function

The audiologist may also take measurements that will provide information about the status of the outer and middle ear. These are called acoustic immittance measures. Tympanometry, one aspect of immittance testing, can assist in the detection of fluid in the middle ear, perforation of the eardrum, or wax blocking the ear canal. Acoustic reflex measurement, another aspect of immittance testing, can add diagnostic information about middle ear function and hearing loss.

After the test battery is completed, the audiologist will review each component of the audiologic evaluation to obtain a profile of hearing abilities and needs. Additional specialized testing may be indicated and recommended on the initial test results. Audiological evaluation may result in recommendations for further follow-up such as medical referral, educational referral, hearing aid/sensory aid assessment,

assessment for assistive listening devices, audiologic rehabilitation assessment, speech and language assessment, and/or counseling.

As you can see, an audiologic evaluation is much more than just a hearing test.

Pure-Tone Audiometry

Pure-tone audiometry is completed in a soundproof booth—a room with special treatment to the walls, ceiling, and floor to ensure that background noise does not affect test results. Only those sounds that the audiologist introduces into the room, either through earphones or through speakers located in the room, will be heard. Sounds may also be sent through a special headset vibrator that has been placed just behind the ear or on the forehead.

In testing hearing for tones, a pure tone air conduction hearing test is given to find out the faintest tones a person can hear at selected pitches (frequencies) from low to high. During this test, earphones are worn and the sound travels through the air in the ear canal to stimulate the eardrum and then the auditory nerve. The person taking the test is instructed to give some type of response such as raising a finger or hand, pressing a button, pointing to the ear where the sound was received, or saying yes to indicate that the sound was heard.

Sometimes children are given a more play-like activity (conditioned play audiometry) to indicate response. They may be instructed to string a peg, drop a block in a bucket, or place a ring on a stick in response to hearing the sound. Infants and toddlers are observed for changes in their behavior such as sucking a pacifier, quieting, or searching for the sound and are rewarded for the correct response by getting to watch an animated toy (visual reinforcement audiometry).

The audiologist uses a calibrated machine called an audiometer to present tones at different frequencies (pitches) and at different intensity (loudness) levels. A signal of a particular frequency (something like a piano note) is presented to one ear, and its intensity is raised and lowered until the person no longer responds consistently. Then another signal of a different frequency is presented to the same ear, and its intensity is varied until there is no consistent response. This procedure is done for at least six frequencies. Then the other ear is tested in the same way.

The frequency or pitch of the sound is referred to in Hertz (Hz). The intensity or loudness of the sound is measured in decibels (dB). The responses are recorded on a chart called an audiogram that provides a graph of intensity levels for each frequency tested.

In some cases, it is necessary to give a pure tone bone conduction hearing test. In this test, the tone is introduced through a small vibrator placed on the temporal bone behind the ear (or on the forehead). This method by-passes blockage, such as wax or fluid, in the outer or middle ears and reaches the auditory nerve through vibration of skull bones. This testing can measure functionality of the inner ear independent of the functionality of the outer and middle ears.

Air conduction test results indicate hearing losses that are either conductive or sensorineural. Bone conduction test results reflect only the sensorineural component. By comparing air conduction and bone conduction test results, the audiologist can determine whether there is a hearing loss due to a problem in the outer or middle ear. If air and bone conduction thresholds are the same, the loss is sensorineural. If there is a difference between air and bone thresholds (an air-bone gap), the loss is conductive or mixed.

Speech Audiometry

Speech audiometry includes determining speech reception threshold (SRT) and testing of word recognition. Speech reception threshold testing determines the faintest level at which a person can hear and correctly repeat easy-to-distinguish two-syllable (spondaic) words. Examples of spondaic words are baseball, ice cream, hot dog, outside, and airplane. Spondaic words have equal stress on each syllable. The individual repeats words (or points to pictures) as the audiologist's voice gets softer and softer. The faintest level, in decibels, at which 50% of the two-syllable words are correctly identified, is recorded as the Speech Reception Threshold (SRT). A separate SRT is determined for each ear.

Tests of word recognition attempt to evaluate how well a person can distinguish words at a comfortable loudness level. It relates to how clearly one can hear single-syllable (monosyllabic) words when speech is comfortably loud. Examples of words used in this test are come, high, knees, chew. In this test, the audiologist's voice (or a recording) stays at the same loudness level throughout. The individual being tested repeats words (or points to pictures). The percentage of words correctly repeated is recorded for each ear.

Thus, a score of 100% would indicate that every word was repeated correctly. A score of 0% would suggest no understanding. Word recognition is typically measured in quiet. For specific purposes, word recognition may also be measured in the presence of recorded background noise that can also be delivered through the audiometer.

How to Interpret an Audiogram

The audiogram is a graph showing the results of the pure-tone hearing tests.

Pitch or Frequency

Each line from left to right represents a pitch or frequency in Hertz (Hz) starting with the lowest pitches on the left side to the very highest frequencies tested on the right side. The range of frequencies tested by the audiologist are 125 Hz, 250 Hz, 500 Hz, 1000 Hz, 2000 Hz, 4000 Hz, and 8000 Hz. If you are familiar with a piano keyboard with the low notes at the left end and the high notes at the right end, the audiogram is similar. 250 Hz on the audiogram is the same as the middle C key on the piano.

Examples of sounds in everyday life that would be considered low frequency are: bass drum, tuba, vowel sounds such as *oo* in who.

Examples of sounds in everyday life that would be considered high frequency are: a bird chirping, a triangle playing, consonant sounds such as *s* in sun.

If we were to compare a flute playing and a tuba playing, we'd say the flute was primarily high frequency (high pitches) and the tuba was primarily low frequency (low pitches).

If we were to compare the sound of *f* as in fly to the sound of *m* as in moon, we'd say the *f* was primarily high frequency (high pitch) and the *m* was primarily low frequency (low pitch).

Loudness or Intensity

Each line on the audiogram from top to bottom represents loudness or intensity in units of decibels (dB). Lines at the top of the chart (small numbers starting at minus 10 dB and 0 dB) represent soft sounds. Lines at the bottom of the chart represent very loud sounds.

Examples of sounds in everyday life that would be considered soft are: a clock ticking, whispering, or the consonant sound *t* in the word too.

Examples of sounds in everyday life that would be considered loud are: a lawnmower, a car horn, or the vowel sound *o* as in the word poke.

If we were to compare the sound of a jackhammer to the sound of a vacuum cleaner, we'd say the jackhammer was loud and the vacuum cleaner was soft.

If we were to compare the sound of *s* as in spot to the sound of *ah* as in spot, we'd say the *s* was soft in comparison to the vowel *ah*.

If we were to compare normal conversational loudness level (typically 60 dB) to whispering (typically 30 dB), we'd say that whispering is soft and conversation is loud.

Some audiograms are also divided into sections showing the severity of hearing loss.

As the audiologist tests your hearing, the results are recorded on the graph. At each frequency tested, the O represents the softest tone you can hear in your right ear and the X represents the softest tone you can hear in your left ear. If the X's and O's all fall in the -10 dB to 15 dB range, your hearing lies in the normal range. If the X's and O's all fall in the 16 dB to 25 dB range, you have a slight/minimal loss. If the X's and O's all fall in the 31 dB to 51 dB range, you have a moderate loss. If the X's and O's all fall in the 91 dB and above range, you have a profound loss.

The audiogram configuration may be flat; sloping down showing better hearing in the low frequencies; rising showing better hearing in the high frequencies. The configuration may be symmetrical, showing the same hearing loss for both ears; or, asymmetrical, showing a different hearing loss configuration for each ear.

Once the audiogram is completed, the audiologist computes the pure tone average for each ear. It is the average of hearing thresholds at 500, 1000, and 2000 Hz, which are considered to be the major frequencies for speech. The pure-tone average represents the degree of hearing loss in decibels. It is not a percentage. Table 20.1 is an example of pure-tone average results.

Other Audiologic Procedures

There are a variety of other audiologic procedures that assess the auditory system and determine the presence of hearing loss. They are sometimes used independently and sometimes used to complement the standard audiologic test battery. They help to supplement information from behavioral testing or to resolve conflicting information

Table 20.1. Pure Tone Average

Frequency	Right Ear Threshold	Left Ear Threshold
500 Hz	20 dB	40 dB
1000 Hz	30 dB	45 dB
2000 Hz	35 dB	50 dB

Average loss = 28 dB (mild loss) 45 dB (moderate loss)

from behavioral testing. They are auditory evoked potentials, oto-acoustic emissions testing, and acoustic immittance measures.

Auditory Evoked Potentials

Electrodiagnostic test procedures give information about the status of neural pathways. These procedures are used with individuals who are difficult to test by conventional behavioral methods. They are also indicated for a person with signs, symptoms, or complaints suggesting a nervous system disease or disorder.

Auditory brainstem response (ABR) is an auditory evoked potential that originates from the auditory nerve. It is often used with babies. Electrodes are placed on the head (similar to electrodes placed around the heart when an electrocardiogram is run), and brain wave activity in response to sound is recorded.

Otoacoustic Emissions (OAE)

Otoacoustic emissions (OAE) are inaudible sounds emitted by the cochlea when the cochlea is stimulated by a sound. When sound stimulates the cochlea, the outer hair cells vibrate. The vibration produces an inaudible sound that echoes back into the middle ear. The sound can be measured with a small probe inserted into the ear canal. Persons with normal hearing produce emissions. Those with hearing loss greater than 25–30 dB do not.

Acoustic Immittance Measures

Acoustic immittance measures are a battery of tests including tympanometry, acoustic reflex, and static acoustic impedance.

Tympanometry introduces air pressure into the ear canal making the eardrum move back and forth. The test measures the mobility of the eardrum. Tympanograms or graphs are produced which show stiffness, flaccidity, or normal eardrum movement.

We all have an acoustic reflex to sounds. A tiny muscle in the ear contracts when a loud sound occurs. The loudness level in decibels at which the acoustic reflex occurs, and/or the absence of the acoustic reflex, gives diagnostic information that aids in identifying location of the problem along the auditory pathway.

Through static acoustic measures, the physical volume of air in the ear canal is measured. This test is useful in identifying a perforated eardrum or the openness of ventilation tubes.

Balance Assessment

Our sense of balance is determined by our visual system, the inner ear, and our sense of movement via muscles (kinesthetic sense). When these systems don't work together and function properly, we become dizzy.

Dizziness is a symptom. Any disturbance in the inner ear, with or without hearing loss or ringing in the ears (tinnitus), may cause a feeling of dizziness. Dizziness can be caused by disease such as Ménière's Disease, by small calcium deposits in the inner ear, drugs which are toxic to the vestibular (balance) system, head trauma, and other conditions not necessarily related to the vestibular system.

Balance system assessment is conducted to detect pathology with the vestibular or balance system; to determine site of lesion; to monitor

Table 20.2. Relationship of Degree of Hearing Loss to Everyday Functioning. Hearing loss affects your quality of life. This table shows how different degrees of hearing loss affect conversation and listening abilities.

Hearing Loss	Effect of Hearing Loss on Listening
Slight/Minimal loss 16-25 dB	Difficulty with faint or distant speech. Difficulty in noise. Difficulty hearing subtle conversational cues.
Mild loss 26-30dB	Will miss consonants. At 30 dB can miss 25-40% of speech signal. Degree of difficulty depends on noise level, distance from speaker, and configuration of the hearing loss. Will benefit from hearing aid.
Moderate loss 31-50 dB	Can understand face-to-face conversation at a distance of 3-5 feet if structure and vocabulary is controlled. May miss 50-75% of a spoken message if the pure tone average is 40 dB. Will benefit from hearing aid.
Moderately/ Severe loss 51-70dB	May miss most or all of the message even if talking face-to-face. Will have great difficulty conversing in a group. Will benefit from hearing aid.
Severe loss 71-90 dB	May not even hear voices, unless speech is very loud. Without amplification, the individual will not recognize any speech through listening alone.
Profound loss 91dB or greater	May not be able to detect the presence of even loud sound without amplification. May perceive vibratory aspects of sound. Will rely on vision communication.

changes in balance function; or, to determine the contribution of visual, vestibular, and proprioceptive systems to functional balance.

Vestibular or balance system assessment is indicated when a person has nystagmus (rapid involuntary eye movement), complaints of vertigo (dizziness), balance dysfunction, gait abnormalities, or when pathology/disease of the vestibular system is suspected.

Chapter 21

Infertility Tests

Infertility is a problem for one out of every six couples trying to have children. If, after a year of trying a couple has not conceived, a basic infertility evaluation may be started. In situations where the female partner is over 30 or has a medical history of irregular periods, pelvic infections, surgery, pregnancy losses, or DES exposure, the infertility evaluation should start earlier.

Couples embarking on an infertility work-up usually do so with some fear and reluctance. Some common concerns are: What is ahead? How painful is it? How expensive is it? And, what will the doctor find out? The whole world of doctors' offices, x-ray departments, and hospitals is stressful for many people. It often helps to know what to expect, to be informed and aware of how it will feel, and what the doctor is hoping to find.

The infertility work-up follows a fairly specific sequence. A complete evaluation of the woman usually takes three or four menstrual cycles to complete because certain tests have to be done at specific times in the cycle. The cost of the complete work-up can be over $5,000 if a laparoscopy is included. Insurance coverage varies; some insurance plans cover various tests relating to infertility, while other do not.

The nature of the infertility evaluation necessitates that it become a priority in your daily life. Suddenly, there are certain days on which

"The Basic Infertility Evaluation," Fact Sheet 47, written by Diane N. Clapp, BSN, RN, Medical Information Director, National RESOLVE. © 2003 The National Infertility Association. All Rights Reserved. For additional information, visit www.resolve.org. Reprinted with permission.

you must have intercourse. For some tests, you may have to report to the doctor's office a specific number of hours after intercourse. As a result, spontaneous lovemaking becomes difficult. Vacations and business trips become low priority.

Personal schedules must be altered to fit the demands of the testing cycle. Many women find it hard to take time off from work, especially if they don't want it known that they are undergoing an infertility evaluation. It is a stressful time. Both husband and wife are being tested; there is a feeling of pass or fail and a real sense of despair if a test comes back showing questionable or undesirable results. Women can often feel frightened and violated by the infertility tests. The male's infertility evaluation is over quickly if the semen analysis is normal. In contrast, a woman may go through various tests which can be painful and frightening. Men often feel like they don't know what to do to comfort their wives at this time. Added to this worry is the uncertainty and lingering fear of what results the doctor will find.

The following is an overview of what is involved in an infertility work-up.

Initial Appointment

Most infertility specialists like to see the couple together at the first appointment. This provides an opportunity for the couple to establish good communication with the doctor. It is also an opportunity to evaluate what, if anything, has been done medically to date and what tests or treatments will be needed in the future. It is important that your infertility specialist has a copy of your medical records that contain reports about any previous testing or treatment done for infertility.

The doctor will take a very careful medical history from the couple including a medical history of the immediate family. Attention will be paid to details concerning previous surgery, infections, chronic illnesses, and hospitalizations. Background information on smoking, alcohol intake, medications, and exposure to environmental or occupational toxins will be requested. Of course, a detailed reproductive history from both partners will be needed. This will include information about when menstrual cycles started, how long they last, quantity, and type of flow, as well as description of menstrual cramps. Details about the birth control, and history of previous pregnancies should be discussed. (Some physicians interview partners separately so that if there are details one partner prefers the other not know, confidentiality can be assured.) Information about previous venereal disease is crucial. The doctor will want to know about the couples' sexual practices including information about lubricants and frequency of intercourse.

Before starting infertility treatment, blood tests are usually done to check for rubella immunity, CMV virus immunity, blood type, toxoplasmosis, and HIV screening. Many doctors will suggest that a woman start on .4 mg of folic acid and a daily multivitamin.

Physical Examination

A physical examination of both partners should be done. For the woman, this includes a physical exam with attention paid to secondary sex characteristics such as breast development and the amount and location of body hair. A pelvic exam will determine the general size, shape, position, and condition of pelvic organs. A Pap smear is routinely taken (to rule out cervical cancer) as well as cultures for chlamydia and mycoplasma, if needed. The physician will also order routine blood and urine tests to check for general health problems.

For the man, the physical exam will include an examination of the genital organs. The doctor will note the size, position, and condition of the penis and testes. A rectal exam is sometimes done to determine the size and consistency of the prostate gland and seminal vesicles. The doctor will also note the development of secondary sex characteristics. Again, routine blood and urine tests will be done.

Medical Evaluation of the Male

Semen Analysis

This important test evaluates the quality of the semen. An analysis can be done anytime because men, unlike women, are not cyclic. Abstaining from ejaculation for 24–48 hours before the analysis is suggested. For the semen analysis, the doctor will ask the man to masturbate the total ejaculate into a clean jar. The total ejaculate may only be a tablespoon, so do not expect to fill the cup. This can be done at home, the specimen must be kept at body temperature and be delivered to the laboratory within a short period of time for evaluation. The lab will examine the specimen under a microscope, looking for the number of sperm present, how fast the sperm swim (motility), and how the sperm are shaped (morphology). The doctor will also check the total volume of the specimen and its thickness (viscosity).

A fertile semen specimen should have at least 20 million sperm per ml, with at least 50% of the sperm motile with good forward progression and 30% with good morphology. Normal volume is 2–5 cc. The strict morphology test, also called the Krueger test, can be used to evaluate the shape of the head of the sperm. At least 4% of the sperm should have normal forms in this test. The semen will be checked for the presence of fructose, a special kind of sugar produced in the epididymis. In addition, the semen will be evaluated for unusual clumping (agglutination) that could indicate an immunologic response, or a so-called sperm antibody condition. The semen will also be evaluated for the presence of white cells. If the semen analysis indicates that there may be an infertility problem, a repeat semen analysis will be done.

It is also a good idea to repeat the semen analysis periodically if the infertility investigation is lengthy, since these levels can change over time.

Other tests that may be done on the semen include: the "zona-free hamster egg test" which evaluates the sperm's ability to penetrate the outer layer of the hamster egg, which is very similar in structure to a human egg. The hemizona assay test uses immature human eggs from in vitro cycles which are mixed with donor sperm and with the husband's sperm. This test documents if the sperm can penetrate the outer layers of the human egg. The ability of the sperm cells to penetrate mucus can be evaluated by using cervical mucus and recording the movement of the sperm cells in this liquid. This is called a cervical mucus penetration test or Penetrak test.

Additional Tests

Blood tests will be done to study the levels of the hormones FSH, LH, testosterone, estradiol, and prolactin.

Evaluation for a varicocele (a varicose vein in the testicle, usually on the left testicle) is done by palpating the scrotum while the man is bearing down or coughing. The link between the presence of a varicocele and infertility is not clearly understood. The most common theory is that the presence of a varicocele causes poor circulation, increased testicular temperature, and increased blood toxins because of poor venous blood flow from the testicle. All of these factors may influence the quantity and quality of the sperm.

In the event of a subfertile semen analysis, a small biopsy of both testicles may be done. This procedure is done in a hospital under local or general anesthesia. The testicular tissue is examined in the laboratory. The doctor can tell if there is an absolute infertile state with no sperm-producing tissue present, or if there is blockage in the vas deferens indicated by the presence of normal testicular tissue yet little or no sperm in the ejaculate.

If blockage in the vas deferens is suspected, a vasography can be done to pinpoint the area of the blockage. Dye is injected into the vas deferens and series of x-rays is taken.

Rectal ultrasound may be used to evaluate the prostate and testes, particularly for the presence of cysts. Doppler ultrasound is also used to evaluate blood flow to the testicles and to rule out a varicocele.

Medical Evaluation of the Female

Ovulation Detection

Some doctors may request 1–2 months of daily BBT (basal body temperature) charts to get a sense of when the woman is ovulating. This involves taking your basal temperature before you get up in the morning. A 0.6° to 0.8° rise above your baseline temperature usually indicates that ovulation has occurred. The doctor will use these charts to schedule certain tests that must be done at special times in the cycle. A better way to predict ovulation and time sexual intercourse is to use a urine test kit which measures the level of the luteinizing hormone (LH) in the urine. LH levels rise just before the ripened egg is released.

A plasma progesterone blood test can be done to document ovulation. A blood test is taken midway between ovulation and menstruation. A serum progesterone of 3–4 ng/ml or greater indicates ovulation has occurred; normally, levels rise to over 10 ng/ml in the mid-luteal part of the cycle. Progesterone, the hormone produced by the ovary after ovulation, is responsible for triggering the build-up of the lining of the uterus, which is essential if the fertilized egg is to implant and grow.

Serial ultrasound films may be taken in specific cycles to monitor the growth of the follicles and ovarian response to the ovulation inducing hormones FSH and LH. In some cases, follicular development is normal but the follicle never ruptures to release the ripened egg(s).

Evaluation of the Uterine Lining

The endometrial biopsy is a test that involves taking a tiny sample of the uterine lining to make sure it is at the proper thickness and development. The endometrial biopsy is uncomfortable because it is necessary to dilate the cervix which causes moderate to strong cramping. Deep breathing using abdominal muscles sometimes relieves this sensation. Most doctors recommend taking ibuprofen 30 minutes before the test. There can be slight vaginal bleeding after this test, but it is usually minimal. Vaginal ultrasound assessment of the uterine lining just prior to ovulation can be useful especially during cycles when ovulation inducing drugs are being used. Color Doppler ultrasound is a technique sometimes used to measure the blood flow volume in the arteries nourishing the uterus and its lining.

Hormonal Evaluation

A series of blood tests, FSH (follicle stimulating hormone) levels, and LH (luteinizing hormone) levels are done to evaluate hormonal levels. Both these hormones are produced in the pituitary gland. Low levels of FSH in mid-cycle may indicate that the pituitary gland is not releasing enough of this vital hormone, which is necessary to stimulate the egg to ripen in the ovary. High levels of FSH, on day three of the cycle, may indicate that the woman is approaching a premenopausal state. Low levels of LH at mid-cycle may indicate that the egg is being stimulated to develop, but because LH levels are low, the egg is never released. Blood tests to check prolactin levels should also be done. Elevated prolactin (over 20 ng/ml) can cause irregular ovulation in some women. Levels of testosterone and androgen (male hormones) will also be checked if a woman's cycle is irregular. Overproduction of either of these hormones from the adrenal gland or ovary can cause irregular ovulation. In addition, levels of TSH and free T4 should be measured in the blood to check for thyroid dysfunction.

Evaluation of the Fallopian Tubes and Uterus

The hysterosalpingogram is a test used to determine whether the fallopian tubes are open. A radiopaque dye is inserted through the dilated cervix into the uterus; x-ray films are taken as the dye flows up and out of the tubes. The hysterosalpingogram is done in the first part of the cycle, before ovulation, to insure that there is no chance of exposing a possible pregnancy to x-ray. The procedure usually lasts 20–30 minutes. This test is uncomfortable because the cervix is dilated, there is cramping and feeling of fullness as the dye flows into the uterine cavity. Some women also experience shoulder pain afterward. Most doctors will order medication for pain, a local cervical block, and/or oral medication to help with relaxation. It is a good idea to have someone come with you when you are having this test because you may not feel like driving home. Ask your doctor about using antibiotics either before or after this test to minimize the risk of infection. In some cases, the hysterosalpingogram is therapeutic because the dye flowing through the tubes may remove tiny mucus plugs, thus increasing the chances for pregnancy in subsequent cycles.

Sonohysterography, also called saline infusion sonography, uses vaginal ultrasound and saline to inflate the uterus to visualize the uterine cavity. This test results in a very accurate assessment of any abnormal conditions inside the uterus, such as polyps or scarring that may not show up on the hysterosalpingogram.

A variety of tests called endoscopy allow the doctor to inspect the internal pelvic organs. There are several types of endoscopy exams. Culdoscopy is a procedure in which a slim telescope is inserted into the abdominal cavity via a small incision made in the vaginal wall. The woman is in a knee-chest position throughout the procedure. Local anesthesia is usually used.

Laparoscopy is the most frequently used technique to evaluate the outside of the uterus, the tubes, and the ovaries. It is the most important test used to check for the presence of endometriosis. For laparoscopy, the woman is under general anesthesia and in the hospital. The laparoscope is inserted through a small incision near the navel. The abdomen is inflated with carbon dioxide gas to allow for the best possible access to the pelvic organs. Two to three additional small incisions may be made near the groin area. Small adhesions or scar tissues can be removed during the laparoscopy and dye can be injected through the cervical canal and observed as it spills out the ends of the tubes, documenting that the tubes are open. Once the woman is fully awake from the anesthesia and can drink clear fluids and urinate, she is sent home. Shoulder and neck pain may be felt as a result of the excess gas left in the abdominal cavity. The gas pushes on the diaphragm and results in referred pain. The incisional pain is minimal. Many women return to full activity within 1–2 days.

New techniques for visualizing the inside of the fallopian tube are being used in some centers. A tiny fiber optic catheter is threaded into the tube itself during the laparoscopy. Another procedure called hysteroscopy is done in combination with laparoscopy or as a separate office procedure when a doctor wants to see the internal cavity of the uterus. A small telescope-like device is inserted through the cervix into the uterus. Any abnormal structures such as a septum, polyp, or scar tissue inside the uterus can be examined and removed using this procedure. Either a CAT (computerized axial tomography) or MRI (magnetic resonance imaging) scan may be done if the hysterosalpingogram shows a pelvic mass such as a fibroid. These expensive, though painless tests, are not routinely used in an infertility evaluation.

Male-Female Interaction Evaluation

The Huhner, or post coital test, is done to ascertain the quality of the woman's mucus and the man's sperm action in the mucus. At the time of ovulation, the couple is instructed to have intercourse, a specified number of hours before coming to the office. (The number of hours can range from two to eight, as doctors vary widely in their practice.) The woman is instructed not to douche or take a bath before seeing the doctor. In the office, a swab of cervical mucus is examined for the presence of active sperm as well as the quality and viscosity of the mucus.

If test results are poor—the mucus is too thick, the sperm are not moving well, or no sperm are present in the cervical mucus—the test should be repeated. It is important to note that the post-coital test does not serve as a substitute for a full semen analysis, as the two tests yield different information. Poor post-coitals may be a clue to the presence of infections, such as chlamydia and T-mycoplasma. Chlamydia can cause tubal damage and mycoplasma may cause early pregnancy loss. T-mycoplasma is a cross between a virus and a bacteria.

Another possible reason for a poor post-coital test is a sperm antibody problem. If antibodies are suspected, the couple should have their blood, and semen checked.

Once an infertility work-up is under way it is important that the couple get the results of each test as it is done. Couples should ask their doctors for explanations if tests are abnormal. It is your body and you have a right to know what is being discovered. It is wise to make a consultation appointment with your doctor if you feel confused or upset about any test results. This is especially important if the work-up has been going on for a long time or if there are both male and female factor problems being treated by different doctors. It is easy to feel helpless and powerless during an infertility work-up. Good communication with your doctor can help alleviate some of these feelings.

Suggested Reading

RESOLVE Staff, *Resolving Infertility*, New York, Harper-Collins, 1999.

Hysterosalpingogram: Facts You Should Know —by Robert Hunt, MD

When being evaluated for infertility, patients are often fearful about hysterosalpingogram (HSG)—and with good reason. This test has the reputation of being painful. However, such discomfort is usually not necessary.

HSG is a valuable procedure. Injected dye outlines the interior of the cervical canal, uterine cavity, and fallopian tubes and determines if the tubes are open. The HSG is extremely useful in assessing the interior of the uterus. For example, significant abnormalities, such as fibroid tumors, polyps, a congenital partition (septum), or scar tissue, may be detected. Conversely, a uterine cavity that appears normal on a properly performed HSG is usually always structurally normal. Similarly, the HSG yields much important information concerning the fallopian tubes, including their internal health, and if and where blockages exist. The greatest weakness of the test is the inability to detect pelvic adhesions and endometriosis.

The study should be done after menses have ceased, but before ovulation has occurred (usually on cycle day 6–10). This timing is to prevent flushing menstrual blood back through the tubes and to avoid exposing a possible pregnancy to irradiation. Provided conception has not yet occurred, the eggs (oocytes) do not appear to be affected by the procedure.

The patient should avoid eating solid food three hours before the procedure and should have someone accompany her to the appointment. She may wish to take an antiprostaglandin, such as ibuprofen (400 mg), one hour before the procedure to reduce uterine cramps.

The procedure involves performing a pelvic examination, injecting an iodine-containing solution through the cervix into the uterus and fallopian tubes, and taking x-rays to document the findings. (If the patient has an allergic history to x-ray dye of any sort, or is just very allergic, she should notify her physician before the procedure, as deaths have occurred from such reactions.) Local cervical anesthesia is often used to reduce uterine contractions, a major source of discomfort.

Initially, a water-soluble dye is injected. Xylocaine, a local anesthetic, can be combined with it to numb the surfaces of the uterus, fallopian tubes, and lining of the abdomen, which reduces pain. To position the tube through which the dye is to be injected, a speculum must be placed in the vagina. The speculum must be removed by the doctor before beginning the injection of the dye as the speculum obscures part of the pelvis on the x-ray and is uncomfortable for the patient.

As the injection of the dye proceeds, the patient should be able to observe the flow of dye on a television monitor connected to the fluoroscopy unit of the x-ray machine. Exposure to x-ray should be kept as brief as possible and a minimum of films taken. Fluoroscopy time should be less than 20 seconds, and seldom should require more that four small x-ray pictures.

If the fallopian tubes are open and the patient is attempting pregnancy, an oil-based dye may be injected into the uterus and fallopian tubes at the conclusion of the study. Several research studies have shown that this practice increases chances of conception for about four cycles, including the cycle in which the study is being performed. Because the oil-based dye is very slowly removed by the body, most physicians use it only after they have determined that the fallopian tubes are open. The water-soluble dye yields more information about the health of the lining of the fallopian tubes than does the oil-based dye.

Sometimes a follow-up x-ray is taken 30 minutes later to see if the dye has distributed throughout the pelvis. For example, if a fallopian tube appears blocked at the end near the ovary, this delayed film will determine whether the tube has emptied or is indeed blocked. Also, if the patient has extensive pelvic adhesions, the dye may not have distributed evenly throughout the pelvis.

Taking an antibiotic, such as doxycycline, either before or after the HSG may lessen chances of infection. With this medication, the patient should avoid exposure to the sun and the medication should be taken with food but not milk products. If a woman is allergic to this antibiotic, another may be prescribed.

If there is any increasing abdominal pain, discharge, or fever over the next several hours or days, she must notify her doctor, as this could be a sign of pelvic infection. The patient may resume trying to conceive as soon as any spotting or bleeding stops.

Sometimes a repeat HSG study is advisable. For example, a follow-up HSG after tubal surgery may determine if the surgery was successful.

How much irradiation does the patient receive with the HSG? According to our calculations the amount received from a study is approximately 0.2 rad. This equals the dose of environmental irradiation each of us receives over eight months. In other words, by the age of 30 years, each of us would have received a quantity of irradiation from the environment that is equivalent to 20 HSG studies.

In summary, HSG is an important procedure and need not be painful. Valuable information can be obtained with little radiation exposure.

About Sperm Analysis —by Diane N. Clapp

Any of the following factors might affect the outcome of the semen analysis.

1. Does the laboratory you are using do at least 50–100 analyses a month?

2. Does the laboratory use the computer assisted method or the microscope to assess the sample?

3. Are you taking any medications, either prescription or non-prescription? If so, have you told your doctor?

4. Have you had a fever in the last three months? If so, have you reported it to your doctor?

5. Did you abstain from ejaculating for at least two days prior to the analysis?

6. Did you collect the whole ejaculate?

7. Did you keep the specimen at body temperature if you had to take it to a lab?

8. Did you get the specimen to the lab within 1–2 hours of collection?

During an infertility evaluation or infertility treatment, it is a good idea to have a repeat semen analysis done periodically even if the initial one was normal.

Additional Information

RESOLVE, The National Infertility Association
1310 Broadway
Somerville, MA 02144
Toll-Free: 888-623-1744
Phone: 617-623-1156
Fax: 617-623-0252
Helpline: 617-623-0744
Website: www.resolve.org
E-mail: info@resolve.org

Chapter 22

Diagnosing Sexually Transmitted Diseases

In the United States, more than 65 million people are currently living with an incurable sexually transmitted disease (STD). An additional 15 million people become infected with one or more STDs each year, roughly half of whom contract lifelong infections (Cates, 1999). Yet, STDs are one of the most under-recognized health problems in the country today. Despite the fact that STDs are extremely widespread, have severe and sometimes deadly consequences, and add billions of dollars to the nation's healthcare costs each year, most people in the United States remain unaware of the risks and consequences of all but the most prominent STD—the human immunodeficiency virus or HIV.

While extremely common, STDs are difficult to track. Many people with these infections do not have symptoms and remain undiagnosed. Even diseases that are diagnosed are frequently not reported and counted. These hidden epidemics are magnified with each new infection that goes unrecognized and untreated.

This chapter includes excerpts from "Tracking the Hidden Epidemics 2000: Introduction," Centers for Disease Control and Prevention (CDC), 2000; "Chlamydial Infection," National Institute of Allergy and Infectious Diseases (NIAID), May 2002; "Genital Herpes," NIAID, March 2002; "Gonorrhea," NIAID, May 2002; "HIV Infection and AIDS: An Overview," NIAID, August 2002; "Human Papillomavirus and Genital Warts," NIAID, March 2001; "Syphilis," NIAID, November 2002; and "HHS Extends Use of Rapid HIV Test to New Sites Nationwide," U.S. Department of Health and Human Services (HHS), January 31, 2003. Also, "Hepatitis B Virus: The Test," © 2003 American Association for Clinical Chemistry. Reprinted with permission. For additional information on clinical lab testing, visit the Lab Tests Online website at www.labtestsonline.org.

Chlamydial Infection

Chlamydial infection is one of the most widespread bacterial STDs in the United States. The U.S. Centers for Disease Control and Prevention (CDC) estimates that more than 4 million people are infected each year. Health economists estimate that chlamydial infections and the other problems they cause cost Americans more than $2 billion a year.

Chlamydial infection is easily confused with gonorrhea because the symptoms of both diseases are similar and the diseases can occur together, though rarely. The most reliable ways to find out whether the infection is chlamydial are through laboratory tests. Usually, a doctor or other health care worker will send a sample of pus from the vagina or penis to a laboratory that will look for the bacteria.

The urine test does not require a pelvic exam or swabbing of the penis. Results from the urine test are available within 24 hours.

Genital Herpes

Genital herpes is an infection caused by the herpes simplex virus or HSV. There are two types of HSV, and both can cause genital herpes. HSV type 1 most commonly infects the lips causing sores known as fever blisters or cold sores, but it also can infect the genital area and produce sores there. HSV type 2 is the usual cause of genital herpes, but it also can infect the mouth during oral sex. A person who has genital herpes infection can easily pass or transmit the virus to an uninfected person during sex.

Because the genital herpes sores may not be visible to the naked eye, a doctor or other health care worker may have to do several laboratory tests to try to prove that any other symptoms are caused by the herpes virus. A person may still have genital herpes, however, even if the laboratory tests don't show the virus in the body.

A blood test cannot show whether a person can infect another person with the herpes virus. A blood test, however, can show if a person has been infected at any time with HSV. There are also newer blood tests that can tell whether a person has been infected with HSV1 and/or 2.

Gonorrhea

Gonorrhea is a curable sexually transmitted disease (STD) caused by a bacterium called *Neisseria gonorrhoeae*. These bacteria can infect the genital tract, the mouth, and the rectum. In women, the opening to the uterus, the cervix, is the first place of infection.

Doctors or other health care workers usually use three laboratory techniques to diagnose gonorrhea: staining samples directly for the bacterium, detection of bacterial genes or DNA in urine, and growing the bacteria in laboratory cultures. Many doctors prefer to use more than one test to increase the chance of an accurate diagnosis.

The staining test involves placing a smear of the discharge from the penis or the cervix on a slide and staining the smear with a dye. Then the doctor uses a microscope to look for bacteria on the slide. You usually can get the test results while in the office or clinic. This test is quite accurate for men but is not good in women. Only one in two women with gonorrhea have a positive stain.

More often, doctors use urine or cervical swabs for a new test that detects the genes of the bacteria. These tests are as accurate or more so than culturing the bacteria, and many doctors use them.

The culture test involves placing a sample of the discharge onto a culture plate and incubating it up to 2 days to allow the bacteria to grow. The sensitivity of this test depends on the site from which the sample is taken. Cultures of cervical samples detect infection approximately 90 percent of the time. The doctor also can take a culture to detect gonorrhea in the throat. Culture allows testing for drug-resistant bacteria.

How Is HIV Infection Diagnosed?

AIDS is caused by the human immunodeficiency virus (HIV). By killing or damaging cells of the body's immune system, HIV progressively destroys the body's ability to fight infections and certain cancers. More than 790,000 cases of AIDS have been reported in the United States since 1981, and as many as 900,000 Americans may be infected with HIV.

Because early HIV infection often causes no symptoms, a doctor or other health care provider usually can diagnose it by testing a person's blood for the presence of antibodies (disease-fighting proteins) to HIV. HIV antibodies generally do not reach detectable levels in the blood for one to three months following infection. It may take the antibodies as long as six months to be produced in quantities large enough to show up in standard blood tests.

People exposed to the virus should get an HIV test as soon as they are likely to develop antibodies to the virus—within 6 weeks to 12 months after possible exposure to the virus. By getting tested early, people with HIV infection can discuss with a health care provider when they should start treatment to help their immune systems combat HIV and help prevent the emergence of certain opportunistic infections. Early testing also alerts HIV-infected people to avoid high-risk behaviors that could spread the virus to others.

Most health care providers can do HIV testing and will usually offer counseling to the patient at the same time. Of course, at many sites individuals can be tested anonymously if they are concerned about confidentiality.

Health care providers diagnose HIV infection by using two different types of antibody tests, ELISA and Western Blot. If a person is highly likely to be infected with HIV and yet both tests are negative, the health care provider may request additional tests. The person also may be told to repeat antibody testing at a later date, when antibodies to HIV are more likely to have developed.

Babies born to mothers infected with HIV may or may not be infected with the virus, but all carry their mothers' antibodies to HIV for several months. If these babies lack symptoms, a doctor cannot make a definitive diagnosis of HIV infection using standard antibody tests until after 15 months of age. By then, babies are unlikely to still carry their mothers' antibodies and will have produced their own, if they are infected. Health care experts are using new technologies to detect HIV itself to more accurately determine HIV infection in infants between ages 3 months and 15 months. They are evaluating a number of blood tests to determine if they can diagnose HIV infection in babies younger than 3 months.

HHS Extends Use of Rapid HIV Test to New Sites Nationwide

On January 31, 2003, the Department of Health and Human Services announced that it has extended the availability of a recently approved rapid HIV test from the current 38,000 laboratories to more than 100,000 sites, including physician offices and HIV counseling centers.

"Ensuring the widespread availability of a rapid HIV test to outreach services in communities where people are at high risk of HIV is vital to the public health," said HHS Secretary Tommy Thompson. "Without today's action, this test would be limited to use in laboratory settings where many high-risk people do not go for testing."

The OraQuick Rapid HIV-1 Antibody Test, manufactured by OraSure Technologies, Inc., of Bethlehem, PA, provides results in as little as 20 minutes. It is performed on a fingerstick sample of blood. Studies show that the test has an accuracy of 99.6 percent. Unlike other antibody tests for HIV, this test can be stored at room temperature, requires no specialized equipment, and can be used outside of traditional laboratory or clinical settings.

HHS' Food and Drug Administration (FDA) approved OraQuick in November 2002 for use in laboratories that perform moderate complexity testing. The expanded use to additional sites was granted by HHS under a Clinical Laboratory Improvement Amendments (CLIA) waiver.

Each year, 8,000 HIV-infected people who go to public clinics for HIV testing do not return a week later to receive their test results. With the new rapid HIV test, results are available on the spot in about 20 minutes. As with all screening tests for HIV, if the OraQuick gives a reactive test result, that result must be confirmed with an additional specific test.

Widespread availability of the rapid HIV test is likely to increase overall HIV testing and decrease the number of people—an estimated 225,000 Americans—who are unaware they are infected with the HIV virus. Early testing enables infected individuals to obtain medical care earlier in the course of their infection, potentially saving lives and limiting the spread of this deadly virus.

FDA approved the OraQuick test in November 2002 as a moderate complexity test. Moderate complexity tests must be performed in a CLIA-approved laboratory by CLIA-certified laboratory staff.

Manufacturers can request a CLIA waiver that allows the test to be used under less stringent controls. CLIA-waived tests can be performed and interpreted in a physician's office or other settings without having to be sent out to a CLIA-certified laboratory. To qualify for a waiver, a test must be simple, accurate, and present no reasonable risk of harm.

OraSure Technologies tested the accuracy and ease of the test by having 102 untrained users administer the test at four sites in the United States, including a local AIDS foundation, a program for homeless and low income people, and a community-based HIV organization. These users were able to obtain results similar to those obtained in the firm's original studies done in laboratories.

Human Papillomavirus and Genital Warts

Human papillomavirus (HPV) is one of the most common causes of sexually transmitted disease (STD) in the world. Health experts estimate that there are more cases of genital HPV infection than of any other STD in the United States. According to the American Social Health

Association, approximately 5.5 million new cases of sexually transmitted HPV infections are reported every year. At least 20 million Americans are already infected.

Diagnosing Genital Warts

A doctor or other health care worker usually can diagnose genital warts by seeing them on a patient. Women with genital warts also should be examined for possible HPV infection of the cervix.

The doctor may be able to identify some otherwise invisible warts in the genital tissue by applying vinegar (acetic acid) to areas of suspected infection. This solution causes infected areas to whiten, which makes them more visible, particularly if a procedure called colposcopy is performed. During colposcopy, the doctor uses a magnifying instrument to look at the vagina and cervix. In some cases, the doctor takes a small piece of tissue from the cervix and examines it under the microscope.

A Pap smear test also may indicate the possible presence of cervical HPV infection. In a Pap smear, a laboratory worker examines cells scraped from the cervix under a microscope to see if they are cancerous. If a woman's Pap smear is abnormal, she might have an HPV infection. If a woman has an abnormal Pap smear, she should have her doctor examine her further to look for and treat any cervical problems.

Syphilis

Syphilis is a sexually transmitted disease (STD), once responsible for devastating epidemics. It is caused by a bacterium called *Treponema pallidum*. The rate of primary and secondary syphilis in the United States declined by 89.2 percent from 1990 to 2000. The number of cases rose, however, from 5,979 in 2000 to 6,103 in 2001. The U.S. Centers for Disease Control and Prevention reported in November 2002 that this was the first increase since 1990.

Of increasing concern is the fact that syphilis increases by 3- to 5-fold the risk of transmitting and acquiring HIV (human immunodeficiency virus), the virus that causes AIDS (acquired immunodeficiency syndrome).

Diagnosing Syphilis

Syphilis is sometimes called the great imitator because its early symptoms are similar to those of many other diseases. Sexually active people should consult a doctor or other health care worker about any rash or sore in the genital area. Those who have been treated for another STD, such as gonorrhea, should be tested to be sure they do not also have syphilis.

There are three ways to diagnose syphilis.

- Recognizing the signs and symptoms
- Examining blood samples
- Identifying syphilis bacteria under a microscope

The doctor usually uses all these approaches to diagnose syphilis and decide upon the stage of infection.

Blood tests also provide evidence of infection, although they may give false-negative results (not show signs of an infection despite its presence) for up to 3 months after infection. False-positive tests (showing signs of an infection when it is not present) also can occur. Therefore, two blood tests are usually used. Interpretation of blood tests for syphilis can be difficult, and repeated tests are sometimes necessary to confirm the diagnosis.

Information from the American Association for Clinical Chemistry about Testing for Hepatitis B

In 2001, an estimated 78,000 persons in the U.S. were infected with HBV. People of all ages get hepatitis B and about 5,000 die per year of sickness caused by HBV. (Source: "Viral Hepatitis B: Frequently Asked Question," Centers for Disease Control and Prevention (CDC), 2003.)

There are several tests used to detect the presence of hepatitis B antibodies. Antibodies are produced by the body to offer protection from antigens (foreign proteins).

The **hepatitis B surface antibody (anti-HBs)** is the most common test. Its presence indicates previous exposure to HBV, but the virus is no longer present and the person cannot pass on the virus to others. The antibody also protects the body from future HBV infection. In addition to exposure to HBV, the antibodies can also be acquired from successful vaccination. This test is done following the completion of vaccination against the disease or following an active infection.

Hepatitis B surface antigen (HBsAg) is a protein antigen produced by HBV. This antigen is the earliest indicator of acute hepatitis B and frequently identifies infected people before symptoms appear. In some people (particularly those infected as children or those with a weak immune system, such as those with AIDS), chronic infection with HBV occurs.

Sometimes, HBV goes into hiding in the liver and other cells and does not produce new viruses that can infect others, or produces them in such low amounts that they cannot be found in the blood. People who have this form are said to be carriers. In other cases, the body continues to make viruses that can further infect the liver and can be spread to other people. In both these cases, HBsAg will be positive. The next test is helpful for distinguishing these two states.

Hepatitis B e-antigen (HBeAg) is a viral protein associated with HBV infections. Unlike the surface antigen, the e-antigen is found in the blood only when there are viruses also present. When the virus goes into "hiding," the e-antigen will no longer be present in the blood. HBeAg is often used as a marker of ability to spread the virus to other people (infectivity).

Measurement of e-antigen may also be used to monitor the effectiveness of HBV treatment; successful treatment will usually eliminate HBeAg from the blood and lead to development of antibodies against e-antigen (anti-HBe). There are some types (strains) of HBV that do not make e-antigen; these are especially common in the Middle East and Asia. In areas where these strains of HBV are common, testing for HBeAg is not very useful.

Anti-hepatitis B core antigen (anti-HBc) is an antibody to the hepatitis B core antigen. The core antigen is found on virus particles but disappears early in the course of infection. This antibody is produced during and after an acute HBV infection and is usually found in chronic HBV carriers as well as those who have cleared the virus, and usually persists for life.

HBV DNA is a more sensitive test than HBeAg for detecting viruses in the blood stream. It is usually used in conjunction with—rather than instead of—the regular serologic tests. It may be used to monitor antiviral therapy in patients with chronic HBV infections.

When Is It Ordered?

These tests are used to determine whether the vaccine has produced the desired level of immunity as well as to diagnose and follow the course of an infection.

In a patient with acute hepatitis, IgM anti-HBc and HBsAg are usually ordered together to detect recent infection by HBV. In persons with chronic hepatitis, or with elevated ALT or AST, HBsAg and anti-HBc are usually done to see if the liver damage is due to HBV. If so, HBsAg and HBeAg are usually measured on a regular basis (every 6 months to a year), since in some people HBeAg (and, less commonly, HBsAg) will go away on their own. In those who are being treated for chronic HBV, HBeAg and HBV DNA can be used to determine whether the treatment is successful. If a person is given the HBV vaccine, anti-HBs is used to see if it successful; if levels of the antibody are over 10 IU/mL, the person is probably protected for life from infection by HBV.

All donated blood is tested for the presence of the HBsAg before being distributed.

What Does the Test Result Mean?

- **Hepatitis B surface antibody (anti-HBs):** a positive result indicates immunity to hepatitis B from the vaccination or recovery from an infection.

- **Hepatitis B surface antigen (HBsAg):** A negative result indicates that a person has recovered from acute hepatitis and has rid themselves of the virus. A positive (or reactive) result indicates an active infection but does not indicate whether the virus can be passed to others.

- **Hepatitis B e-antigen (HBeAg):** A positive (or reactive) result indicates the presence of virus that can be passed to others. A negative result usually means the virus cannot be spread to others, except in parts of the world where infection with strains that cannot make this protein are common.

- **Anti-hepatitis B core antigen (anti-HBc):** If it is present with a positive anti-HBs, it usually indicates recovery from an infection and the person is not a carrier. In acute infection, the first type of antibody to HBc to appear is an IgM antibody. Testing for this type of antibody can prove whether a person has recently been infected by HBV (where IgM anti-HBc would be positive) or has been infected for some time (where IgM anti-HBc would be negative).

- **HBV DNA:** A positive (or reactive) result indicates the presence of virus that can be passed to others. A negative result usually means the virus cannot be spread to others, especially if tests that can pick up as few as 1,000 viruses (copies) in one mL of blood are used.

In most cases, test results are reported as numerical values rather than as high or low, positive or negative, or normal. In these instances, it is necessary to know the reference range for the particular test. However, reference ranges may vary by the patient's age, sex, as well as the instrumentation or kit used to perform the test.

Is There Anything Else I Should Know?

While the tests described are specific for HBV, other liver function tests such as AST, ALT, and gamma-glutamyl transferase (GGT) may be used to monitor the progress of the disease. In some cases, a liver biopsy may be performed for confirmation.

Part Four

Home-Use
Tests and Assessments

Chapter 23

Home-Use Tests:
What You Need to Know

What Are Home-Use Tests?

Home-use tests allow easy access to medical information about your health status. They can be cost-effective, quick, and confidential. Home tests can help:

1. Detect possible health conditions when you have no symptoms, so that you can get early treatment and lower your chance of developing later complications (i.e., cholesterol testing, hepatitis testing).

2. Detect specific conditions when there are no signs so that you can take immediate action (i.e., pregnancy testing).

3. Monitor conditions to allow frequent changes in treatment (i.e., glucose testing to monitor blood sugar levels in diabetes).

Despite the benefits of home testing, you should take precautions when using home-use tests. Home-use tests are intended to help you with your health care, but they should not replace periodic visits to your doctor. Many times, you should talk to your doctor even if you get normal test results. Most tests are best evaluated together with your medical history, a physical exam, and other testing. Always see your doctor if you are feeling sick, are worried about

"Consumer Information: Home-Use Tests," U.S. Food and Drug Administration (FDA), updated 4/2003.

a possible medical condition, or if the test instructions recommend you do so.

How Can You Get the Best Results with Home-Use Tests?

Follow the tips listed here to use home-use tests as safely and effectively as possible.

- Read the label and instructions carefully. Review all instructions and pictures carefully to make sure you understand how to perform the test. Be sure you know:
  - what the test is for and what it is not for
  - how to store the test before you use it
  - how to collect and store the sample
  - when and how to run the test, including timing instructions
  - how to interpret the test
  - what might interfere with the test
  - the manufacturer's phone number if you have questions

- Only use tests regulated by FDA. There are several ways to find out if a home-use test is regulated by FDA. You can ask your pharmacist or the vendor selling the test. You can also search for the product in FDA's databases. If a test is not regulated by FDA, the U.S. government has not determined the product to be reasonably safe or effective, or substantially equivalent to another legally marketed device.

- Follow all instructions. You must follow all test instructions to get an accurate result. Most home tests require specific timing, materials, and sample amounts. You should also check the expiration dates and storage conditions before performing a test to make sure the components still work correctly.

- Keep good records of your testing.

- Call the 800 telephone number listed on your home-use test if you have any questions.

- When in doubt, contact your doctor. All tests can give false results. You should see your doctor if you believe your test results are wrong.

- Don't change medications or dosages based on a home test without talking to your doctor.

How Can You Know If a Home-Use Test Is Regulated by FDA?

To find out if a home-use test is regulated by FDA, you must first know if it is test kit or a collection kit.

- Test Kit: you take your own sample, test the sample, and read your own results.

- Collection Kit: you take your own sample, mail it to a laboratory, and get your results over the phone or in the mail.

Test Kits. To find out if a test kit is regulated by FDA, you can look for it in FDA's CLIA database on the Internet at http://www.access data.fda.gov/scripts/cdrh/cfdocs/cfCLIA/search.cfm. To search the CLIA database:

- Enter the exact name of the test kit in the first space on the page where it says "Manufacture Test System Name."

- You do not need to enter any other information.

- Select Search at the bottom of the screen to submit your request.

The database will search for records that match your request. It will list the records, and you can select any that interest you. If the database finds no record of the test kit you requested, the test may not be regulated by FDA.

Collection Kits. FDA is developing a database of home collection kits, but it is not available yet for the public. If you do not know whether or not a particular collection kit is regulated by FDA, you can contact them.

How Can You Get Consumer Information about Home-Use Tests?

Home-use tests can be used to screen for different types of diseases or conditions. Some tests require a doctor's prescription, but most are available over-the-counter (OTC) at your local pharmacy.

How Does FDA Evaluate Home-Use Tests?

Before home-use tests come to market, FDA receives a submission from the manufacturer describing the product. FDA reviews these submissions to determine if:

239

- the user will get acceptable results from the test compared to the results obtained when a professional performs the test;

- the user will be able to interpret test results correctly; and

- the benefits of the test outweigh its risks.

How Can You Find Out about Problems Reported to FDA for Medical Tests?

FDA keeps data on medical devices that have malfunctioned or caused a death or serious injury in the Manufacturer and User Facility Device Experience (MAUDE) database.

How Can You Report Your Own Problems with a Test?

If your symptoms don't seem to agree with your test results, or if your test or device does not seem to be working properly, you can report it to FDA's MedWatch program at http://www.fda.gov/medwatch/report/consumer/consumer.htm.

If you want to notify OIVD (Office of In Vitro Diagnostic Device Evaluation and Safety) directly of a problem with a home-use test, contact them at fdalabtest@cdrh.fda.gov.

Additional Information

U.S. Food and Drug Administration
5600 Fishers Lane
Rockville MD 20857-0001
Toll-Free: 888-INFO-FDA (888-463-6332)
Website: www.fda.gov

FDA's MedWatch Program
Toll-Free: 800-3323-1088
Website: www.fda.gov/medwatch/report/consumer/consumer.htm

Office of In Vitro Diagnostic Device Evaluation and Safety (OIVD)
HFZ 440
2098 Gaither Road
Rockville, MD 20850
Phone: 301-594-3084
Fax: 301-594-5941
E-mail: fdalabtest@cdrh.fda.gov

Chapter 24

Home Tests: A Physician's Perspective

The last thirty years have seen a great deal of democratization of health care for patients. Today's patients are more assertive, expect more information from their doctors, and a greater role in making decisions about their care. It is therefore no surprise that an increasing number of tests have become available directly to patients, without requiring a physician as an intermediary. These new home test kits represent progressive advancements in medical technology and a new understanding of the relationship between physicians and patients in managing their health.

At the same time, the availability of home testing raises new issues for patients and doctors. It is now possible to get tested for a variety of conditions without consulting a physician. However, understanding the results of these tests and their implications remains a challenge for most patients. More often than not, patients find themselves consulting their physicians after self-testing for guidance on how to make use of their results.

I certainly cannot claim to represent all physicians in writing about doctors' attitudes towards home testing. Like any other group, we are a diverse lot, with a variety of opinions. However, I can help to explain some of the issues that most physicians are concerned about when a patient comes to an office appointment with results from home test kits.

"Home Tests: A Physician's Perspective," by David A. Cooke, M.D., Diplomate, American Board of Internal Medicine. © 2004 Omnigraphics, Inc.

For most physicians, the biggest issue will be *can I trust this test result?* When we perform tests in our offices or through professional laboratories, we generally have a good sense of the accuracy and limitations of the tests we are ordering. With home tests, this is often less clear. The test may be performed by an unfamiliar method. Or, there may be an outside lab involved of uncertain reliability. This, more than any other issue, accounts for the unease many physicians feel about making decisions based on home testing. However, this varies considerably depending upon the test involved. The following gives an overview of the issues as they pertain to some common home tests.

Pregnancy Tests

Home pregnancy tests are readily available and widely used. Because of their simplicity, it is very unlikely that a patient will perform the test incorrectly. The tests sold in stores are almost identical to the rapid pregnancy tests used in doctors' offices.

As a rule, if a patient reports a positive pregnancy test, I will trust this result. Since the test is highly specific, it will almost never give a positive result in a non-pregnant patient. Furthermore, if a patient is not truly pregnant, this will usually become apparent over time.

However, I will not always believe a negative test result. This is because of limitations in the sensitivity of home pregnancy tests. In other words, home tests will sometimes miss pregnancy. This mostly happens if the testing is done very early in pregnancy. While tests vary somewhat by brand, generally they are not reliable until a woman has been pregnant for at least two to four weeks. If a woman needs to know with certainty that she is not pregnant, I usually tell her to retest in one to two weeks, or else have a more sensitive test performed in a professional laboratory.

Ovulation Prediction Tests

These tests fall into a slightly different category than most other home tests. These tests allow for testing that would be otherwise be impractical. Predicting ovulation requires daily testing; to do so otherwise would require constant visits to a lab or doctor's office. Home testing allows for testing that would probably not be otherwise done due to the inconvenience and expense.

Like home pregnancy tests, home ovulation kits are simple to perform, and relatively fool proof. There is a bit more skill required in their interpretation, but most individuals can quickly learn, and results can be forwarded to a physician.

Generally, these tests are accurate and reliable, and their results will usually be accepted by a physician.

Blood Glucose Tests

Glucose testing is an invaluable tool for the management of diabetic patients. Like the home ovulation kits, they allow for frequent testing that would otherwise be impractical.

Current tests require the use of an electronic meter. While they are slightly less accurate than professional laboratory testing, they are certainly good enough for determining insulin dosing. However, they are not considered accurate enough for making a diagnosis of diabetes.

HIV Tests

If a patient were to bring me a home HIV test result, I would almost certainly repeat it through a professional laboratory. Why? In the case of HIV, there is too much riding on the result. A positive test has huge implications. A patient who has HIV has a life-threatening disease, and will need to undergo extensive further testing, consultation, and treatment. I would not start a patient down that road without reasonable certainty that this patient is truly HIV infected. I would also repeat a negative test. While a negative test has somewhat less riding on it, it is still important to ensure this is an accurate result. A false negative test will give a patient false reassurance, and may delay treatment. Additionally, since HIV is an infectious disease, this could also put others at risk.

Hepatitis C

From my point of view, home tests for Hepatitis C fall into the same category as HIV testing. Hepatitis C is also a serious infectious disease that requires confirmation and follow-up testing. I would find it difficult to accept either a positive or a negative result from a home test for this condition because of the seriousness of the disease.

Home Testing: The Bottom Line

Home medical tests have the potential to provide information to patients and their doctors that would be difficult or inconvenient to obtain otherwise. However, they are not good replacements for testing through professional labs. Their utility depends greatly on the condition being tested for, as well as the inherent accuracy of the home tests.

Like most medical issues, it would probably be best to discuss home testing with your physician first. This will help maximize benefits and avoid misunderstandings about the significance of your results.

Chapter 25

Buying Diagnostic Tests from the Internet: Buyer Beware!

Sally was afraid that she had been exposed to HIV. She didn't want to buy a test in the local pharmacy because someone she knew might see her. She didn't want to go to a clinic for the same reason. So, like many other consumers, Sally decided to purchase her HIV test from an Internet source. She took the test and was distraught to find that the result was positive. After several agonizing weeks, she went to her doctor who did a confirmatory test with a more sophisticated testing method—and the result was negative. Sally did not have HIV. The test she purchased from the Internet had not been approved or cleared by the Food and Drug Administration (FDA), so it did not include the required labeling for a confirmatory test and counseling after a positive result.

Tests such as Sally bought are called in vitro diagnostic (IVD for short) tests. They use a sample of blood, urine, or other specimen taken from the human body. A doctor uses IVD tests along with a physical examination and a medical history to get a picture of a patient's health status. Rarely does one IVD test provide a diagnosis.

Although many quality IVD tests are being sold over the Internet, other tests sold on-line may not work or be harmful. Some tests are illegal, that is, being sold without clearance or approval by the FDA. Examples of some types of IVD tests available from the Internet are:

"Buying Diagnostic Tests from the Internet: Buyer Beware!" U.S. Food and Drug Administration (FDA), updated October 31, 2001.

- pregnancy

- hepatitis

- fertility

- cholesterol

- drugs of abuse

- blood sugar

- HIV

- antibodies to silicone

While some of the above tests are approved or cleared for sale directly to the consumer (called over-the-counter or OTC), most IVD tests are not. FDA has cleared or approved many tests for use in a doctor's office or for professional use only, but Internet marketers are selling them OTC or for unapproved uses.

Misleading advertising is another problem. Ads promise in-home results, but most IVD tests should be followed with a second, more sophisticated laboratory test to confirm the results. For example, tests to detect prostate cancer, called PSA (prostate surface antigen) test, are for screening only and should be used in conjunction with a rectal exam performed by a doctor. Elevated PSA test results often are further evaluated using additional tests such as free PSAs or complexed PSA.

Internet sources also heavily advertise tests for detecting the presence of drugs such as marijuana, nicotine, amphetamine, and methamphetamine in children and employees. Again, to be sure of their accuracy, the positive results for these tests must be confirmed by additional laboratory tests. Another example of false advertising is claiming that disposable supplies, such as test strips for blood glucose monitors, will work in any meter.

So what precautions can a consumer take? If you think that you have a medical condition or disease, see your doctor or healthcare professional. Don't try to diagnose yourself with questionable products obtained over the Internet. If you still want to buy an IVD test over the Internet, how can you tell if it is a legitimate product? First, ask if FDA has cleared or approved the product for use at home. Second, be wary if you see that the test:

- Claims to diagnose more than one illness, e.g., cancer, arthritis, and anemia.

- Is made in a country other than the United States. If so, check to see if FDA has cleared or approved the test for use at home.

- Is made by only one laboratory and sold directly to the public. This is a *home-brew* test and is not intended for OTC sale.

The following general precautions apply to any healthcare purchase on the Internet:

- Don't be fooled by a professional-looking website. Anyone can hire a webpage designer to create an appealing site.

- Avoid websites with only a post office number and no telephone number.

- Avoid websites that use the words *new cure* or *miracle cure*.

- Avoid products with impressive-sounding terminology that can hide bad science.

- Avoid products that claim the government, medical profession, or research scientists have conspired to suppress the product.

- Beware of claims that the test complies with all regulatory agencies.

- Beware of tests labeled for export only. This usually means that the test is not cleared or approved for sale in the U.S.

Although FDA's resources are limited, the agency is taking action against Internet websites with misleading marketing or unsafe products. FDA has sent warning letters that demand the owners of these websites stop selling medical devices until they can prove FDA has cleared or approved the devices for sale. In a warning letter, FDA typically requests that the firm send to FDA (by a certain date) a description of the corrective action that it plans to take. FDA is working with the Federal Trade Commission (FTC) whose laws allow it to quickly regulate practices that are unfair and deceptive. FDA also sends information about deceptive companies to the National Consumer League's Fraud Information Center.

If you have questions or complaints about a particular medical device or website, you can call FDA or your local FDA district office. They will be able to tell you if FDA has cleared or approved the medical device in question. Finally, if you want to purchase an IVD test promising a diagnosis for treatment of a serious illness, talk to your healthcare provider before using it to find out if additional tests will be needed.

Additional Information

You can report false claims to the Federal Trade Commission (FTC) at:

Consumer Response Center
Federal Trade Commission
600 Pennsylvania Ave. N.W.
Washington, DC 20850
Toll-Free: 877-FTC-HELP (877-382-4357)
TDD/TTY: 866-653-4261
Phone: 202-326-2222
Website: www.ftc.gov

Food and Drug Administration (FDA)
MedWatch Office
5600 Fishers Lane, HFD-410
Rockville, MD 20857
Toll-Free: 800-FDA-1088 (800-332-1088)
Phone: 301-827-7240
Fax: 301-827-7241
Website: www.fda.gov/medwatch.

Chapter 26

Home-Use Tests of Blood, Body Fluids, and Specimens

Chapter Contents

Section 26.1

Cholesterol

"Home-Use Tests: Cholesterol," Center for Devices and Radiological
Health (CDRH), U.S. Food and Drug Administration (FDA), updated
February 2003.

There are home-use test kits to measure total cholesterol. Cholesterol is a fat (lipid) in your blood. High-density lipoprotein (HDL) (good
cholesterol) helps protect your heart, but low-density lipoprotein
(LDL) (bad cholesterol) can clog the arteries of your heart. Some cholesterol tests also measure triglycerides, another type of fat in the
blood. This is a quantitative test—you find out the amount of total
cholesterol present in your sample.

You should do this test to find out if you have high total cholesterol. High cholesterol increases your risk of heart disease. When the
blood vessels of your heart become clogged by cholesterol, your heart
does not receive enough oxygen. This can cause heart disease.

If you are more than 20 years old, you should test your cholesterol
about every 5 years. If your doctor has you on a special diet or drugs
to control your cholesterol, you may need to check your cholesterol
more frequently. Follow your doctor's recommendations about how
often you test your cholesterol.

Cholesterol Levels

Your total cholesterol level should be 200 mg/dL or less, according
to recommendations in the National Cholesterol Education Program
(NCEP) Third Adult Treatment Panel (ATP III). You should try to keep
your LDL values less than 100 mg/dL, your HDL values greater or
equal to 40 mg/dL, and your triglyceride values less than 150 mg/dL.

Test Accuracy

This test is about as accurate as the test your doctor uses, but you
must follow the directions carefully. Total cholesterol tests vary in
accuracy from brand to brand. Information about the test's accuracy

is printed on its package. Tests that say they are traceable to a program of the Centers for Disease Control and Prevention (CDC) may be more accurate than others.

The FDA has cleared home tests for HDL cholesterol and for triglycerides.

If Your Test Shows High Cholesterol

Talk to your doctor if your test shows that your cholesterol is higher than 200 mg/dL. Many things can cause high cholesterol levels including diet, exercise, and other factors. Your doctor may want you to test your cholesterol again.

How Do You Do This Test?

You prick your finger with a lancet to get a drop of blood. Then put the drop of blood on a piece of paper that contains special chemicals. The paper will change color depending on how much cholesterol is in your blood. Some testing kits use a small machine to tell you how much cholesterol there is in the sample.

Section 26.2

Two-Step Test for Drug Use

"Home-Use Tests: Drugs of Abuse (Two-Step Test)," Center for Devices
and Radiological Health (CDRH), U.S. Food and Drug Administration
(FDA), updated February 1, 2003.

This is a two-step test to indicate if one or more drugs of abuse
are present in urine. First, you do a quick home test, then if the test
suggests that one or more drugs may be present, you send the sample
to a laboratory for additional testing. There are many different tests
on the market. You must buy a test that checks for the drug or drugs
you are looking for.

Examples of drugs of abuse include marijuana, cocaine, opiates (including heroin), amphetamines (including Ecstasy or MDMA), and
PCP (angel dust). Prescription drugs, such as codeine or other painkillers, also may be abused.

This is a qualitative test—you find out whether or not a particular drug is in the urine, not how much is present. You should use this
test when you think someone you care about might be abusing drugs.

Test Accuracy

The at-home testing part of this test is fairly sensitive to the presence of drugs in the urine. This means that if drugs are present, you
will usually get a preliminary (or presumptive) positive test result.
If you get a preliminary positive result, you should send the urine
sample to the laboratory for a second, more accurate, test.

It is very important to send the urine sample to the laboratory,
because at-home tests often give positive results when no drugs are
actually present. Some tests are wrong more than half of the time.
Certain foods, food supplements, beverages, diet pills, or over-the-
counter medicines can cause a reaction with the tests.

Laboratories use a very reliable test, with very few errors, to determine whether or not your sample contains drugs of abuse. Note
that all amphetamine results should be considered carefully, even
those from the laboratory. Some over-the-counter medications contain

amphetamines that cannot be distinguished from illegally abused amphetamines.

Many things can affect the accuracy of this test, including (but not limited to):

- the way you did the test
- the way you stored the test or urine
- what the person ate or drank before taking the test
- any prescription or over-the-counter drugs the person may have taken before the test

Test Results

Does a positive test mean that you found drugs of abuse? No. Take no serious actions until you get the laboratory's result. Remember that many factors may cause a false positive result in the home test.

If the test results are negative, can you be sure that the person you tested did not take drugs? No. There are several factors that can make the test results negative even though the person is using drugs. First, you may have tested for the wrong drugs. Or, you may not have tested the urine when it contained drugs. It takes time for drugs to appear in the urine after a person takes them, and they do not stay in the urine indefinitely; you may have gotten the urine too soon or too late. It is also possible that the chemicals in the test went bad because they were stored incorrectly or they passed their expiration date.

If you get a negative test result, but still suspect that someone is abusing drugs, you can test again at a later time. You should also consider using a test that looks for other types of drugs. Talk to your doctor if you need more help deciding what steps to take next.

The drug clearance rate tells how soon a person will have a positive test after taking a particular drug. It also tells how long the person will continue to test positive after the last time he or she took the drug. Clearance rates for common drugs of abuse are given in Table 26.1. These are only guidelines, however, and the times can vary significantly from these estimates based on how long the person has been taking the drug, the amount of drug they use, or the person's metabolism.

How Do You Do the Two-Step Test?

You first get a urine sample. Depending on the test, you add a few drops of urine to a test card or other device, or you dip a test strip onto the urine sample. The test cards or strips contain chemicals that react with the drug and show some visible result. Often a visible change may mean the drug of abuse is not present. Read and follow the directions carefully and exactly. The kit should have the containers you need for sending the sample to the laboratory for additional testing. The price of the kit should include the cost of the laboratory analysis.

Table 26.1. Drug Clearance Rates for Common Drugs of Abuse

Drug	How soon after taking drug will there be a positive drug test?	How long after taking drug will there continue to be a positive drug test?
Marijuana/Pot	1-3 hours	1-7 days
Crack (Cocaine)	2-6 hours	2-3 days
Heroin (Opiates)	2-6 hours	1-3 days
Speed/Uppers (Amphetamine, methamphetamine)	4-6 hours	2-3 days
Angel Dust/PCP	4-6 hours	7-14 days

Section 26.3

Collection Kit for Drug Use

"Home-Use Tests: Collection Kit," Center for Devices and Radiological Health (CDRH), U.S. Food and Drug Administration (FDA), updated February 2003.

With a home collection kit for drugs of abuse, you collect a sample of urine, hair, saliva, or other human material and send it to a laboratory for analysis. The laboratory does a quick screening test for drugs, then, if the test suggests that one or more drugs may be present, it performs additional testing.

Examples of drugs of abuse include marijuana, cocaine, opiates (including heroin), amphetamines (including Ecstasy or MDMA), and PCP (angel dust). Prescription drugs, such as codeine or other painkillers, also may be abused.

This is a qualitative test—you find out whether or not the person tested took drugs of abuse, not how much is present. You should use this test when you think someone you care about might be using drugs of abuse.

Test Accuracy

Laboratories use a very reliable test, with very few errors, to determine whether or not your sample contains drugs of abuse. Note that all amphetamine results should be considered carefully, even those from the laboratory. Some over-the-counter medications contain amphetamines that cannot be distinguished from illegally abused amphetamines. Many things can affect the accuracy of this test, including (but not limited to):

- the way you did the test
- the way you stored the test or urine
- what the person ate or drank before taking the test
- any prescription or over-the-counter drugs the person may have taken before the test

Test Results

If the test results are negative, can you be sure that the person you tested did not take drugs? No. You may not have taken a sample when it contained drugs. It takes time for drugs to appear in urine, hair, saliva, or other human materials, and they do not stay in the in the materials indefinitely; you may have gotten the sample too soon or too late.

If you get a negative test result, but still suspect that someone is abusing drugs, you can test again at a later time. Talk to your doctor if you need more help deciding what steps to take next.

Collecting a Sample

You do not do the testing yourself. You simply collect a sample of urine, hair, saliva, or other human material and send it to a laboratory for analysis. The laboratory does a preliminary analysis to see if the sample might contain drugs of abuse. If the result is positive, they will do a more complete analysis of the sample and report the results to you. These collection kits contain the sample containers, instructions, and shipping containers. The price you pay for the kit usually pays for the analysis.

Section 26.4

Fecal Occult Blood

"Home-Use Tests: Fecal Occult Blood," Center for Devices and Radiological Health (CDRH), U.S. Food and Drug Administration (FDA), updated February 2003.

This is a home-use test kit to measure the presence of hidden (occult) blood in your stool (feces). Fecal occult blood is blood in your feces that you cannot see in your stool or on your toilet paper after you use the toilet. This is a qualitative test—you find out whether or not you have occult blood in your feces, not how much is present.

You should do this test, because blood in your feces may be an early sign of a digestive condition, for example abnormal growths (polyps) or cancer in your colon. The American Cancer Society recommends that you test for fecal occult blood every year after you turn 50. Some doctors suggest that you start testing at age 40, if your family is thought to be at increased risk. Follow your doctor's recommendations about how often you test for fecal occult blood.

Test Accuracy

This test is about as accurate as the test your doctor uses, but you must follow the directions carefully. For accurate results, you must prepare properly for the test and get a good stool sample. A positive result means that the test has detected blood. This does not mean you have tested positive for cancer or any other illness. False positive results may be caused by diet or medications. Further testing and examinations should be performed by the physician to determine the exact cause and source of the occult blood in the stool. If the test results are negative, you could still have a bowel condition that you should know about. You should use this test again in a year.

Testing Methods

There are several different methods for detecting hidden blood in the stool. In one method, you collect stool samples and smear them onto paper cards in a holder. You then either send these cards to a laboratory for testing or test them at home. If you test them at home, you add a special solution from your test kit to the paper cards to see if they change color. If the paper cards change color, it means there was blood in the stool.

In another method, you put special paper in the toilet after a bowel movement. If the special paper changes color, it indicates there was blood in the toilet. You will need to test your feces from three separate bowel movements. These bowel movements should be three in a row, closely spaced in time to minimize the time you need to be on the special diet. This is necessary because if you have polyps, they may not bleed all the time. You improve your chances of catching any bleeding if you sample three different bowel movements.

Unless you use the method where you put a test solution into the toilet, it is best to catch your feces before it enters the toilet. You can do this by holding a piece of toilet paper in your hand. After you catch it, cut it apart in two places with the little wooden stick you get in the kit. Take a little bit of the feces from each place where you cut it apart and put these bits on one place in the cardboard in the kit. You use the second and third spots on the cardboard for other bowel movements.

Test Results

To get good results with this test, you have to follow the instructions. You may find it difficult because you need to do things you do not ordinarily do. Because the test is for blood, any source of blood will give a positive test. Blood from another source, like bleeding hemorrhoids or your menstrual period will interfere with the test, so you won't be able to tell what made the test positive.

Pay attention to your diet before the test:

- Eat a high fiber diet, such as one that has cereals and breads with bran.

- Cook your fruits and vegetables well.

- Don't eat raw turnips, radishes, broccoli, or horseradish. These foods can make it look like you have hidden blood when you don't.

- Don't eat red meat. (You may eat poultry or fish). Red meat in your diet can make it look like you have hidden blood when you don't.

Avoid the following drugs for the 7 days before the test—they can make it look like you have hidden blood when you don't:

- Aspirin
- Anti-inflammatory drugs, such as Motrin

Don't take vitamin C supplements for the 7 days before the test. They can prevent the test from detecting your hidden blood.

Section 26.5

Glucose

"Home-Use Tests: Glucose," Center for Devices and Radiological Health (CDRH), U.S. Food and Drug Administration (FDA), updated February 2003.

This is a home-use test kit to measure blood sugar (glucose) in your blood. Glucose is blood sugar that your body uses as a source of energy. Unless you have diabetes, your body regulates the amount of glucose in your blood. People with diabetes have poorly-controlled blood glucose. This is a quantitative test—you find out the amount of glucose present in your sample.

You should do this test if you have diabetes and you need to monitor your blood sugar (glucose) levels. You can use the results to help you determine your daily adjustments in treatment, know if you have dangerously high or low levels of glucose, and understand how your diet and exercise change your glucose levels. The Diabetes Control and Complications Trial (1993) showed that good glucose control using home monitors led to fewer complications.

Follow your doctor's recommendations about how often you test your glucose. You may need to test yourself several times each day to determine adjustments in your treatment.

Glucose Levels

Your fasting blood glucose level (after not eating for 8–10 hours) should be lower than 126 mg/dL. Your blood glucose level immediately after eating should be lower than 200 mg/dL.

Test Accuracy

The accuracy of this test depends on many factors including:

- The quality of your meter.

- The quality of your test strips.

- How well you are trained to do the test.

- Your hematocrit (the amount of red blood cells in the blood). If you have a high hematocrit, you may test low for blood glucose. Or, if you have a low hematocrit, you may test high for glucose. If you know your hematocrit is low or high, discuss with your health care provider how it may affect your glucose testing.

- Interfering substances (some substances, such as vitamin C and uric acid, may interfere with your glucose testing). Check the package insert for your meter and test strips to find out what substances may affect the testing accuracy.

- Altitude, temperature, and humidity (high altitude, low and high temperatures, and humidity can cause unpredictable effects on glucose results). Check the meter and test strip package inserts for more information. Store and handle the meter and strips according to instructions.

Testing Blood Glucose

Before you self-monitor your blood glucose, you must read and understand the instructions for your meter. In general, you prick your finger with a lancet to get a drop of blood. Place the blood on a disposable test strip that is coated with chemicals that react with glucose. Then place the test strip in your meter. Some meters measure the amount of electricity that passes through the test strip. Others measure how much light reflects from it. In the U.S. meters report results in milligrams of glucose per deciliter of blood or mg/dL.

You can get information about your meter and test strips from several different sources including the toll-free number in the user manual or the manufacturer's website. If you have an urgent problem, always contact your health care provider or a local emergency room for advice.

Glucose Meter Selection

You can purchase more than 25 different types of meters. They differ in several ways including:

- amount of blood needed for each test
- how easy it is to use
- pain associated with using the product
- accuracy
- testing speed
- overall size
- ability to store test results in memory
- cost of the meter
- cost of the test strips used
- doctor's recommendation
- technical support provided by the manufacturer
- special features such as automatic timing, error codes, large display screen, spoken instructions, or results

Talk to your health care practitioner about glucose meters and how to use them.

Home Test Glucose Values Versus Laboratory Values

Most home blood glucose meters in the U.S. measure glucose in whole blood. Most lab tests, in contrast, measure glucose in plasma. Plasma is blood without the cells. A lab test of your blood glucose will be about 10–15% higher than the value given by your meter. Look at the instructions for your meter to find out if it gives its results as whole blood or plasma equivalent. Many meters now sold give values that are plasma equivalent, which means they can be compared more directly to lab test values.

Test Strips

You may choose test strips that are made by a different company than the one that made your meter. Sometimes, generic test strips are cheaper. If you choose generic test strips:

- Make sure the generic strips will work with your meter. Check the label of the test strips to make sure they will work with the make and model of your meter. Just because the generic test strip looks like it will work does not mean that it will work.

- Watch for inconsistent results. If you get poor results, try strips made or recommended by the maker of your meter until you again get consistent results.

Meter Performance

There are three ways to make sure your meter works properly:

1. Use liquid control solution

   - every time you open a new container of test strips
   - occasionally as you use the container of test strips
   - whenever you get unusual results

   You test a drop of these solutions just like you test a drop of your blood. The value you get should match that written on the liquid control solution bottle.

2. Use electronic checks. Every time you turn on your meter, it does an electronic check. If it detects a problem it will give you an error code. Look in your owner's manual to see what the error codes mean and how to fix the problem.

3. Compare your meter with a laboratory meter. Take your meter with you to your next appointment with your health care provider. Ask your provider to watch your technique to make sure you are using the meter correctly. Ask your health care provider to have your blood tested with a routine laboratory method. If the values you obtain on your glucose meter match the laboratory values, then your meter is working well and you are using good technique. If your meter malfunctions, you should tell your health care professional and the company that made your meter and strips.

Some new meters allow you to test blood from the base of your thumb, upper arm, forearm, thigh, or calf. If your glucose changes rapidly, these other sites may not give you accurate results. You should probably use your fingers to get your blood for testing if any of the following applies:

- you have just taken insulin
- you think your blood sugar is low
- you are not aware of symptoms when you become hypo-glycemic

- the site results do not agree with the way you feel
- you have just eaten
- you have just exercised
- you are ill
- you are under stress

Researchers have been trying to find ways to test glucose without finger sticks, but none are available yet. Some new methods may make it easier for some people to monitor their glucose levels between finger sticks, such as Cygnus GlucoWatch Automatic Glucose Biographer or the MiniMed Continuous Glucose Monitoring System (CGMS). Several reports in the literature describe methods where you shine a beam of light on the skin and interpret the way the glucose under the skin responds to the light. FDA has not yet approved any of these methods.

Section 26.6

Glycated Hemoglobin Test

"Home Glycated Hemoglobin Test for People with Diabetes," FDA Updates, *FDA Consumer*, March-April 2003, U.S. Food and Drug Administration.

Home Glycated Hemoglobin Test for People with Diabetes

The FDA has cleared the first over-the-counter test that measures glycated hemoglobin in people with diabetes to help monitor how well they are managing their disease.

The test, called Metrika A1cNow, had been available previously only by prescription and most often performed by lab technicians. Over-the-counter status means that consumers now can buy the test without a prescription and use it at home with results available immediately. The test is manufactured by Metrika Inc. of Sunnyvale, California.

People with diabetes should check their glycated hemoglobin level two to four times a year to monitor long-term control over blood glucose (sugar) levels. The level of glycated hemoglobin provides information on the average level of glucose in the body over a 90- to 120-day period.

This test provides information to complement that obtained from daily finger-stick blood glucose tests, which measure glucose at a single point in time.

Diabetes is a chronic disease in which blood glucose levels are too high. Abnormally high levels of glucose can damage the small and large blood vessels, possibly leading to blindness, kidney disease, amputation of limbs, stroke, and heart disease. About 17 million Americans have diabetes. Many of them may find the new home glycated hemoglobin test helpful.

Additional Information

Metrika A1cNow
510 Oakmead Parkway
Sunnyvale, CA 94085
Toll-Free: 877-638-7452
Phone: 408-524-2255
Fax: 408-524-2252
Website: metrika.com
E-mail: A1cNowMail@Metrika.com

Section 26.7

Hepatitis C

"Home-Use Tests: Hepatitis C," Center for Devices and Radiological Health (CDRH), U.S. Food and Drug Administration (FDA), updated February 2003.

This is a home-use collection kit to determine if you may have a hepatitis C infection now or had one in the past. You collect a blood sample and send it to a testing laboratory for analysis. Hepatitis C infection is caused by the hepatitis C virus (HCV). Untreated, hepatitis C can cause liver disease. This is a qualitative test—you find out whether or not you may have this infection, not how advanced your disease is.

You should do this test if you think you may have been infected with HCV. If you are infected with HCV, you should take steps to avoid spreading the disease to others. At least 8 out of 10 people with acute hepatitis C develop chronic liver infection, and 2 to 3 out of 10 develop cirrhosis. A small number of people may also develop liver cancer. Hepatitis C infection is the number 1 cause for liver transplantation in the U.S.

The Centers for Disease Control (CDC) recommend that you do this test if you:

- have ever injected illegal drugs,
- received clotting factor concentrates produced before 1987,
- were ever on long-term dialysis,
- received a blood transfusion before July 1992,
- received an organ transplant before July 1992, or
- are a health care, emergency medicine, or public safety worker who contacted HCV-positive blood through needlesticks, sharps, or mucosal exposure.

Test Accuracy

This test is about as accurate as the test your doctor uses, but you must carefully follow the directions about getting the sample and sending it the testing laboratory. Proper sample collection is important for obtaining accurate results.

Researchers found that about 90 of 100 home users were able to obtain acceptable samples to send to the laboratory. After the laboratory got these 90 samples, it could get results for about 81 of them. Of these 81 samples, the laboratory got correct results in 77 and incorrect results in 4.

If you have a positive test, you either are infected with HCV now or you have been infected with HCV in the past. You need to see your doctor to find out if you have an active infection and what therapy you should have. Some people who become infected with HCV develop antibodies and then are no longer infected.

A negative test does not guarantee that you don't have HCV infection since it takes some time for you to develop antibodies after you are infected with this virus. If you think you were exposed to the virus and might be infected, you should see your doctor for a more accurate laboratory test.

How to Do This Test

The test kit comes with a small piece of filter paper, a lancet, and instructions for obtaining a blood sample and placing it on the filter paper. You first prick your finger with the lancet to get a drop of blood. Then, you put your drop of blood on a piece of filter paper and send it in a special container to the testing laboratory. You get the results of your test by phone from the laboratory.

The laboratory performs a preliminary (screening) test that separates the samples into three groups:

- Samples that are clearly positive,
- Samples that might be positive, and
- Samples that are negative.

All samples that might be positive receive a more specific (confirmatory) test to find those that are truly positive. All the clearly positives from the preliminary test and the truly positives from the more specific test are reported to you as positive.

You should note that a positive result does not mean that you are infected with HCV. If you receive a positive result from this test, you should see your doctor for further testing and information.

Section 26.8

Human Immunodeficiency Virus (HIV)

"Home-Use Tests: HIV," Center for Devices and Radiological
Health (CDRH), U.S. Food and Drug Administration (FDA), updated
February 2003.

This is a home-use collection kit to detect whether or not you have
antibodies to HIV (Human Immunodeficiency Virus). HIV is the virus that causes AIDS (acquired immunodeficiency syndrome). This is
a qualitative test—you find out whether or not you have this infection, not how advanced your disease is.

You should do this test to find out if you have an HIV infection. If
you know that you have an HIV infection, you can obtain medical
treatment that helps slow the course of the disease, and you can take
precautions to keep from infecting others. Untreated, HIV destroys
your immune system. The most advanced stage of HIV infection is
AIDS, an often-fatal disease.

You should do this test if you believe there is a chance you may
have an HIV infection. You are at greatest risk for HIV if you:

- Have ever shared injection drug needles and syringes or "works."

- Have ever had sex without a condom with someone who had HIV.

- Have ever had a sexually transmitted disease, like chlamydia or
  gonorrhea.

- Received a blood transfusion or a blood-clotting factor between
  1978 and 1985.

- Have ever had sex with someone who has done any of those things.

If you use this test, no one but you will know you were tested for
HIV or what the results showed.

Test Accuracy

This test is similar to the test your doctor would use. Researchers have
found that about 90 of 100 home users were able to obtain acceptable

samples for sending to the laboratory. After the laboratory got these 90 samples, they could get results for about 81 of 100 of them. Of these 81 samples, the laboratory almost always shows whether or not the person tested had HIV infection.

If you test positive in this test, you are infected with the HIV virus. You should take precautions so you do not spread this infection to your sexual partners or others who might be at risk. You should not donate blood because this infection could spread to others. Having HIV infection does not necessarily mean you have AIDS. You should see your doctor so you can learn the status of your disease and decide what therapy, if any, you need.

If you test negative for HIV, it means you did not have antibodies to HIV at the time of the test. However, if you are newly infected, it will take time for you to make antibodies. It is uncertain how long it may take you to develop antibodies—it may take more than 3 months. So, although you may be infected, the results of your testing will not verify that you are infected for several months. If you think you were exposed to the virus and might be infected, you should test yourself again in a few months.

How to Do This Test

The test comes with sterile lancets, an alcohol pad, gauze pads, a blood specimen collection card, a bandage, a lancet disposal container, a shipping pouch, and instructions. To do the test, you:

- call a specified telephone number,
- register a code number that is included with the specimen collection kit,
- prick your finger with a lancet to get a drop of blood,
- place drops of blood on the card,
- send the shipping pouch by express courier service to the central testing laboratory,
- receive results by phone after 3–7 business days later, and
- if you test positive for HIV, you get counseling on what to do about your infection.

Section 26.9

Male Infertility Test

"Home Male Infertility Test ," FDA Updates, *FDA Consumer*, January-February 2002, U.S. Food and Drug Administration (FDA).

The first male infertility home test kit available without a prescription has been cleared for marketing by the FDA. The test indicates when sperm cell counts fall below a certain level—a potential indicator for male infertility.

The FertilMARQ Home Diagnostic Screening Test for Male Infertility stains cells in the sperm sample to produce a color. The color is then compared to a reference (chart/guide) on the test kit. The color comparison tells the user whether the sperm cells in the sample are positive—above 20 million per milliliter (/mL) or negative—below 20 million/mL. However, because this is a screening test, a positive test is no guarantee of infertility, meaning that other factors may be involved. Users should confirm test results with their physicians.

Embryotech Laboratories Inc., of Wilmington, Mass., makes the FertilMARQ test kit, which was cleared for marketing in August 2001.

Section 26.10

Menopause

"Home-Use Tests: Menopause," Center for Devices and Radiological Health (CDRH), U.S. Food and Drug Administration (FDA), updated February 2003.

This is a home-use test kit to measure follicle stimulating hormone (FSH) in your urine. This may help indicate if you are in menopause or perimenopause. Menopause is the stage in your life when menstruation stops for at least 12 months. The time before this is called perimenopause and could last for several years. You may reach menopause in your early 40s or as late as your 60s.

Follicle stimulating hormone (FSH) is a hormone produced by your pituitary gland. FSH levels increase temporarily each month to stimulate your ovaries to produce eggs. When you enter menopause and your ovaries stop working, your FSH levels also increase. This is a qualitative test—you find out whether or not you have elevated FSH levels, not if you definitely are in menopause or perimenopause.

You should use this test if you want to know if your symptoms, such as irregular periods, hot flashes, vaginal dryness, or sleep problems are part of menopause. While many women may have little or no trouble when going through the stages of menopause, others may have moderate to severe discomfort and may want treatment to alleviate their symptoms. This test may help you be better informed about your current condition when you see your doctor.

Test Accuracy

These tests will accurately detect FSH about 9 out of 10 times. This test does not detect menopause or perimenopause. As you grow older, your FSH levels may rise and fall during your menstrual cycle. While your hormone levels are changing, your ovaries continue to release eggs and you can still become pregnant.

Your test will depend on whether you:

- used your first morning urine,

- drank large amounts of water before the test,
- use, or recently stopped using, oral or patch contraceptives, hormone replacement therapy, or estrogen supplements.

How This Test Is Done

In this test, you put a few drops of your urine on a test device, put the end of the testing device in your urine stream, or dip the test device into a cup of urine. Chemicals in the test device react with FSH and produce a color. Read the instructions with the test you buy to learn exactly what to look for in this test.

Some home menopause tests are identical to the one your doctor uses. However, doctors would not use this test by itself. Your doctor would use your medical history, physical exam, and other laboratory tests to get a more thorough assessment of your condition.

A positive test indicates that you may be in a stage of menopause. If you have a positive test, or if you have any symptoms of menopause, you should see your doctor. Do not stop taking contraceptives based on the results of these tests because they are not foolproof and you could become pregnant.

If you have a negative test result, but you have symptoms of menopause, you may be in perimenopause or menopause. You should not assume that a negative test means you have not reached menopause, there could be other reasons for the negative result. You should always discuss your symptoms and your test results with your doctor. Do not use these tests to determine if you are fertile or can become pregnant. These tests will not give you a reliable answer on your ability to become pregnant.

Section 26.11

Ovulation (Urine Test)

"Home-Use Tests: Ovulation (Urine Test)," Center for Devices and Radiological Health (CDRH), U.S. Food and Drug Administration (FDA), updated February 2003.

This is a home-use test kit to measure luteinizing hormone (LH) in your urine. This helps detect the LH surge that happens in the middle of your menstrual cycle, about 1–1½ days before ovulation. Some tests also measure another hormone—estrone-3-glucuronide (E3G). Luteinizing hormone (LH) is a hormone produced by your pituitary gland. Your body always makes a small amount of LH, but just before you ovulate, you make much more LH. This test can detect this LH surge, which usually happens 1–1½ days before you ovulate. E3G is produced when estrogen breaks down in your body. It accumulates in your urine around the time of ovulation and causes your cervical mucus to become thin and slippery. Sperm may swim more easily in your thin and slippery cervical mucus, increasing your chances of getting pregnant. This is a qualitative test—you find out whether or not you have elevated LH or E3G levels, not if you will definitely become pregnant.

You should do this test if you want to know when you expect to ovulate and be in the most fertile part of your menstrual cycle. This test can be used to help you plan to become pregnant. You should not use this test to help prevent pregnancy because it is not reliable for that purpose.

Test Accuracy

How well this test will predict your fertile period depends on how well you follow the instructions. These tests can detect LH and E3G reliably about 9 times out of 10, but you must do the test carefully.

How to Do This Test?

You add a few drops of your urine to the test, hold the tip of the test in your urine stream, or dip the test in a cup of your urine. You either read the test by looking for colored lines on the test or you put the test device into a monitor. You can get results in about 5 minutes. The details of what the color looks like, or how to use the monitor varies among the different brands.

Most kits come with multiple tests to allow you to take measurements over several days. This can help you find your most fertile period, the time during your cycle when you can expect to ovulate based on your hormone levels. Follow the instructions carefully to get good results. You will need to start your testing at the proper time during your cycle, otherwise the test will be unreliable, and you will not find your hormonal surges or your fertile period.

The fertility tests your doctor uses are automated, and they may give more consistent results. Your doctor may use other tests that are not yet available for home use (i.e., blood and urine laboratory tests) and information about your history to get a better view of your fertility status.

Section 26.12

Ovulation (Saliva Test)

"Home-Use Tests: Ovulation (Saliva Test)," Center for Devices and Radiological Health (CDRH), U.S. Food and Drug Administration (FDA), updated February 2003.

This is a home-use test kit to predict ovulation by looking at patterns formed by your saliva. When your estrogen increases near your time of ovulation, your dried saliva may form a fern-shaped pattern. This is a qualitative test—you find out whether or not you may be near your ovulation time, not if you will definitely become pregnant.

You should do this test if you want to know when you expect to ovulate and be in the most fertile part of your menstrual cycle. This test can be used to help you plan to become pregnant. You should not use this test to help prevent pregnancy because it is not reliable for that purpose.

Test Accuracy

This test may not work well for you. Some of the reasons are:

- not all women fern
- you may not be able to see the fern
- women who fern on some days of their fertile period, don't necessarily fern on all of their fertile days
- ferning may be disrupted by
  - smoking
  - eating
  - drinking
  - brushing your teeth
  - how you put your saliva on the slide
  - where you were when you did the test

How to Do This Test

In this test, you get a small microscope with built-in or removable slides. You put some of your saliva on a glass slide, allow it to dry, and look at the pattern it makes. You will see dots and circles, a fern (full or partial), or a combination depending on where you are in your monthly cycle.

You will get your best results when you use the test within the 5-day period around your expected ovulation. This period includes the 2 days before and the 2 days after your expected day of ovulation. The test is not perfect, though, and you might fern outside of this time period or when you are pregnant. Even some men will fern.

The fertility tests your doctor uses are automated, and they may give more consistent results. Your doctor may use other tests that are not yet available for home use (i.e., blood and urine laboratory tests) and information about your history to get a better view of your fertility status.

A positive test indicates that you may be near ovulation. It does not mean that you will definitely become pregnant.

Negative test results do not mean that you are not ovulating. There may be many reasons why you did not detect your time of ovulation. You should not use this test to help prevent pregnancy because it is not reliable for that purpose.

Section 26.13

Pregnancy

"Home-Use Tests: Pregnancy," Center for Devices and Radiological
Health (CDRH), U.S. Food and Drug Administration (FDA), updated
February 2003.

This is a home-use test kit to measure human chorionic gonadotropin (hCG) in your urine. You produce this hormone only when you
are pregnant. The hCG is a hormone produced by your placenta when
you are pregnant. It appears shortly after the embryo attaches to the
wall of the uterus. If you are pregnant, this hormone increases very
rapidly. If you have a 28 day menstrual cycle, you can detect hCG in
your urine 12–15 days after ovulation. This is a qualitative test—you
find out whether or not you have elevated hCG levels indicating that
you are pregnant. You should use this test to find out if you are pregnant.

Test Accuracy

The accuracy of this test depends on how well you follow the instructions and interpret the results. If you mishandle or misunder-
stand the test kit, you may get poor results. Most pregnancy tests have
about the same ability to detect hCG, but their ability to show whether
or not you are pregnant depends on how much hCG you are producing. If you test too early in your cycle or too close to the time you became pregnant, your placenta may not have had enough time to
produce hCG. This would mean that you are pregnant, but you got a
negative test result. Because many women have irregular periods, and
women may miscalculate when their period is due, 10 to 20 pregnant
women out of every 100 will not detect their pregnancy on the first
day of their missed period.

How to Do This Test

For most home pregnancy tests, you either hold a test strip in your
urine stream or you collect your urine in a cup and dip your test strip

into the cup. If you are pregnant, most test strips produce a colored line, but this will depend on the brand you purchased. Read the instructions for the test you bought and follow them carefully. Make sure you know how to get good results. The test usually takes only about 5 minutes.

The different tests for sale vary in their abilities to detect low levels of hCG. For the most reliable results, test 1–2 weeks after you miss your period. There are some tests for sale that are sensitive enough to show you are pregnant before you miss your period.

You can improve your chances for an accurate result by using your first morning urine for the test. If you are pregnant, it will have more hCG in it than later urines. If you think you are pregnant, but your first test was negative, you can take the test again after several days. Since the amount of hCG increases rapidly when you are pregnant, you may get a positive test on later days. Some test kits come with more than one test in them to allow you to repeat the test.

The home pregnancy test and the test your doctor uses are similar in their abilities to detect hCG, however your doctor is probably more experienced in running the test. If you produce only a small amount of hCG, your doctor may not be able to detect it any better than you could. Your doctor may also use a blood test to see if you are pregnant. Finally, your doctor may have more information about you from your history, physical exam, and other tests that may give a more reliable result. A positive test usually means you are pregnant, but you must be sure to read and interpret the results correctly.

Negative test results do not mean you are not pregnant. There are several reasons why you could receive false negative test results. If you tested too early in your cycle, your placenta may not have had time to produce enough hCG for the test to detect. Or, you may not have waited long enough before you took this test.

Section 26.14

Prothrombin Time

"Home-Use Tests: Prothrombin Time," Center for Devices and Radiological Health (CDRH), U.S. Food and Drug Administration (FDA), updated February 2003.

This is a home-use test kit to measure how long it takes for your blood to clot. This is a quantitative test—you find out the length of time it takes your blood to clot.

If you take blood-thinning drugs such as Coumadin or Warfarin, you may need to test your blood regularly to make sure it clots properly. Doctors often prescribe these drugs to prevent blood clots in patients who have artificial heart valves, irregular heart beats, or inherited clotting tendencies. Your doctor will prescribe this test for you if you need to do it.

You should follow your doctor's instructions about how often you do this test. Your doctor may ask you to use the results to adjust the amount of drugs you to take to control your blood clotting. Never change the drugs you take without your doctor's permission.

The Test

You prick your finger with a lancet to get a drop of blood. Place the drop of blood on a test strip or cartridge, and insert it into your test meter. Your meter will measure how long it takes for the blood to form a clot and how much anticoagulant effect there is.

Meter Operation

Your meter has some built-in features that allow it to test itself and detect problems in its operation. Your meter comes with sample solutions to use instead of your blood to assure that it is working properly. Look in your meter's operator manual to see how to check on its accuracy.

Take your meter with you to your doctor's office. Have your doctor watch you do your testing. Your doctor may want to take a sample of your blood and compare the clotting time of that sample with the time your meter gives. If the value you get matches your doctor's value, then you will know your meter is working well and that you are doing the test correctly.

Section 26.15

Vaginal pH

"Home-Use Tests: Vaginal pH," Center for Devices and Radiological Health (CDRH), U.S. Food and Drug Administration (FDA), updated February 2003.

This is a home-use test kit to measure the pH of your vaginal secretions—pH is a way to describe how acidic a substance is. It is given by a number on a scale of 1–14. The lower the number, the more acidic the substance. This is a quantitative test—you find out how acidic your vaginal secretions are.

You should do this test to help evaluate if your vaginal symptoms (i.e., itching, burning, unpleasant odor, or unusual discharge) are likely caused by an infection that needs medical treatment. The test is not intended for HIV, chlamydia, herpes, gonorrhea, syphilis, or group B streptococcus.

Test Accuracy

Home vaginal pH tests showed good agreement with a doctor's diagnosis. However, just because you find changes in your vaginal pH, doesn't always mean that you have a vaginal infection. pH changes also do not help or differentiate one type of infection from another. Your doctor diagnoses a vaginal infection by using a combination of: pH, microscopic examination of the vaginal discharge, amine odor, culture, wet preparation, and Gram stain.

A positive test does not mean you have a vaginal infection. A positive test (elevated pH) could occur for other reasons. If you detect elevated pH, you should see your doctor for further testing and treatment. There are no over-the-counter medications for treatment of an elevated vaginal pH.

A negative test does not guarantee that you do not have a vaginal infection. You may have an infection that does not show up in these tests. If you have no symptoms, your negative test could suggest the possibility of chemical, allergic, or other noninfectious irritation of the vagina. Or, a negative test could indicate the possibility of a yeast infection. You should see your doctor if you find changes in your vaginal pH or if you continue to have symptoms.

How to Do This Test

You hold a piece of pH paper against the wall of your vagina for a few seconds, then compare the color of the pH paper to the color on the chart provided with the test kit. The number on the chart for the color that best matches the color on the pH paper is the vaginal pH number.

The test is similar to your doctor's test. The home vaginal pH tests are practically identical to the ones sold to doctors. But your doctor can provide a more thorough assessment of your vaginal status through your history, physical exam, and other laboratory tests than you can using a single pH test in your home.

Chapter 27

Home Vision Tests

Alternative names: Visual acuity test—home; Amsler grid test

Definition: Measurement of the ability to see fine detail.

How the test is performed: There are 3 vision tests that can be done at home; distance vision, near vision, and Amsler grid testing.

Distance Vision

This is the standard eye chart used by doctors adapted for use at home. The chart is attached to a wall at eye level. Stand 10 feet away from the chart. If you wear glasses or contact lenses for distance vision, wear them for the test. Each eye is checked separately, first the right and then the left. Keep both eyes open and cover one eye with the palm of the hand. Read the chart beginning with the top line and moving down the lines until it is too difficult read the letters. Record the number of the smallest line that was read correctly. Repeat with the other eye. Record the number of the smallest line that you were able to read accurately.

Near Vision

This is similar to the distance vision test above, but for use at 14 inches. If glasses are worn for reading, wear them for the test. Hold

"Home Vision Tests," © 2003 A.D.A.M., Inc. Reprinted with permission. And "Amsler Grid" graphics, National Eye Institute, National Institutes of Health.

the near vision test card about 14 inches from the eyes. Do not bring the card any closer. Read the chart using each eye separately as described. Record the size of the smallest line which you were able to read accurately.

Amsler Grid Test

This test helps detect macular degeneration, a disease that may cause blurred vision, distortion, or blank spots. If you normally wear glasses for reading, wear them for this test. If you wear bifocals, look through the bottom reading portion. Do the test with each eye separately, first the right and then the left. Hold the test grid directly in front of you, 14 inches away from your eye, and look at the dot in the center of the grid. You should look only at the dot in the center, and not look around the grid pattern. While looking at the dot, you will see the rest of the grid in your peripheral vision. All the lines, both vertical and horizontal, should appear straight and unbroken, and meet at all the crossing points with no missing areas. If any lines appear distorted or broken you should note the location of these on the grid.

How to Prepare for the Test

A well-lit area at least 10 feet long is needed for the distance vision test. Measuring tape or yardstick, eye charts, tape or tack to hang the eye charts on the wall, pencil to record results, and if possible another person to help are needed. The vision chart needs to be tacked to the wall at eye level. Exactly 10 feet from the chart should be marked on the floor with a piece of tape.

Children: The physical and psychological preparation you can provide for this or any test or procedure depends on your child's age, interests, previous experiences, and level of trust.

How the Test Will Feel

The test cause no discomfort.

Why the Test Is Performed

Vision may change gradually, and you adjust to the change without being aware of it. Home vision tests are useful in early detection of eye and vision problems. Perform home vision tests every year.

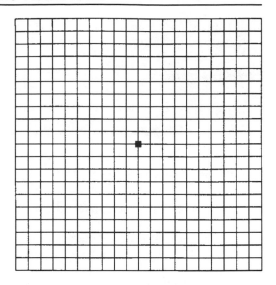

Figure 27.1. Amsler Grid (Source: National Eye Institute, National Institutes of Health.)

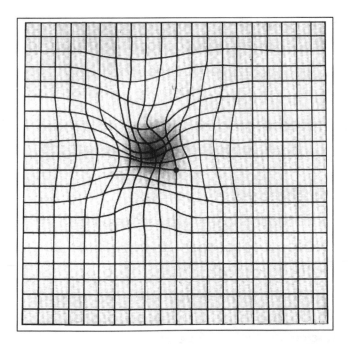

Figure 27.2. Amsler Grid as it might appear to someone with age-related macular degeneration.(Source: National Eye Institute, National Institutes of Health.)

Many people at risk for macular degeneration may be told by their ophthalmologist to perform the Amsler grid test more frequently.

Normal Values

- Distance vision test: All letters on the 20/20 line read correctly.
- Near vision test: The ability to read line labeled 20/20 or J-1.
- Amsler grid test: All lines appear straight and unbroken with no distorted or missing areas.

What Abnormal Results Mean

Abnormal results may mean there is a vision problem or eye disease and that you should have a professional eye examination.

Distance-vision test: If the 20/20 line is not correctly read, it may be a sign of nearsightedness (myopia), farsightedness (hyperopia), astigmatism, or other eye abnormality.

Near-vision test: Not being able to read the small type may be a sign of aging vision (presbyopia).

Amsler grid test: If the grid appears distorted or broken, there may be a problem with the retina.

What the Risks Are

The tests have no risks.

Special Considerations

If there are any of the following symptoms, have a professional eye examination:

- difficulty focusing on near objects
- objects or faces looking blurred or foggy
- double vision
- impression of "skin" or "film" over the eye
- frequent changing of glasses
- trouble seeing at night, trouble adjusting to darkened rooms

- light flashes, dark spots, or ghostlike images
- rainbow-colored rings around lights
- straight lines look wavy
- eye pain
- experiencing a blotting out of vision (curtainlike)

If children have any of the following symptoms, they should also have a professional eye examination.

- getting too close to an object (for example, television) in order to see it
- eyes watering
- crossed eyes
- head tilting
- excessive blinking
- squinting
- difficulty in school

Additional Information

National Eye Institute
31 Center Drive MSC 2510
Bethesda, MD 20892-2510
Phone: 301-496-5248
Website: www.nei.nih.gov

The National Eye Institute has eye charts and free publications that you may send for or download from their website.

Chapter 28

Bystander Stroke Diagnosis

A team of stroke researchers has devised a one-minute test that can be used by ordinary people to diagnose stroke—and the test is so simple that even a child can use it. Such an easy, quick test could potentially save thousands of stroke sufferers from the disabling effects by allowing faster treatment.

"It is just three simple steps," says Jane Brice, MD, assistant professor of emergency medicine at the University of North Carolina-Chapel Hill School of Medicine. Brice tells WebMD that the test is based on a scale developed by researchers at the University of Cincinnati. The three-part test, called the Cincinnati Pre-Hospital Stroke Scale (CPSS), can be used to diagnose most strokes, says Brice.

Brice and her colleagues measured the accuracy of the test by first teaching it to 100 healthy bystanders. The bystanders then performed the test on stroke survivors. To diagnose a stroke, the bystanders performed the following three steps:

1. Bystander told the patients, "Show me your teeth." The "smile test" is used to check for one-sided facial weakness—a classic sign of stroke.

2. Then the patients were told to close their eyes and raise their arms. Stroke patients usually cannot raise both arms to the same height, a sign of arm weakness.

Reprinted with permission from "Got a Minute? You Could Diagnose Stroke," by Peggy Peck, WebMD Medical News, February 13, 2003. © 2003 WebMD Corporation. All rights reserved.

3. Finally, the patients were asked to repeat a simple sentence to check for slurring of speech, which is another classic sign of stroke. "In Cincinnati, the researchers asked patients to say, 'The sky is blue in Cincinnati,'" says Brice. But in the study, the researchers varied four simple phrases such as "Don't cry over spilled milk."

Overall, 97% of the bystanders were able to accurately follow the directions for giving the test, says Amy S. Hurwitz, a medical student at UNC who helped design the study.

The bystanders were 96% accurate at detecting speech problems and 97% accurate at spotting one-sided arm weakness. They were less accurate at detecting facial weakness—with only a 72% accuracy rate for this test. But Hurwitz says, "It is difficult to detect differences in the smile of a stranger. We are hoping that in most cases the 'bystander' will actually be someone who knows the patient and so an unusual smile will be apparent."

"This is all about time," says Edgar J. Kenton III, professor of clinical neurology at Thomas Jefferson University in Wynnewood, Pennsylvania. Kenton, who wasn't involved in the study, says that clot-busting drugs used to treat most strokes can only be given within the first three hours after a stroke. Thus, he and other stroke specialists constantly seek ways to speed treatment.

"This is so simple that even a child could use it. Look at how many children have saved their parents by doing CPR, and this is so much simpler," says Kenton. He says he thinks the test should be promoted for use by the general public.

Brice agrees with this assessment, saying that it could be like the Stop, Drop, and Roll campaign to avoid burn injuries. "We call it: Talk, Wave, Smile."

Sources: American Stroke Association 28th International Stroke Conference; Jane Brice, MD, assistant professor of emergency medicine, University of North Carolina-Chapel Hill School of Medicine; Amy S. Hurwitz, medical student, University of North Carolina-Chapel Hill; and Edgar J. Kenton III, professor of clinical neurology, Thomas Jefferson University, Wynnewood, Pennsylvania.

Chapter 29

Online Screening Tests

Chapter Contents

Section 29.1

Tests for Mental Illness

This section includes "Confidential Depression-Screening Test," and "Results and Recommendations," © 1999, reprinted with permission. Copyrighted and published by the National Mental Health Association. No part of these documents may be reproduced without written consent. Also, "Florida Obsessive Compulsive Inventory (FOCO)–Parts A and B," Copyright © 1994 Wayne K. Goodman, M.D. Dr. Goodman is Professor and Chair of the Department of Psychiatry, University of Florida College of Medicine. Reprinted with permission.

Confidential Depression Screening Test

Available on the Internet at http://www.depression-screening.org/ screeningtest/screeningtestMain.htm

Taking a depression-screening test is one of the quickest and easiest ways to determine whether you are experiencing symptoms of clinical depression. The depression-screening test on the Internet at www .depression-screening.org/screeningtest/screeningtestMain.htm is completely anonymous and confidential.

The depression-screening.org website is not designed to respond to suicide crisis. If you believe you are at risk for suicide, dial 911 or go immediately to the nearest hospital emergency room for an evaluation.

The screening test on the website is intended solely for the purpose of identifying the symptoms of depressive disorders, and is not designed to provide a diagnosis for clinical depression. An accurate diagnosis for depression and other psychiatric disorders can only be made by a physician or qualified mental health professional after a complete evaluation, including a physical exam to rule out any medical illnesses or conditions.

The screening test on the site is not appropriate for, and should not be completed by, persons under age 18. Persons under age 18 with symptoms of depression are advised to talk with their parents or guardians about seeing a physician or qualified mental health professional for a complete evaluation.

Depression Screening Test

Over the past two weeks, how often have you:

1. Been feeling low in energy or slowed down?

2. Been blaming yourself for things?

3. Had poor appetite?

4. Had difficulty falling asleep or staying asleep?

5. Been feeling hopeless about the future?

6. Been feeling blue?

7. Been feeling no interest in things?

8. Had feelings of worthlessness?

9. Thought about wanting to commit suicide?

10. Had difficulty concentrating or making decisions?

Results and Recommendations

The online test will evaluate your answers giving results in terms of the likelihood that you could be suffering from depression.

This screening is not a substitute for a complete clinical evaluation. If you are still concerned about some of your symptoms, see your doctor or a mental health professional for a complete evaluation.

The sponsor of the website, the National Mental Health Association (NMHA) provides a listing of the screening site locator service of the National Mental Illness Screening Project for information only. NMHA is not responsible for the clinical diagnosis or treatment procedures of any provider of services listed in the site locator service. NMHA has not made any independent investigation of any provider listed and has not verified the credentials of any provider. NMHA does not endorse any provider in the referral network. Each user should independently and carefully investigate and verify the credentials of any provider before seeking consultation or treatment.

Florida Obsessive Compulsive Inventory (FOCI)

Available on the Internet at http://www.ufocd.org/foci.htm

General Instructions: These questions are designed to identify some of the common symptoms of obsessive compulsive disorder (OCD). Keep in mind, a high score on this questionnaire does not necessarily mean you have OCD. Only an evaluation by a health professional can make this determination. Answer these questions as accurately as you can.

Part A Instructions: Please answer yes or no for the following questions, based on your experience in the past month.

Have you been bothered by unpleasant thoughts or images that repeatedly enter your mind, such as:

1. Concerns with contamination (dirt, germs, chemicals, radiation) or acquiring a serious illness such as AIDS?

2. Overconcern with keeping objects (clothing, tools, etc.) in perfect order or arranged exactly?

3. Images of death or other horrible events?

4. Personally unacceptable religious or sexual thoughts?

Have you worried a lot about terrible things happening, such as:

5. Fire, burglary, or flooding of the house?

6. Accidentally hitting a pedestrian with your car or letting it roll down a hill?

7. Spreading an illness (giving someone AIDS)?

8. Losing something valuable?

9. Harm coming to a loved one because you weren't careful enough?

Have you worried about acting on an unwanted and senseless urge or impulse, such as:

10. Physically harming a loved one, pushing a stranger in front of a bus, steering your car into oncoming traffic; inappropriate sexual contact; or poisoning dinner guests?

Have you felt driven to perform certain acts over and over again, such as:

11. Excessive or ritualized washing, cleaning, or grooming?

12. Checking light switches, water faucets, the stove, door locks, or the emergency brake.

13. Counting, arranging; evening-up behaviors (making sure socks are at same height)?

14. Collecting useless objects or inspecting the garbage before it is thrown out?

15. Repeating routine actions (in/out of chair, going through doorway, relighting cigarette) a certain number of times or until it feels just right?

16. Needing to touch objects or people?

17. Unnecessary rereading or rewriting; reopening envelopes before they are mailed?

18. Examining your body for signs of illness?

19. Avoiding colors ("red" means blood), numbers ("13" is unlucky) or names (those that start with "D" signify death) that are associated with dreaded events or unpleasant thoughts?

20. Needing to "confess" or repeatedly asking for reassurance that you said or did something correctly?

If you answered yes to 3 or more of these questions, please continue with Part B.

Part B

Part B Instructions: The following questions refer to the repeated thoughts, images, urges, or behaviors identified in Part A. Consider your experience during the past 30 days when selecting an answer.

Choose the number, from 0 to 4, that represents the most appropriate answer.

After answering the questions in Part B, total your score, the range is from 0 to a maximum of 20. If you score 8 or more, it is recommended that you consider consulting a mental health professional.

In the past month:

1. On average, how much time is occupied by these thoughts or behaviors each day?

    0   None
    1   Mild (less than 1 hour)
    2   Moderate (1 to 3 hours)
    3   Severe (3 to 8 hours)
    4   Extreme (more than 8 hours)   _____

2. How much distress do they cause you?

    0   None
    1   Mild
    2   Moderate
    3   Severe
    4   Extreme (disabling)   _____

3. How hard is it for you to control them?

    0   Complete control
    1   Much control
    2   Moderate control
    3   Little control
    4   No control   _____

4. How much do they cause you to avoid doing anything, going
    anyplace or being with anyone?

    0   No avoidance
    1   Occasional avoidance
    2   Moderate avoidance
    3   Frequent and extensive avoidance
    4   Extreme avoidance (house-bound)   _____

5. How much do they interfere with school, work or your social
    or family life?

    0   None
    1   Slight interference
    2   Definitely interferes with functioning
    3   Much interference
    4   Extreme interference (disabling)   _____

Total   _____

Section 29.2

Tests for Alcohol Abuse

This section includes: *Are You Troubled by Someone's Drinking?* Copyright © 1980 by Al-Anon Family Group Headquarters, Inc. Reprinted with permission of Al-Anon Family Group Headquarters, Inc., Virginia Beach, VA; "How Are Alcohol and Drugs Affecting Your Life? (A Self-Test for Teenagers)" © 2001 National Council on Alcoholism and Drug Dependence Inc., (NCADD). Reprinted with permission. For additional information, visit the NCADD website at www.ncadd.org.; The "Alcohol Screening Test." This information is reprinted with permission from the Alcohol Research Group, www.arg.org. © 2003 Alcohol Research Group. The Rapid Alcohol Problems Screen (RAPS4) was developed by ARG Senior Scientist Cheryl J. Cherpitel, Dr. P.H., R.N.; Also, Ewing, J.A. (1984). Detecting alcoholism: The CAGE questionnaire. *Journal of the American Medical Association,* 252 (14), 1905-1907. Copyright © 1984 American Medical Association. All rights reserved. Reprinted with permission; and excerpted with permission from Babor, T.F.; Higgins-Biddle, J.C.; Saunders, J.B.; and Monteiro, M.G. AUDIT. *The Alcohol Use Disorders Identification Test. Guidelines for use in primary health care.* Second Edition. Geneva, Switzerland: World Health Organization. © 2001 World Health Organization.

Are You Troubled by Someone's Drinking? Al-Anon Is for You!

Available on the Internet at http://www.al-anon.alateen.org/quiz.html

Millions of people are affected by the excessive drinking of someone close.

These 20 questions are designed to help you decide whether or not you need Al-Anon.

1. Do you worry about how much someone else drinks?

2. Do you have money problems because of someone else's drinking?

3. Do you tell lies to cover up for someone else's drinking?

4. Do you feel that if the drinker cared about you, he or she would stop drinking to please you?

5. Do you blame the drinker's behavior on his or her companions?

6. Are plans frequently upset or canceled or meals delayed because of the drinker?

7. Do you make threats, such as, "If you don't stop drinking, I'll leave you"?

8. Do you secretly try to smell the drinker's breath?

9. Are you afraid to upset someone for fear it will set off a drinking bout?

10. Have you been hurt or embarrassed by a drinker's behavior?

11. Are holidays and gatherings spoiled because of drinking?

12. Have you considered calling the police for help in fear of abuse?

13. Do you search for hidden alcohol?

14. Do you ever ride in a car with a driver who has been drinking?

15. Have you refused social invitations out of fear or anxiety?

16. Do you feel like a failure because you can't control the drinking?

17. Do you think that if the drinker stopped drinking, your other problems would be solved?

18. Do you ever threaten to hurt yourself to scare the drinker?

19. Do you feel angry, confused, or depressed most of the time?

20. Do you feel there is no one who understands your problems?

If you answered yes to any of these questions, Al-Anon or Alateen may be able to help you.

Al-Anon Family Group Headquarters, Inc.
1600 Corporate Landing Parkway
Virginia Beach, VA 23454-5617
Toll-Free: 888-425-2666
Phone: 757-563-1600
Fax: 757-563-1655
Website: www.al-anon.alateen.org
E-mail: WSO@al-anon.org

How Are Alcohol and Drugs Affecting Your Life? A Self-Test for Teenagers

Available on the Internet at http://www.ncadd.org/facts/youth1.html

Please answer yes or no to each of the following questions.

1. Do you use alcohol or other drugs to build self-confidence?

2. Do you ever drink or get high immediately after you have a problem at home or at school?

3. Have you ever missed school due to alcohol or other drugs?

4. Does it bother you if someone says that you use too much alcohol or other drugs?

5. Have you started hanging out with a heavy drinking or drug using crowd?

6. Are alcohol or other drugs affecting your reputation?

7. Do you feel guilty or bummed out after using alcohol or other drugs?

8. Do you feel more at ease on a date when drinking or using other drugs?

9. Have you gotten into trouble at home for using alcohol or other drugs?

10. Do you borrow money or "do without" other things to buy alcohol and other drugs?

11. Do you feel a sense of power when you use alcohol or other drugs?

12. Have you lost friends since you started using alcohol or other drugs?

13. Do your friends use less alcohol or other drugs than you do?

14. Do you drink or use other drugs until your supply is all gone?

15. Do you ever wake up and wonder what happened the night before?

16. Have you ever been busted or hospitalized due to alcohol or use of illicit drugs?

17. Do you "turn off" any studies or lectures about alcohol or illicit drug use?

18. Do you think you have a problem with alcohol or other drugs?

19. Has there ever been someone in your family with a drinking or other drug problem?

20. Could you have a problem with alcohol or other drugs?

Purchase or public possession of alcohol is illegal for anyone under the age of 21 everywhere in the United States. Aside from the fact that you may be breaking the law by using alcohol and/or illicit drugs, if you answer yes to any three of the above questions, you may be at risk for developing alcoholism and/or dependence on another drug. If you answer yes to five of these questions, you should seek professional help immediately.

The Alcohol Research Group Alcohol Screening Test

Available on the Internet at http://www.arg.org/RAPS4-1.html

Please answer these 4 questions with either a yes or no:

- During the last year have you had a feeling of guilt or remorse after drinking?

- During the last year has a friend or a family member ever told you about things you said or did while you were drinking that you could not remember?

- During the last year have you failed to do what was normally expected from you because of drinking?

- Do you sometimes take a drink when you first get up in the morning?

Disclaimer

This test does not provide a diagnosis of alcohol abuse, alcohol dependence, or any other medical condition. The information provided here cannot substitute for a full evaluation by a health professional, and should only be used as a guide to understanding your alcohol use and the potential health issues involved with it.

You Answered Yes to at Least One of the Four Questions

Your response suggests that your drinking is harmful to your health and well-being and may adversely affect your work and those around you.

Because the screening test is only a scientific estimate of likelihood, you may want to consider seeking further guidance from a local treatment program where a qualified health professional can answer your questions.

You Answered No to All Four Questions

Your drinking pattern is considered safe for most people and your results do not suggest that alcohol is harming your health.

You should be aware, however, that it is not safe to drink any alcohol in some situations and that some people should not drink at all. Certain medical conditions and medications interact with alcohol, for instance. Also, women who are pregnant or trying to become pregnant may be risking the health of their fetus. Drinking before driving, flying, or operating machinery poses a hazard to oneself and others. Familial disposition to alcohol problems has been recognized and it may be prudent to restrict alcohol consumption. Finally, drinking by minors is not only illegal, but it is also harmful to developing bodies and minds.

About the Test

This test is called the Rapid Alcohol Problems Screen (RAPS4) and was developed by ARG Senior Scientist Cheryl J. Cherpitel, Dr.P.H., R.N. The name is also an acronym for Remorse–Amnesia–Perform–Starter. For technical information see the following:

Cherpitel, C. J. (1995). Screening for alcohol problems in the emergency room: A rapid alcohol problems screen. *Drug and Alcohol Dependence* 40, 133-137.

Cherpitel, C. J. (1997). Brief screening instruments for alcoholism. *Alcohol Health & Research World* 21 (4), 348-351.

Cherpitel, C. J. (2000) A brief screening instrument for problem drinking in the emergency room: the RAPS4. *Journal of Studies on Alcohol* 61, 447-449.

Cherpitel, C. J. (2002) Screening for alcohol problems in the U.S. general population: comparison of the CAGE, RAPS4, and RAPS4-QF by gender, ethnicity, and services utilization. *Alcoholism: Clinical & Experimental Research* 26 (11), 1686-1691.

The CAGE Questionnaire

Available on the Internet at http://www.addiction-medicine.org/files/4doc.htm

Have you ever felt you should **C**ut down on your drinking?

Have people **A**nnoyed you by criticizing your drinking?

Have you ever felt bad or **G**uilty about your drinking?

Have you ever had a drink first thing in the morning to steady your nerves or to get rid of a hangover (**E**ye opener)?

Item responses on the CAGE are scored 0 for "no" answers and 1 for "yes" answers, with a higher score an indication of alcohol problems. A total score of 2 or greater is considered clinically significant.

The Alcohol Use Disorders Identification Test (AUDIT): Self-Report Version

Available on the Internet at http://www.who.int/substance_abuse/PDFfiles/auditbro.pdf

In some settings there may be advantages to administering the AUDIT as a questionnaire completed by the patient rather than as an oral interview. Such an approach often saves time, costs less, and may produce more accurate answers by the patient. These advantages may also result from administration via computer.

Scoring instructions: Each response is scored using the numbers at the top of each response column. Write the appropriate number associated with each answer in the column at the right. Then add all numbers in that column to obtain the total score.

If your score is eight or more, you are at risk for alcohol-related problems. For a more in-depth assessment, see your health care provider.

Table 29.1. The Alcohol Use Disorders Identification Test: Self-Report Version (continued on next page)

1. How often do you have a drink containing alcohol?
    0   Never
    1   Monthly or less
    2   2 to 4 times a month
    3   2 to 3 times a week
    4   4 or more times a week   _____

2. How many drinks containing alcohol do you have on a typical day when you are drinking?
    0   1 or 2
    1   3 or 4
    2   5 or 6
    3   7 to 9
    4   10 or more   _____

3. How often do you have six or more drinks on one occasion?
    0   Never
    1   Less than monthly
    2   Monthly
    3   Weekly
    4   Daily or almost daily   _____

4. How often during the last year have you found that you were not able to stop drinking once you had started?
    0   Never
    1   Less than monthly
    2   Monthly
    3   Weekly
    4   Daily or almost daily   _____

5. How often during the last year have you failed to do what was normally expected of you because of drinking?
    0   Never
    1   Less than monthly
    2   Monthly
    3   Weekly
    4   Daily or almost daily   _____

6. How often during the last year have you needed a first drink in the morning to get yourself going after a heavy drinking session?
    0   Never
    1   Less than monthly
    2   Monthly
    3   Weekly
    4   Daily or almost daily   _____

Table 29.1. The Alcohol Use Disorders Identification Test: Self-Report Version (continued from previous page)

7. How often during the last year have you had a feeling of guilt or remorse after drinking?

   0   Never
   1   Less than monthly
   2   Monthly
   3   Weekly
   4   Daily or almost daily   _____

8. How often during the last year have you been unable to remember what happened the night before because of your drinking?

   0   Never
   1   Less than monthly
   2   Monthly
   3   Weekly
   4   Daily or almost daily   _____

9. Have you or someone else been injured because of your drinking?

   0   No
   2   Yes, but not in the last year
   4   Yes, during the last year   _____

10. Has a relative, friend, doctor, or other health care worker been concerned about your drinking or suggested you cut down?

   0   No
   2   Yes, but not in the last year
   4   Yes, during the last year   _____

Total   _____

Additional Information

Al-Anon Family Group Headquarters, Inc.
1600 Corporate Landing Parkway
Virginia Beach, VA 23454-5617
Toll-Free: 888-425-2666
Phone: 757-563-1600
Fax: 757-563-1655
Website: www.al-anon.alateen.org
E-mail: WSO@al-anon.org

Alcoholics Anonymous (AA) World Services, Inc.
Grand Central Station
P.O. Box 459
New York, NY 10163
Phone: 212-870-3400
Fax: 212-870-3003
Website: www.aa.org

National Council on Alcoholism and Drug Dependence, Inc. (NCADD)
20 Exchange Place, Suite 2902
New York, NY 10005
Toll-Free Hopeline: 800-NCA-CALL (24-hour Affiliate referral)
Phone: 212-269-7797
Fax: 212-269-7510
Website: www.ncadd.org
E-mail: national@ncadd.org

National Institute on Alcohol Abuse and Alcoholism (NIAAA)
Scientific Communications Branch
6000 Executive Boulevard
Willco Building, Suite 409
Bethesda, MD 20892-7003
Phone: 301-443-3860
Fax: 301-480-1726
Website: www.niaaa.nih.gov
E-mail: niaaaweb-r@exchange.nih.gov

Chapter 30

Assess Your Risk for Developing Obesity-Associated Diseases

According to the National Heart, Lung, and Blood Institute (NHLBI) guidelines, assessment of overweight involves using three key measures:

- body mass index (BMI),
- waist circumference, and
- risk factors for diseases and conditions associated with obesity.

The BMI is a measure of your weight relative to your height and waist circumference which measures abdominal fat. Combining these with information about your additional risk factors yields your risk for developing obesity-associated diseases.

What Is Your Risk?

Body Mass Index (BMI)

BMI is a reliable indicator of total body fat, which is related to the risk of disease and death. The score is valid for both men and women but it does have some limits.

- It may overestimate body fat in athletes and others who have a muscular build.
- It may underestimate body fat in older persons and others who have lost muscle mass.

"Aim for a Healthy Weight," Patient and Public Education Materials, National Heart, Lung, and Blood Institute (NHLBI), 2001.

Use the BMI table (Table 30.1) to estimate your total body fat. To use the table, find the appropriate height in the left-hand column labeled height. Move across to a given weight. The number at the top of the column is the BMI at that height and weight. Pounds have been rounded off.

Waist Circumference

Determine your waist circumference by placing a measuring tape snugly around your waist. It is a good indicator of your abdominal fat which is another predictor of your risk for developing risk factors for heart disease and other diseases. This risk increases with a waist measurement of over 40 inches in men and over 35 inches in women. Table 30.3, Risks of Obesity-Associated Diseases by BMI and Waist Circumference, provides you with an idea of whether your BMI combined with your waist circumference increases your risk for developing obesity associated diseases or conditions.

Other Risk Factors

Besides being overweight or obese, there are additional risk factors to consider:

- high blood pressure (hypertension)
- high LDL-cholesterol (bad cholesterol)
- low HDL-cholesterol (good cholesterol)
- high triglycerides
- high blood glucose (sugar)
- family history of premature heart disease
- physical inactivity
- cigarette smoking

Assessment

For people who are considered obese (BMI greater than or equal to 30), or those who are overweight (BMI of 25 to 29.9) and have two or more risk factors, the guidelines recommend weight loss. Even a small weight loss (just 10 percent of your current weight) will help to lower your risk of developing diseases associated with obesity. Patients who are overweight, do not have a high waist measurement, and have

Table 30.1. Body Mass Index Table.

BMI	19	20	21	22	23	24	25	26	27	28	29	30	31	32	33	34	35
Height (inches)	Body Weight (pounds)																
58	91	96	100	105	110	115	119	124	129	134	138	143	148	153	158	163	167
59	94	99	104	109	114	119	124	128	133	138	143	148	153	158	163	168	173
60	97	102	107	112	118	123	128	133	138	143	148	153	158	163	168	174	179
61	100	106	111	116	122	127	132	137	143	148	153	158	164	169	174	180	185
62	104	109	115	120	126	131	136	142	147	153	158	164	169	175	180	186	191
63	107	113	118	124	130	135	141	146	152	158	163	169	175	180	186	191	197
64	110	116	122	128	134	140	145	151	157	163	169	174	180	186	192	197	204
65	114	120	126	132	138	144	150	156	162	168	174	180	186	192	198	204	210
66	118	124	130	136	142	148	155	161	167	173	179	186	192	198	204	210	216
67	121	127	134	140	146	153	159	166	172	178	185	191	198	204	211	217	223
68	125	131	138	144	151	158	164	171	177	184	190	197	203	210	216	223	230
69	128	135	142	149	155	162	169	176	182	189	196	203	209	216	223	230	236
70	132	139	146	153	160	167	174	181	188	195	202	209	216	222	229	236	243
71	136	143	150	157	165	172	179	186	193	200	208	215	222	229	236	243	250
72	140	147	153	162	169	177	184	191	199	206	213	221	228	235	242	250	258
73	144	151	159	166	174	182	189	197	204	212	219	227	235	242	250	257	265
74	148	155	163	171	179	186	194	202	210	218	225	233	241	249	256	264	272
75	152	160	168	176	184	192	200	208	216	224	232	240	248	256	264	272	279
76	156	164	172	180	189	197	205	213	221	230	238	246	254	263	271	279	287

less than 2 risk factors may need to prevent further weight gain rather than lose weight.

Talk to your doctor to see if you are at an increased risk and if you should lose weight. Your doctor will evaluate your BMI, waist measurement, and others risk factors for heart disease. People who are overweight or obese have a greater chance of developing high blood pressure, high blood cholesterol or other lipid disorders, type 2 diabetes, heart disease, stroke, and certain cancers.

Table 30.2. BMI Score Meaning

Underweight	Below 18.5
Normal	18.5–24.9
Overweight	25.0–29.9
Obesity	30.0 and above

Table 30.3. Classification of Overweight and Obesity by BMI, Waist Circumference, and Associated Disease Risks

Weight	BMI (kg/m²)	Obesity Class	Disease Risk* Relative to Normal Weight and Waist Circumference	
			Men 102 cm (40 in) or less, Women 88 cm (35 in) or less	Men greater than 102 cm (40 in), Women greater than 88 cm (35 in)
Underweight	less than 18.5			
Normal	18.5–24.9			
Overweight	25.0–29.9		Increased	High
Obesity	30.0–34.9	I	High	Very High
	35.0–39.9	II	Very High	Very High
Extreme Obesity	40.0 +	III	Extremely High	Extremely High

*Disease risk for type 2 diabetes, hypertension, and CVD.

+ Increased waist circumference can also be a marker for increased risk even in persons of normal weight.

Part Five

Testing of Blood, Body Fluids, and Specimens

Chapter 31

How to Interpret
Your Blood Test Results

Laboratory tests are tools helpful in evaluating the health status of an individual. It is important to realize that laboratory results may be outside of the so-called normal range for many reasons. These variations may be due to such things as race, dietetic preference, age, sex, menstrual cycle, degree of physical activity, problems with collection and/or handling of the specimen, non-prescription drugs (aspirin, cold medications, vitamins, etc.), prescription drugs, alcohol intake, and a number of non-illness-related factors. Any unusual or abnormal results should be discussed with your physician. It is not possible to diagnose or treat any disease or problem with a blood test alone. It can, however, help you to learn more about your body and detect potential problems in early stages when treatment or changes in personal habits can be most effective.

Almost all labs set the normal result range for a particular test so that 95% of the healthy patients fall within the normal range. That means that 5% of the healthy patients fall outside of the normal range, even when there is nothing wrong with them. Thus an abnormal test does not necessarily mean that there is something wrong with you. Statistically if you have 20 or 30 individual tests run as part of a panel, 1 or 2 may be slightly outside the normal range. Part of what you see your doctor for is to interpret whether or not these changes are significant.

This chapter is a brief summary and is not intended to be comprehensive or replace discussion of your results with your health care team.

"How to Interpret Your Blood Test Results," is reprinted with permission from Amarillo Medical Specialists, LLP, Amarillo, TX, www.amarillomed.com. © 2003 Amarillo Medical Specialists. All rights reserved.

Glucose

This is a measure of the sugar level in your blood. High values are associated with eating before the test, and diabetes.

The normal range for a fasting glucose is 60–109 mg/dL. According the 1999 ADA criteria, diabetes is diagnosed with a fasting plasma glucose of 126 or more. A precursor, impaired fasting glucose (IFG), is defined as a reading of fasting glucose levels of 110–125. Sometimes a glucose tolerance test, which involves giving you a sugary drink followed by several blood glucose tests, is necessary to properly sort out normal from IFG or diabetes.

Be aware that variations in lab normals exist. Also, Europeans tend to use a 2 hour after eating definition of diabetes rather than a fasting glucose. Using the European standards tends to increase the number of people who are classified as having diabetes.

Electrolytes

These are your potassium, sodium, chloride, and carbon dioxide (CO_2) levels.

Potassium is controlled very carefully by the kidneys. It is important for the proper functioning of the nerves and muscles, particularly the heart. Any value outside the expected range, high or low, requires medical evaluation. This is especially important if you are taking a diuretic (water pill) or heart pill (digitalis, Lanoxin, etc.).

Sodium is also regulated by the kidneys and adrenal glands. There are numerous causes of high and low sodium levels, but the most common causes of low sodium are diuretic usage, diabetes drugs like chlorpropamide, and excessive water intake in patients with heart or liver disease.

CO_2 reflects the acid status of your blood. Low CO_2 levels can be due to either increased acidity from uncontrolled diabetes, kidney disease, metabolic disorders, or low CO_2 can be due to chronic hyperventilation.

Waste products

Blood Urea Nitrogen (BUN) is a waste product produced in the liver and excreted by the kidneys. High values may mean that the kidneys are not working as well as they should. BUN is also affected by high protein diets and/or strenuous exercise which raise levels, and by pregnancy which lowers it.

312

Creatinine is a waste product largely from muscle breakdown. High values, especially with high BUN levels, may indicate problems with the kidneys.

Uric Acid is normally excreted in urine. High values are associated with gout, arthritis, kidney problems, and the use of some diuretics.

Enzymes

Aspartate aminotransferase (AST), alanine aminotransferase (ALT), serum glutamic-oxaloacetic transaminase (SGOT), serum glutamic pyruvate transaminase (SGPT), gamma glutamyl transpeptidase (GGT), and alkaline phosphatase (ALP) are names of proteins called enzymes which help all the chemical activities within cells to take place. Injuries to cells release these enzymes into the blood. They are found in muscles, the liver, and heart. Damage from alcohol and a number of diseases are reflected in high values.

ALP is an enzyme found primarily in bones and the liver. Expected values are higher for those who are growing (children and pregnant women) or when damage to bones or liver has occurred or with gallstones. Low values are probably not significant.

GGT is also elevated in liver disease, particularly with obstruction of bile ducts. Unlike the alkaline phosphatase it is not elevated with bone growth or damage.

AST/SGOT and ALT/SGPT are also liver and muscle enzymes. They may be elevated from liver problems, hepatitis, excess alcohol ingestion, muscle injury, and recent heart attack.

Lactate dehydrogenase (LDH) is the enzyme present in all the cells in the body. Anything which damages cells, including blood drawing itself, will raise amounts in the blood. If blood is not processed promptly and properly, high levels may occur. If all values except LDH are within expected ranges, a processing error was probably made and the results do not require further evaluation.

Bilirubin is a pigment removed from the blood by the liver. Low values are of no concern. If slightly elevated above the expected ranges, but with all other enzymes (LDH, GOT, GPT, and GGT) within expected values, it is probably a condition known as Gilbert's syndrome and is not significant.

313

Creatine kinase or creatine phosphokinase (CK or CPK) is an enzyme which is very useful for diagnosing diseases of the heart and skeletal muscle. This enzyme is the first to be elevated after a heart attack (3 to 4 hours). If CPK is high in the absence of heart muscle injury, this is a strong indication of skeletal muscle disease.

Proteins

Albumin and globulin measure the amount and type of protein in your blood. They are a general index of overall health and nutrition. Globulin is the antibody protein important for fighting disease. A/G ratio is the mathematical relationship between albumin and globulin.

Blood Fats

Cholesterol is a fat-like substance in the blood which, if elevated, has been associated with heart disease. A level less than 200 is recommended by the National Heart, Lung, and Blood Institute.

Total cholesterol: High cholesterol in the blood is a major risk factor for heart and blood vessel disease. Cholesterol is not all bad; in fact, our bodies need a certain amount of this substance to function properly. However, when the level gets too high, serious problems can result. Levels of 200 or more are too high for good health. Levels of 240 and above are considered high risk, and may indicate the need for cholesterol lowering medication. A low-fat diet and regular exercise are recommended. As the level of blood cholesterol increases, so does the possibility of plugging the arteries due to cholesterol plaque build-up. Such a disease process is called hardening of the arteries or atherosclerosis. When the arteries feeding the heart become plugged, a heart attack may occur. If the arteries that go to the brain are affected, then the result is a stroke.

There are three major kinds of cholesterol: high density lipoprotein (HDL), low density lipoprotein (LDL), and very low density lipoprotein (VLDL).

LDL cholesterol is considered bad cholesterol because cholesterol deposits form in the arteries when LDL levels are high. An LDL level of less than 130 is recommended, 100 is ideal. Values greater than 160 are considered high risk and should be followed by your physician. Those persons who have established coronary or vascular disease may be instructed by their doctor to get their LDL cholesterol well below 100. You should ask your doctor which LDL target he or she wants for you. There are two ways to report LDL. The most common is simply an estimate calculated from the total cholesterol, HDL, and triglycerides results. This may say *LDL Calc*. A directly measured LDL cholesterol is usually more accurate but more expensive and may require that your doctor specify the direct LDL.

HDL cholesterol is good cholesterol as it protects against heart disease by helping remove excess cholesterol deposited in the arteries. High levels seem to be associated with low incidence of coronary heart disease.

Triglyceride is fat in the blood which, if elevated, has been associated with heart disease, especially if over 500 mg. High triglycerides are also associated with pancreatitis. Triglyceride levels over 150 mg/dl may be associated with problems other than heart disease. Ways to lower triglycerides are:

- weight reduction, if overweight;
- reduce animal fats in the diet: eat more fish;
- take certain medications your physician can prescribe;
- get regular aerobic exercise;
- decrease alcohol and sugar consumption—alcohol and sugar are not fats, but the body can convert them into fats then dump those fats into your blood stream;
- restrict calories—carbohydrates are converted to triglycerides when eaten to excess.

VLDL (very low density lipoprotein) is another carrier of fat in the blood.

Cardiac Risk Factors

C reactive protein: This is a marker for inflammation. Traditionally it has been used to assess inflammation in response to infection. A highly sensitive C reactive protein blood test is useful in predicting vascular disease.

Homocysteine: Homocysteine is an amino acid that is normally found in small amounts in the blood. Higher levels are associated with increased risk of heart attack and other vascular diseases. Homocysteine levels may be high due to a deficiency of folic acid or vitamin

B_{12}, due to heredity, older age, kidney disease, or certain medications. Men tend to have higher levels. Normal lab values are 4–15 micromole/l, but if you have had previous vascular disease medications may be recommended to reduce it below 10.

Minerals

Calcium is controlled in the blood by the parathyroid glands and the kidneys. Calcium is found mostly in bone and is important for proper blood clotting, nerve, and cell activity. Elevated calcium can be due to medications such as thiazide-type diuretics, inherited disorders of calcium handling in the kidneys, excess parathyroid gland activity, or vitamin D. Low calcium can be due to certain metabolic disorders such as insufficient parathyroid hormone; or drugs like Fosamax or furosemide-type diuretics.

Phosphorus is also largely stored in the bone. It is regulated by the kidneys. High levels of phosphorus may be due to kidney disease. When low levels are seen with high calcium levels it suggests parathyroid disease, however there are other causes. Low phosphorus, in combination with high calcium, may suggest an overactive parathyroid gland.

Thyroid

There are 2 types of thyroid hormones easily measured in the blood, thyroxine (T4) and triiodothyronine (T3). For technical reasons, it is easier and less expensive to measure the T4 level, so T3 is usually not measured on screening tests.

Please be clear about which test you are looking at. The total T3, free T3, and T3 uptake tests are not the same test.

Thyroxine (T4): This shows the total amount of T4. High levels may be due to hyperthyroidism, however high levels may occur when estrogen levels are higher from pregnancy, birth control pills, or estrogen replacement therapy. A free T4 can avoid this interference.

T3 resin uptake or thyroid uptake: First, this is not a thyroid test, but a test of the proteins that carry thyroid hormone around in your blood stream. A high test number may indicate a low level of the protein. The method of reporting varies from lab to lab. The proper use of the test is to compute the free thyroxine index.

Free thyroxine index (FTI or T7): A mathematical computation allows the lab to estimate the free thyroxine index from the T4 and T3 uptake tests. The results tell how much thyroid hormone is free in the blood stream to work in the body. Unlike the T4 alone, it is not affected by estrogen levels.

Free T4: This test directly measures the free T4 in the blood rather than estimating it like the FTI. It is a more reliable test, but a little more expensive. Some labs now do the free T4 routinely rather than the total T4.

Total T3: This is usually not ordered as a screening test, but rather when thyroid disease is being evaluated. T3 is the more potent and shorter lived version of thyroid hormone. Some people with high thyroid levels secrete more T3 than T4. In these (overactive) hyperthyroid cases the T4 can be normal, the T3 high, and the TSH low. The total T3 reports the total amount of T3 in the bloodstream, including T3 bound to carrier proteins plus freely circulating T3.

Free T3: This test measures only the portion of thyroid hormone T3 that is free, not bound to carrier proteins.

Thyroid stimulating hormone (TSH): This protein hormone is secreted by the pituitary gland and regulates the thyroid gland. A high level suggests the thyroid is underactive, and a low level suggests the thyroid is overactive.

Glycohemoglobin (hemoglobin A1 or A1c, HbA1c): Glycohemoglobin measures the amount of glucose chemically attached to your red blood cells. Since blood cells live about 3 months, it tells your average glucose for the last 6–8 weeks. A high level suggests poor diabetes control. Standardization for glycohemoglobin from lab to lab is poor, and you cannot compare tests from different labs unless you can verify the technique for measuring glycohemoglobin is the same. The only exception is if your lab is standardized to the national DCCT referenced method. You can ask your lab if they use a DCCT referenced method.

Complete Blood Count (CBC)

The CBC typically has several parameters that are created from an automated cell counter. Following are the most common values tested.

317

White blood count (WBC) is the number of white cells. High WBC can be a sign of infection. WBC is also increased in certain types of leukemia. Low white counts can be a sign of bone marrow diseases or an enlarged spleen. In some cases, low WBC is found in HIV infection; however, the vast majority of low white blood counts in the U.S. population are not HIV-related.

Hemoglobin (Hgb) and hematocrit (Hct): Hemoglobin is the amount of oxygen carrying protein contained within the red blood cells. Hematocrit is the percentage of the blood volume occupied by red blood cells. In most labs the Hgb is actually measured, while the Hct is computed using the red blood count (RBC) measurement and the mean corpuscular volume (MCV) measurement. Thus purists prefer to use the Hgb measurement as more reliable. Low Hgb or Hct suggest an anemia. Anemia can be due to nutritional deficiencies, blood loss, destruction of blood cells internally, or failure to produce blood in the bone marrow. High Hgb can occur due to lung disease, living at high altitude, or excessive bone marrow production of blood cells.

Mean corpuscular volume (MCV): This helps diagnose a cause of an anemia. Low values suggest an iron deficiency; high values suggest either deficiencies of B12 or folate, ineffective production in the bone marrow, or recent blood loss with replacement by newer (and larger) cells from the bone marrow.

Platelet count (PLT): This is the number of cells that plug up holes in your blood vessels and prevent bleeding. High values can occur with bleeding, cigarette smoking, or excess production by the bone marrow. Low values can occur from premature destruction states such as immune thrombocytopenia (ITP), acute blood loss, drug effects (such as heparin), infections with sepsis, entrapment of platelets in an enlarged spleen, or bone marrow failure from diseases such as myelofibrosis or leukemia.

Chapter 32

Blood Tests

Chapter Contents

Section 32.1

Calcium Test

"Calcium Test," © 2003 American Association for Clinical Chemistry. Reprinted with permission. For additional information on clinical lab testing, visit the Lab Tests Online website at www.labtestsonline.org.

How Is It Used?

Blood calcium is tested to screen for, diagnose, and monitor a range of conditions relating to the bones, heart, nerves, kidneys, and teeth. Blood calcium levels do not directly tell how much calcium is in the bones, but rather, how much total calcium or ionized calcium is circulating in the blood.

Doctors can get a better picture of your health by comparing your calcium result with the results of other tests. Calcium levels in the blood are regulated and stabilized by a feedback loop that includes: calcium, parathyroid hormone (PTH), vitamin D, phosphorus, and magnesium. Your doctor is looking at the balance among all of these elements. Conditions and diseases that disrupt this feedback loop can cause inappropriate elevations or decreases in calcium and lead to symptoms of hyper- or hypocalcemia. For example, when parathyroid hormone (PTH) from the parathyroid gland is released, PTH level rises, calcium also rises, and phosphorus drops. In some kidney problems, a high phosphorus level in blood can depress calcium levels. Depending on the levels you have, these two tests can help your doctor discover whether you have a parathyroid problem or another condition.

Directly measuring free or ionized calcium is important during major surgery (particularly if blood or blood products are transfused), in critically ill patients, and when protein levels are very abnormal. Large fluctuations in free calcium can cause the heart to slow down or beat too rapidly, can cause muscles to go into spasm (tetany), and can cause confusion or even coma.

When Is It Ordered?

Calcium is often used as a screening test as part of a general medical examination. It is typically included in the comprehensive metabolic panel.

Calcium can be used as a diagnostic test if you go to your doctor with symptoms that suggest:

- kidney stones,

- bone disease, or

- neurologic (nerve-related) disorders.

Your doctor also may order a calcium test if:

- you have kidney disease, because low calcium is especially common in those with kidney failure;

- you have symptoms of too much calcium, such as fatigue, weakness, loss of appetite, nausea, vomiting, constipation, abdominal pain, urinary frequency, and increased thirst;

- you have symptoms of low calcium, such as cramps in your abdomen, muscle cramps, or tingling fingers; or

- you have other diseases that can be associated with abnormal blood calcium, such as thyroid disease, intestinal disease, cancer, or poor nutrition.

Your doctor may order an ionized calcium test if you have numbness around the mouth and in the hands and feet and muscle spasms in the same areas, which are symptoms of low levels of ionized calcium. If calcium levels fall slowly, however, many people have no symptoms at all.

You may need calcium monitoring as part of your regular laboratory tests if you have certain kinds of cancer (particularly breast, lung, head and neck, kidney, and multiple myeloma) or kidney disease or transplant. You may also need to be monitored for calcium levels if it is clear that you have abnormal calcium levels or if you are receiving calcium or vitamin D supplements.

What Does the Test Result Mean?

A normal calcium result with other normal lab results means that you have no problems with calcium metabolism (use by the body).

Because about half of the calcium in your blood is bound by albumin (a protein), these two tests are usually ordered together. Calcium values must be interpreted in combination with albumin to determine if the calcium concentration of serum is appropriate. As albumin levels rise, calcium rises as well, and vice versa.

A high calcium level is called hypercalcemia. You have too much calcium in your blood and will need treatment for the underlying condition. This usually is caused by:

- **Hyperparathyroidism** (increase in parathyroid gland function): This condition is usually caused by a benign (not cancerous) tumor on the parathyroid gland. This form of hypercalcemia is usually mild and can be present for many years before being noticed.

- **Cancer:** Cancer can cause hypercalcemia when it spreads to the bones, which releases calcium into the blood, or when cancer causes a hormone similar to PTH to increase calcium levels.

Other causes of hypercalcemia include:

- hyperthyroidism,
- sarcoidosis,
- tuberculosis,
- bone breaks combined with bed rest or not moving for long periods of time,
- excess vitamin D intake,
- kidney transplant, and
- high protein levels (for example, if a tourniquet is used for too long while blood is collected). In this case, free or ionized calcium remains normal.

High levels of ionized calcium occur with all the listed causes of hypercalcemia except high protein levels.

Low calcium levels, called hypocalcemia, mean that you do not have enough calcium in your blood or that you don't have enough protein in your blood. The most common cause of low total calcium is low protein levels, especially low albumin. When low protein is the problem, the ionized calcium level remains normal.

Low calcium, known as hypocalcemia, is caused by many conditions:

- low protein levels,
- underactive parathyroid gland (hypoparathyroidism),
- decreased dietary intake of calcium,
- decreased levels of vitamin D,

- magnesium deficiency,
- too much phosphorus,
- acute inflammation of the pancreas,
- chronic renal failure,
- calcium ions becoming bound to protein (alkalosis),
- bone disease,
- malnutrition, and
- alcoholism.

Causes of low ionized calcium levels include all these, except low protein levels.

In most cases, test results are reported as numerical values rather than as high or low, positive or negative, or normal. In these instances, it is necessary to know the reference range for the particular test. However, reference ranges may vary by the patient's age, sex, as well as the instrumentation or kit used to perform the test.

Is There Anything Else I Should Know?

Two hormones control blood calcium within a small range of values. Parathyroid hormone (PTH) is produced by a group of small glands in the neck (near the thyroid gland), stimulated by a decrease in ionized calcium. PTH causes the release of calcium from bone and decreases calcium losses from the kidneys, so that calcium levels rise. PTH also stimulates activation of vitamin D by the kidneys.

Vitamin D, in turn, increases calcium absorption in the intestine, but decreases calcium lost from the kidneys in urine. Overall, as vitamin D levels rise, calcium levels rise, and PTH falls. In healthy people, these two hormones keep blood calcium at normal levels, even though maintaining that balance in the blood may cause calcium to be released from bones.

Newborns, especially premature and low birth weight infants, often are monitored during the first few days of life for neonatal hypocalcemia. This can occur because of an immature parathyroid gland and doesn't always cause symptoms. The condition may resolve itself or may require treatment with supplemental calcium, given orally or intravenously.

Blood and urine calcium measurements cannot tell how much calcium is in the bones. A test similar to an x-ray, called a bone density or Dexa scan, is needed for this purpose.

Taking thiazide diuretic drugs (drugs that encourage urination) is the most common drug-induced reason for a high calcium level.

Section 32.2

Electrolyte Tests: Sodium Test, Potassium Test, Carbon Dioxide (CO$_2$) Test, and Chloride Test

This section includes "Sodium Test," "Potassium Test," "CO$_2$ Test," and "Chloride Test," © 2003 American Association for Clinical Chemistry. Reprinted with permission. For additional information on clinical lab testing, visit the Lab Tests Online website at www.labtestsonline.org.

Sodium Test

How Is It Used?

Blood sodium is used to detect the cause and help monitor treatment in persons with dehydration, edema, or with a variety of symptoms. Blood sodium is often abnormal with many diseases; your doctor may order this test if you have symptoms of illness involving the brain, lungs, liver, heart, kidney, thyroid, or adrenal glands.

Urine sodium levels are typically tested in patients who have abnormal blood sodium levels, to help determine whether an imbalance is from taking in too much sodium or losing too much sodium. Urine sodium is also used to see if a person with high blood pressure is eating too much salt. It is often used in persons with abnormal kidney tests to help the doctor determine the cause of kidney damage, which can help guide treatment.

When Is It Ordered?

This test is a part of the routine lab evaluation of most patients. It is one of the blood electrolytes, which are often ordered as a group. It is also included in the basic metabolic panel, widely used when someone has non-specific health complaints, in monitoring treatment involving IV fluids, or when there is a possibility of developing dehydration.

Electrolytes or the basic metabolic panel are commonly used to monitor treatment of certain problems, including high blood pressure, heart failure, liver disease, and kidney disease.

What Does the Test Result Mean?

A low level of blood sodium means you have hyponatremia, which is usually due to too much sodium loss, too much water intake or retention, or to fluid accumulation in the body (edema). If sodium falls quickly, you may feel weak and fatigued; in severe cases, you may experience confusion or even fall into a coma. However, when sodium falls slowly there may be no symptoms. That is why sodium levels are often checked even if you don't have any symptoms.

Hyponatremia is rarely due to decreased sodium intake (deficient dietary intake or deficient sodium in IV fluids). Most commonly, it is due to sodium loss (Addison's disease, diarrhea, vomiting, excessive sweating, diuretic administration, or kidney disease). In some cases, it is due to increased water (drinking too much water, heart failure, cirrhosis, kidney diseases that cause protein loss [nephrotic syndrome]) and malnutrition. In a number of diseases (particularly those involving the brain and the lungs, many kinds of cancer, and with some drugs), your body makes too much anti-diuretic hormone, causing you to keep too much water in your body.

A high blood sodium level means you have hypernatremia, almost always due to excessive loss of water (dehydration) without taking in enough water. Symptoms include dry mucous membranes, thirst, agitation, restlessness, acting irrationally, and coma or convulsions if levels rise extremely high. In rare cases, hypernatremia may be due to increased salt intake without enough water, Cushing's syndrome, or too little anti-diuretic hormone (called diabetes insipidus).

In most cases, test results are reported as numerical values rather than as high or low, positive or negative, or normal. In these instances, it is necessary to know the reference range for the particular test. However, reference ranges may vary by the patient's age, sex, as well as the instrumentation or kit used to perform the test.

Is There Anything Else I Should Know?

Recent trauma, surgery, or shock may increase sodium levels because blood flow to the kidneys is decreased. Drugs such as lithium and anabolic steroids may increase sodium levels; this is not common with most other drugs.

Drugs such as diuretics, sulfonylureas (used to treat diabetes), ACE inhibitors (such as captopril), heparin, NSAIDs (such as ibuprofen), tricyclic antidepressants, and vasopressin, among others, can decrease sodium levels. Check with your doctor if you have any concerns about drugs you are taking and their effect on your body.

Potassium Test

How Is It Used?

Serum or plasma tests are performed to diagnose levels of potassium that are too high (hyperkalemia) or too low (hypokalemia). The most common cause of hyperkalemia is kidney disease, but many drugs can decrease potassium excretion from the body and result in this condition. Hypokalemia can occur if you have diarrhea and vomiting, or if you are sweating excessively. Potassium can be lost through your kidneys in urine; in rare cases, potassium may be low because you are not getting enough in your diet. Drugs can cause your kidneys to lose potassium, particularly diuretics (water pills), resulting in hypokalemia. Once your doctor discovers the reason for the too-high or -low potassium levels, she/he can start treating you.

When Is It Ordered?

Serum or plasma tests for potassium levels are routinely performed in most patients investigated for any type of serious illness. Also, because potassium is so important to heart function, it is a part of all complete routine evaluations, especially in those who take diuretics or heart medications, and in the investigation of high blood pressure and kidney disease. It is also used to monitor the patient receiving dialysis, diuretic therapy, or intravenous therapy.

What Does the Test Result Mean?

Increased potassium levels indicate hyperkalemia. Increased levels may also indicate the following health conditions:

- excessive dietary potassium intake (for example, fruits are particularly high in potassium, so excessive intake of fruits or juices may contribute to high potassium);
- excessive intravenous potassium intake;
- acute or chronic kidney failure;
- Addison's disease;

- hypoaldosteronism;
- injury to tissue;
- infection;
- diabetes; or
- dehydration.

Certain drugs can also cause hyperkalemia in a small percent of patients. Among them are non-steroidal anti-inflammatory drugs (such as Advil, Motrin, and Nuprin); beta-blockers (such as propanolol and atenolol), angiotensin-converting inhibitors (such as captopril, enalapril, and lisinopril), and potassium-sparing diuretics (such as triamterene, amiloride, and spironolactone). Decreased levels of potassium indicate hypokalemia. Decreased levels may occur in a number of conditions, particularly:

- dehydration,
- vomiting,
- diarrhea, or
- deficient potassium intake (this is rare).

In diabetes, your potassium may fall after you take insulin, particularly if your diabetes had been out of control for a while. Low potassium is commonly due to water pills (diuretics); if you are taking these, your doctor will check your potassium level regularly.

In most cases, test results are reported as numerical values rather than as high or low, positive or negative, or normal. In these instances, it is necessary to know the reference range for the particular test. However, reference ranges may vary by the patient's age, sex, as well as the instrumentation or kit used to perform the test.

Is There Anything Else I Should Know?

The way that your blood is drawn and handled may cause the potassium level in the sample to be falsely high. If you clench and relax your fist a lot while your blood is drawn, this will make potassium rise. If blood comes out of your veins too fast or too slow, the blood cells can break and increase potassium. Sometimes, if more than one tube of blood is drawn at the same time, some potassium from the tubes with the purple tops can get into the other tubes and increase the potassium. If the specimen does not get from your doctor's office to the laboratory quickly, the potassium can also increase.

If there are any questions as to how your blood was collected, your doctor may request that the test be repeated before starting any treatment.

Carbon Dioxide (CO₂) Test

How Is It Used?

Carbon dioxide levels are almost always done as part of an electrolyte panel to tell your doctor whether your sodium, potassium, chloride, and bicarbonate (H_2CO_3—measured as total CO_2) are in balance. They may be done as part of an annual screen, included as part of a basic or comprehensive metabolic panel, or done when your doctor suspects an imbalance. The CO_2 test is also done when your doctor is evaluating your acid-base balance, to screen for an imbalance, and to monitor a known problem during treatment.

When Is It Ordered?

Carbon dioxide testing may be ordered, usually as part of an electrolyte panel when:

- you are having a routine annual blood screen;

- your doctor suspects that you may be retaining water or are dehydrated, upsetting your electrolyte balance;

- to evaluate your body's acid-base balance (pH); or

- to monitor a condition or treatment that might cause an electrolyte imbalance.

What Does the Test Result Mean?

When CO_2 levels are higher than normal; it suggests that your body is having trouble maintaining its pH balance by releasing excess carbon dioxide, or that you have upset your electrolyte balance, perhaps by losing or retaining fluid. Both of these imbalances may be due to a wide range of dysfunctions. CO_2 elevations may be seen with chronic lung-related problems such as emphysema and metabolic problems such as severe diarrhea or prolonged vomiting (which can cause metabolic alkalosis—an excessive loss of body acidity).

Low CO_2 levels may be seen with respiratory alkalosis (which can be caused by hyperventilation), metabolic acidosis, shock, starvation, and during kidney failure.

In most cases, test results are reported as numerical values rather than as high or low, positive or negative, or normal. In these instances, it is necessary to know the reference range for the particular test. However, reference ranges may vary by the patient's age, sex, as well as the instrumentation or kit used to perform the test.

Is There Anything Else I Should Know?

Some drugs may increase blood carbon dioxide levels including: aldosterone, barbiturates, bicarbonates, hydrocortisone, loop diuretics, and steroids.

Drugs that may decrease blood carbon dioxide levels include methicillin, nitrofurantoin, tetracycline, thiazide diuretics, and triamterene.

Chloride Test

How Is It Used?

Blood chloride is used, along with sodium, to evaluate problems with the acid-base balance in the body and to monitor treatment. In persons with too much base, urine chloride measurements can tell the doctor whether the cause is loss of salt (in cases of dehydration, vomiting, or use of diuretics, where urine chloride would be very low), or an excess of certain hormones such as cortisol or aldosterone (where urine chloride would be high). Urine tests for chloride are also used, along with sodium, to monitor persons put on a low-salt diet. If sodium and chloride levels are high, the doctor knows that the patient is not following the diet.

When Is It Ordered?

A blood chloride test is usually ordered as part of an electrolyte panel or a basic metabolic panel. It is almost never ordered by itself. If your sodium measurement is abnormal, the doctor will look at whether the chloride measurement changes in the same way. This helps the doctor know if there is also a problem with acid or base and helps him/her to guide treatment. Urine chloride is usually performed along with sodium in evaluating the cause of low or high blood levels. It is also helpful in persons with too much base (alkalosis) to help determine the cause.

What Does the Test Result Mean?

A severe elevation or loss of this electrolyte indicates a serious fluid and electrolyte imbalance. Medical staff must take immediate action to restore the electrolyte balance. The type of medical treatment depends on the cause of the problem.

Increased levels of chloride (called hyperchloremia) usually indicate dehydration, but can also occur with any other problem that causes high blood sodium. Hyperchloremia also occurs when too much base is lost from the body (producing metabolic acidosis), or when a person hyperventilates (causing respiratory alkalosis).

Decreased levels of chloride (called hypochloremia) occur with any disorder that causes low blood sodium. Hypochloremia also occurs with prolonged vomiting or gastric suction, chronic diarrhea, emphysema, or other chronic lung disease (causing respiratory acidosis), and with loss of base from the body (called metabolic alkalosis).

In most cases, test results are reported as numerical values rather than as high or low, positive or negative, or normal. In these instances, it is necessary to know the reference range for the particular test. However, reference ranges may vary by the patient's age, sex, as well as the instrumentation or kit used to perform the test.

Is There Anything Else I Should Know?

Drugs that affect sodium will also cause changes in chloride. In addition, swallowing large amounts of baking soda or substantially more than the recommended dosage of antacids can also cause low chloride. Some instructions for routine testing advise patients to stop all food and fluids for eight hours before the test to prevent the normal drop in chloride value after eating.

Section 32.3

Glucose Tests and Testing for Pre-Diabetes

This section includes "Glucose Tests," and "Testing for Pre-Diabetes Encouraged," © 2003 American Association for Clinical Chemistry. Reprinted with permission. For additional information on clinical lab testing, visit the Lab Tests Online website at www.labtestsonline.org.

Glucose Tests

The glucose test is a snapshot, a still photograph of a moving picture. It tells what the blood glucose level was at the moment it was collected. The fasting blood glucose level (collected after an 8 to 10 hour fast) is used to screen for and diagnose diabetes and pre-diabetes. An oral glucose tolerance test (OGTT/GTT) may also be used to diagnose diabetes and pre-diabetes, but according to the American Diabetes Association, two tests (either the fasting glucose or the OGTT) should be done at different times in order to confirm the diagnosis. The OGTT involves a fasting glucose, followed by the patient drinking a standard amount of a glucose solution to challenge their system, followed by another glucose test two hours later.

Gestational diabetes is a temporary type of hyperglycemia seen in some pregnant women, usually late in their pregnancy. Almost all pregnant women are screened for gestational diabetes between their 24th and 28th week of pregnancy using a one hour glucose challenge. If the blood glucose is high, they are considered at risk of developing gestational diabetes and they will undergo further testing.

Diabetics must monitor their own blood glucose levels, often several times a day, to determine how far above or below normal their glucose is and to determine what oral medications or insulin they may need. This is usually done by placing a drop of blood from a finger prick onto a plastic indicator strip and then inserting the strip into a glucometer, a small machine that provides a digital readout of the blood glucose. In those with suspected hypoglycemia, glucose levels are used as part of the Whipple triad to confirm a diagnosis.

331

When Is It Ordered?

This test can be used to screen healthy individuals for diabetes and pre-diabetes because diabetes is a common disease that begins with few symptoms. Screening for glucose may occur at public health fairs or as part of workplace health programs. It may also be ordered as part of a routine physical exam. Screening is especially important for people at high risk of developing diabetes—those with a family history of diabetes, those who are overweight, and those who are more than 40 to 45 years old.

The glucose test may also be ordered to help diagnose diabetes and hypoglycemia when someone has symptoms of hyperglycemia such as:

- Increased thirst
- Increased urination
- Fatigue
- Blurred vision
- Slow-healing infections

or of hypoglycemia, such as:

- Sweating
- Hunger
- Trembling
- Anxiety
- Confusion
- Blurred Vision

Glucose testing is also done in emergency settings to determine if low or high glucose is contributing to symptoms such as fainting and unconsciousness.

If a patient has pre-diabetes (characterized by fasting or OGTT levels that are higher than normal, but lower than those defined as diabetic), their doctor will order a glucose test at regular intervals to monitor their progress. With known diabetics, doctors will order glucose levels in conjunction with other tests such as: insulin and C-Peptide to monitor insulin production, and hemoglobin A1c to monitor glucose control over a period of time.

Diabetics will self check their glucose, once or several times a day, to monitor glucose levels and to determine treatment options.

Pregnant women are usually screened for gestational diabetes late in their pregnancies, unless they have symptoms earlier or have had gestational diabetes with a previous child. When a woman has gestational diabetes, her doctor will usually order glucose levels throughout the rest of her pregnancy and after delivery to monitor her condition.

What Does the Test Result Mean?

High levels of glucose most frequently indicate diabetes, but many other diseases and conditions can also cause elevated glucose. The following information summarizes the meaning of the test results. These are based on the clinical practice recommendations of the American Diabetes Association.

Table 32.1. Fasting Blood Glucose

From 70 to 109 mg/dL	normal glucose tolerance
From 110 to 125 mg/dL	impaired fasting glucose (pre-diabetes)
126 mg/dL and above	probable diabetes

Table 32.2. Oral Glucose Tolerance Test (OGTT) Results (2 hours after a 75-gram glucose drink)

Less than 140 mg/dL	normal glucose tolerance
From 140 to 200 mg/dL	impaired fasting glucose (pre-diabetes)
Over 200 mg/dL	probable diabetes

Table 32.3. Gestational Diabetes (screening at 1 hour after a 50-gram glucose drink*)

Less than 140 mg/dL	normal glucose tolerance
140 mg/dL and over	abnormal, needs oral glucose tolerance test

*Practices may vary regarding the use of the glucose drink; screening 1 hour after eating is sometimes deemed acceptable. However, testing 1 hour after consuming the 50-gram glucose drink has been shown to produce the most reliable test result.

Some of the other diseases and conditions that can result in elevated glucose levels include:

- Acromegaly
- Acute stress (response to trauma, heart attack, and stroke for instance)
- Chronic renal failure
- Cushing's syndrome
- Drugs, including: corticosteroids, tricyclic antidepressants, diuretics, epinephrine, estrogens (birth control pills and hormone replacement), lithium, phenytoin (Dilantin), and salicylates
- Excessive food intake
- Hyperthyroidism
- Pancreatic cancer
- Pancreatitis

Moderately increased levels may be seen with pre-diabetes. This condition, if left un-addressed, often leads to type 2 diabetes.

Low glucose levels (hypoglycemia) are also seen with:

- Adrenal insufficiency
- Drinking alcohol
- Drugs, such as: acetaminophen, and anabolic steroids
- Extensive liver disease
- Hypopituitarism
- Hypothyroidism
- Insulin overdose
- Insulinomas (insulin-producing pancreatic tumors)
- Starvation

In most cases, test results are reported as numerical values rather than as high or low, positive or negative, or normal. In these instances, it is necessary to know the reference range for the particular test. However, reference ranges may vary by the patient's age, sex, as well as the instrumentation or kit used to perform the test.

Is There Anything Else I Should Know?

Hypoglycemia is characterized by a drop in blood glucose to a level where first it causes nervous system symptoms (sweating, palpitations, hunger, trembling, and anxiety), then begins to affect the brain (causing confusion, hallucinations, blurred vision, and sometimes even coma and death). An actual diagnosis of hypoglycemia requires satisfying the Whipple triad. These three criteria include:

- Documented low glucose levels (less than 40 mg/dL often tested along with insulin levels and sometimes with C-peptide levels).

- Symptoms of hypoglycemia.

- Reversal of the symptoms when blood glucose levels are returned to normal.

Primary hypoglycemia is rare. People may have symptoms of hypoglycemia without really having low blood sugar. In such cases, dietary changes such as eating frequent small meals and several snacks a day, and choosing complex carbohydrates over simple sugars may be enough to ease symptoms. Those with fasting hypoglycemia may require IV (intravenous) glucose if dietary measures are insufficient.

Testing for Pre-Diabetes Encouraged

As of April 3, 2002, the figures are staggering: 17 million Americans have diabetes and 16 million more may have pre-diabetes, a new name for impaired glucose tolerance, which is an early indicator of developing diabetes. Those who have pre-diabetes probably don't experience any symptoms, but their blood glucose levels are higher than normal. If nothing is done to reduce these levels, diabetes will most likely develop within 10 years. Diabetes is associated with increased risk of heart disease, including heart attack and stroke, as well as complications that can lead to blindness, kidney failure, and limb amputations. Now, the U.S. Department of Health and Human Services (HHS) and the American Diabetes Association (ADA) are encouraging people to be tested for this pre-diabetic condition.

A simple blood glucose test that can be done at a regular doctor's office visit is all that's needed. The test can be done in two ways: a fasting plasma glucose test, which looks at the level of glucose in the blood after the patient fasts for 8 hours, or an oral glucose tolerance test, which measures the blood glucose level two hours after the patient drinks a solution with a fixed amount of sugar in it.

As part of this educational campaign, guidelines from an expert panel at HHS and ADA were released. They recommend:

- Testing everyone 45 years of age and older, especially if overweight.

- Testing younger adults if they have risk factors, such as obesity, low HDL (or good) cholesterol and high triglycerides, high blood pressure, family history of diabetes, history of diabetes developed during pregnancy, or belong to a racial minority group at increased risk for type 2 diabetes.

- Repeat testing every 3 years if the test results are normal.

- For those with a high glucose test result, encouraging preventive measures, such as walking 30 minutes per day 5 days a week, and losing weight, which can significantly reduce the risk.

The panel is hopeful that physicians and patients will heed this warning and take advantage of the easy steps available to prevent the disease: a simple blood test to determine risk of developing diabetes and lifestyle changes that can be made to reduce that risk.

Section 32.4

Kidney Function Tests: Blood Urea Nitrogen (BUN) Test and Creatinine Test

This section includes "BUN Test," and "Creatinine Test," © 2003 American Association for Clinical Chemistry. Reprinted with permission. For additional information on clinical lab testing, visit the Lab Tests Online website at www.labtestsonline.org.

The BUN Test

The BUN level, usually ordered with tests for creatinine, is used to evaluate kidney function and to monitor patients with kidney failure or those receiving dialysis therapy.

When Is It Ordered?

BUN is part of the basic metabolic panel, widely used:

- when someone has non-specific complaints,
- as part of a routine testing panel, or
- to check how the kidneys are functioning before starting to take certain drugs.

BUN is often ordered with creatinine:

- if kidney problems are suspected,
- to monitor treatment of kidney disease, or
- to monitor kidney function while someone is on certain drugs.

What Does the Test Result Mean?

High BUN levels suggest impaired kidney function. This may be due to acute or chronic kidney disease. However, there are many things besides kidney disease that can affect BUN levels such as decreased blood flow to the kidneys as in congestive heart failure, shock, stress, recent heart attack, or severe burns; conditions that cause obstruction of urine flow; or dehydration.

Low BUN levels are not common and are not usually a cause for concern. They can be seen in severe liver disease or malnutrition, but are not used to diagnose or monitor these conditions. Low BUN is also seen in normal pregnancy.

In most cases, test results are reported as numerical values rather than as high or low, positive or negative, or normal. In these instances, it is necessary to know the reference range for the particular test. However, reference ranges may vary by the patient's age, sex, as well as the instrumentation or kit used to perform the test.

Is There Anything Else I Should Know?

BUN levels increase with age and also with the amount of protein in your diet. High-protein diets may cause abnormally high BUN levels. Very low-protein diets can cause abnormally low BUN. Lower BUN levels are also seen in infants and small children. Drugs that impair kidney function may increase BUN levels. Your BUN and creatinine may be monitored if you are on certain drugs.

Creatinine Test

The creatinine test is used to determine whether your kidneys are functioning normally (in this case the amount of creatinine in your blood will be very low). A combination of blood and urine creatinine levels may be used to calculate a creatinine clearance. This measures how effectively your kidneys are filtering small molecules like creatinine out of your blood.

When Is It Ordered?

Creatinine may be part of a basic metabolic panel, widely used when someone has non-specific health complaints, or it may be ordered if your doctor suspects kidney problems. The test is also used to monitor treatment of kidney disease or to monitor kidney function while you are on certain drugs.

What Does the Test Result Mean?

Increased creatinine levels in the blood suggest diseases that affect kidney function. These can include:

- glomerulonephritis (swelling of the kidney's blood vessels);
- pyelonephritis (pus-forming infection of the kidneys);

- acute tubular necrosis (death of cells in the kidneys' small tubes);
- urinary tract obstruction; or
- reduced blood flow to the kidney due to shock, dehydration, congestive heart failure, atherosclerosis, or complications of diabetes.

Creatinine can also increase as a result of muscle injury. Low levels of creatinine are not common and are not usually a cause for concern. They can be due to lack of height, decreased muscle mass, and some severe liver disease.

In most cases, test results are reported as numerical values rather than as high or low, positive or negative, or normal. In these instances, it is necessary to know the reference range for the particular test. However, reference ranges may vary by the patient's age, sex, as well as the instrumentation or kit used to perform the test.

Is There Anything Else I Should Know?

Since creatinine levels are in proportion to muscle mass, women tend to have lower levels than men. In general, creatinine levels will stay the same if you eat a normal diet. However, eating large amounts of meat may cause short-lived increases in blood creatinine levels. Taking creatine supplements may also increase creatinine.

There are very few drugs that interfere with the creatinine test, although there are some drugs that can cause some impairment in kidney function. Your creatinine levels may be monitored if you are taking one of these drugs.

Section 32.5

Lipid Profile: Cholesterol, High Density Lipoprotein (HDL), Low Density Lipoprotein (LDL), Triglycerides

This section includes "Lipid Profile," "Cholesterol Test," "HDL Cholesterol Test," "LDL Cholesterol Test," and "Triglycerides Test," © 2003 American Association for Clinical Chemistry. Reprinted with permission. For additional information on clinical lab testing, visit the Lab Tests Online website at www.labtestsonline.org.

Lipid Profile

The lipid profile is a group of tests that are often ordered together to determine risk of coronary heart disease. The tests that make up a lipid profile are tests that have been shown to be good indicators of whether someone is likely to have a heart attack or stroke caused by blockage of blood vessels (hardening of the arteries).

What Tests Are Included in a Lipid Profile?

The lipid profile includes total cholesterol, HDL cholesterol (often called good cholesterol), LDL cholesterol (often called bad cholesterol), and triglycerides. Sometimes the report will include additional calculated values such as HDL/cholesterol ratio or a risk score based on lipid profile results, age, sex, and other risk factors.

How Is a Lipid Profile Used?

The lipid profile is used to guide providers in deciding how a person at risk should be treated. The results of the lipid profile are considered along with other known risk factors of heart disease to develop a plan of treatment and follow-up.

Cholesterol Test

The cholesterol test is different from most tests in that it is not used to diagnose or monitor a disease, but is used to estimate risk of

340

developing a disease—specifically heart disease. Because high blood cholesterol has been associated with hardening of the arteries, heart disease, and a raised risk of death from heart attacks, cholesterol testing is considered a routine part of preventive health care.

When Is It Ordered?

Cholesterol testing is recommended as a screening test to be done on all adults at least once every five years. It is usually ordered as part of a routine physical exam. It may be ordered alone or in combination with other tests including HDL, LDL, and triglycerides often called a lipid profile.

Cholesterol is tested at more frequent intervals (often several times per year) in patients who have been prescribed diet and/or drugs to lower their cholesterol. The test is used to track how well these measures are succeeding in lowering cholesterol to desired levels, and, in turn, lowering the risk of developing heart disease.

What Does the Test Result Mean?

In a routine setting where testing is done to screen for risk, the test results are grouped in three categories of risk:

- Desirable: Cholesterol below 200 mg/dL is considered desirable and reflects a low risk of heart disease.

- Borderline high: Cholesterol of 200 to 240 mg/dL is considered to reflect moderate risk. Your doctor may decide to order a lipid profile to see if your high cholesterol is bad cholesterol (high LDL) or good cholesterol (high HDL). Depending on the results of the lipid profile (and any other risk factors you may have) your doctor will decide what to do.

- High Risk: Cholesterol above 240 mg/dL is considered high risk. Your doctor may order a lipid profile (as well as other tests) to try to determine the cause of your high cholesterol. Once the cause is known, an appropriate treatment will be prescribed.

In a treatment setting, testing is used to see how much cholesterol is decreasing as a result of treatment. The goal for the amount of change or the final (target) value will be set by your doctor. The target value is usually based on LDL.

In most cases, test results are reported as numerical values rather than as high or low, positive or negative, or normal. In these instances, it is necessary to know the reference range for the particular test. However, reference ranges may vary by the patient's age, sex, as well as the instrumentation or kit used to perform the test.

Is There Anything Else I Should Know?

Cholesterol should be measured when a person is healthy. Blood cholesterol is temporarily low during acute illness, immediately following a heart attack, or during stress (like from surgery or an accident). You should wait at least 6 weeks after any illness to have cholesterol measured.

It is not necessary to fast when you have a cholesterol test. Cholesterol does not change in response to a single meal. Cholesterol does change in response to changes in long term patterns of eating—like changing from a high fat diet to a low fat diet—but it takes several weeks to see changes in blood cholesterol in response to changes in diet.

There is some debate about whether very low cholesterol is bad. Low cholesterol (less than 100 mg/dL) is often seen when there is an existing problem like malnutrition, liver disease, or cancer. However there is no evidence that low cholesterol causes any of these problems.

Cholesterol is high during pregnancy. Women should wait at least six weeks after the baby is born to have cholesterol measured.

Some drugs that are known to increase cholesterol levels include anabolic steroids, beta blockers, epinephrine, oral contraceptives and vitamin D.

High Density Lipoprotein (HDL) Cholesterol Test

The test of HDL cholesterol is used to determine your risk of heart disease. If high cholesterol is due to high HDL, a person is probably at low risk and further testing or treatment for high cholesterol is not advised.

When Is It Ordered?

HDL is usually ordered with other tests, either with cholesterol or as part of a lipid profile, including LDL and triglycerides. The combination of total cholesterol and HDL is very useful for screening for heart disease since it is not necessary to fast for these two tests. In contrast, a more complete lipid profile requires fasting for at least 12 hours.

What Does the Test Result Mean?

High HDL is better than low HDL. There are two ways that HDL cholesterol values are interpreted—as a percent of total cholesterol or as a measured value.

- **Percent:** If HDL is 20% of the total cholesterol, risk of heart disease is average. If HDL is more than 20% of the total cholesterol, risk of heart disease is less than average. This is usually expressed as a ratio of cholesterol to HDL. It is desirable for the cholesterol/HDL ratio to be less than 5.

- **Measured Value:** If HDL is less than 40 mg/dl, there is an increased risk of heart disease. A desirable level of HDL is greater than 40 mg/dL and is associated with average risk of heart disease. A good level of HDL is 60 mg/dL or more and is associated with a less than average risk of heart disease.

HDL should be interpreted in the context of the overall findings from the lipid profile and in consultation with your doctor.

In most cases, test results are reported as numerical values rather than as high or low, positive or negative, or normal. In these instances, it is necessary to know the reference range for the particular test. However, reference ranges may vary by the patient's age, sex, as well as the instrumentation or kit used to perform the test.

Is There Anything Else I Should Know?

HDL cholesterol should be measured when a person is healthy. Cholesterol is temporarily low during acute illness, immediately following a heart attack, or during stress (as from surgery or an accident). You should wait at least 6 weeks after any illness to have cholesterol measured.

In women, HDL cholesterol may change during pregnancy. You should wait at least six weeks after your baby is born to have your HDL-cholesterol measured.

Low Density Lipoprotein (LDL) Cholesterol Test

The test for LDL is used to predict your risk of developing heart disease. Of all the forms of cholesterol in the blood, the LDL cholesterol is considered the most important form in determining risk of heart disease. Treatment decisions are based on LDL values.

When Is It Ordered?

LDL levels are ordered as part a lipid profile, along with total cholesterol, HDL, and triglycerides. This profile may be ordered as a screening profile in a healthy person as part of a routine physical exam. A lipid profile may be ordered on someone who has had high screening cholesterol to see if the total cholesterol is high because of too much LDL.

What Does the Test Result Mean?

Elevated levels of LDL indicate risk for heart disease. Treatment (with diet or drugs) for high LDL aims to lower LDL to a target value based on your overall risk of heart disease. Your target value is:

- LDL less than 100 mg/dL if you have heart disease or diabetes.
- LDL less than 130 mg/dL if you have 2 or more risk factors.
- LDL less than 160 mg/dL if you have 0 or 1 risk factor.

Risk factors include cigarette smoking, hypertension, low HDL (less than 40 mg/dL), family history, age (male 55 or older; female 65 or older), being overweight, and failure to exercise regularly.

In most cases, test results are reported as numerical values rather than as high or low, positive or negative, or normal. In these instances, it is necessary to know the reference range for the particular test. However, reference ranges may vary by the patient's age, sex, as well as the instrumentation or kit used to perform the test.

Is There Anything Else I Should Know?

Measurement of LDL generally requires a 12-hour fast—meaning that you must not eat or drink anything that has calories for 12 hours before your blood is drawn. This is because LDL is usually calculated from the results of other tests, including triglycerides, which require fasting. This result may be reported as calculated LDL. Some laboratories can measure LDL directly using a special technology and fasting is not necessary. This test is usually called direct LDL. LDL cholesterol should be measured when a person is healthy.

LDL cholesterol is temporarily low during acute illness, immediately following a heart attack, or during stress (as from surgery or an accident). You should wait at least six weeks after any illness to have LDL cholesterol measured.

In women, cholesterol is high during pregnancy. Women should wait at least six weeks after the baby is born to have LDL cholesterol measured.

Triglycerides Test

Blood tests for triglycerides are usually part of a lipid profile used to identify the risk of developing heart disease. If you are diabetic, it is especially important to have triglycerides measured as part of any lipid testing since triglycerides increase significantly when blood sugar is out of control.

When Is It Ordered?

Lipid profiles, including triglycerides, are recommended as routine tests to evaluate risk of heart disease in healthy adults. The test for triglycerides is not often ordered alone since risk of heart disease is based on cholesterol levels not triglycerides. However, if you have been found to have high triglycerides and are being treated for it, a triglyceride test may be ordered to see if treatment is working.

What Does the Test Result Mean?

A normal level for fasting triglycerides is less than 150 mg/dL. It is unusual to have high triglycerides without also having high cholesterol. Most treatments for heart disease risk will be aimed at lowering cholesterol. However, the type of treatment used to lower cholesterol may differ depending on whether triglycerides are high or normal.

When triglycerides are very high (greater than 1000 mg/dL), there is a risk of developing pancreatitis. Treatment to lower triglycerides should be started as soon as possible.

In most cases, test results are reported as numerical values rather than as high or low, positive or negative, or normal. In these instances, it is necessary to know the reference range for the particular test. However, reference ranges may vary by the patient's age, sex, as well as the instrumentation or kit used to perform the test.

Is There Anything Else I Should Know?

Testing should be done when you are fasting. For 12 to 14 hours before the test, only water is permitted. In addition, alcohol should not be consumed for the 24 hours just before the test. If you are diabetic and your blood sugar is out of control, triglycerides will be very high.

Triglycerides change dramatically in response to meals, increasing as much as 5 to 10 times higher than fasting levels just a few hours after eating. Even fasting levels vary considerably day to day. Therefore modest changes in fasting triglycerides measured on different days are not considered to be abnormal.

Section 32.6

Liver Function Tests: Alkaline Phosphatase (ALP or ALK PHOS) Test, Alanine Aminotransferase (ALT) Test, Aspartate Aminotransferase (AST) Test, and Bilirubin Test

This section includes "ALP Test," "ALT Test," "AST Test," and "Bilirubin Test," © 2003 American Association for Clinical Chemistry. Reprinted with permission. For additional information on clinical lab testing, visit the Lab Tests Online website at www.labtestsonline.org.

Alkaline Phosphatase (ALP or ALK PHOS) Test

When a person has evidence of liver disease, very high ALP levels can tell the doctor that the person's bile ducts are somehow blocked. Often, ALP is high in persons who have cancer that has spread to the liver or the bones, and doctors can do further testing to see if this has happened. If a person with bone or liver cancer responds to treatment, ALP levels will decrease. When a person has high levels of ALP, and the doctor is not sure why, she/he may also order ALP isoenzyme tests to try to determine the cause.

When Is It Ordered?

ALP is generally part of a routine lab testing profile, often with a group of other tests called a liver panel. Also, it is usually ordered along with several other tests if a patient seems to have symptoms of a liver or bone disorder.

What Does the Test Result Mean?

High ALP usually means that the bone or liver has been damaged. If other liver tests such as bilirubin, aspartate aminotransferase (AST), or alanine aminotransferase (ALT) are also high, the ALP is usually coming from the liver. If calcium and phosphate measurements are abnormal, the ALP is usually coming from bone.

In some forms of liver disease, such as hepatitis, ALP is usually much less elevated than AST and ALT. When the bile ducts are blocked (usually by gallstones, scars from previous gallstones or surgery, or by cancers), ALP and bilirubin may be increased much more than AST or ALT. In a few liver diseases, ALP may be the only test that is high.

In some bone diseases, such as a disorder called Paget's disease (where bones become enlarged and deformed), or in certain cancers that spread to bone, ALP may be the only test result that is high.

Sometimes doctors don't know why ALP is high, and they need to order other tests to determine the exact cause. In such cases, your doctor may order a gamma glutamyl transpeptidase (GGT) test, another enzyme that is made by the liver in the same places as is ALP, but which is not made by bone.

In most cases, test results are reported as numerical values rather than as high or low, positive or negative, or normal. In these instances, it is necessary to know the reference range for the particular test. However, reference ranges may vary by the patient's age, sex, as well as the instrumentation or kit used to perform the test.

Is There Anything Else I Should Know?

Pregnancy can increase ALP levels. Children have higher ALP levels because their bones are growing, and ALP is often very high during the growth spurt, which occurs at different ages in males and females.

Eating a meal can increase the ALP level slightly for a few hours in some people. It is usually better to do the test after fasting overnight. Some drugs may increase ALP levels, especially some of the drugs used to treat psychiatric problems, but this is rare. Fasting is preferred, but not required for this test.

Alanine Aminotransferase (ALT) Test

The ALT test detects liver injury. ALT values are usually compared to the levels of other enzymes, such as alkaline phosphatase (ALP) and aspartate aminotransferase (AST), to help determine which form of liver disease is present.

When Is It Ordered?

A physician usually orders an ALT test (and several others) to evaluate a patient who has symptoms of a liver disorder. Some of these symptoms include jaundice, dark urine, nausea, vomiting, abdominal swelling, unusual weight gain, and abdominal pain. ALT can also be ordered, either by itself or with other tests, for:

- persons who have a history of known or possible exposure to hepatitis viruses,
- those who drink too much alcohol,
- individuals whose families have a history of liver disease, or
- persons who take drugs that might occasionally damage the liver.

In persons with mild symptoms, such as fatigue or loss of energy, ALT may be tested to make sure they do not have chronic liver disease. ALT is often used to monitor the treatment of persons who have liver disease, to see if the treatment is working, and may be ordered either alone or along with other tests.

What Does the Test Result Mean?

Very high levels of ALT (more than 10 times the highest normal level) are usually due to acute hepatitis, often due to a virus infection. In acute hepatitis, ALT levels usually stay high for about 1–2 months, but can take as long as 3–6 months to come back to normal.

ALT levels are usually not as high in chronic hepatitis, often less than 4 times the highest normal level: in this case, ALT levels often vary between normal and slightly increased, so doctors typically will order the test frequently to see if there is a pattern. In some liver diseases, especially when the bile ducts are blocked, when a person has cirrhosis, and when other types of liver cancer are present, ALT may be close to normal levels.

In most cases, test results are reported as numerical values rather than as high or low, positive or negative, or normal. In these instances, it is necessary to know the reference range for the particular test. However, reference ranges may vary by the patient's age, sex, as well as the instrumentation or kit used to perform the test.

Is There Anything Else I Should Know?

A shot or injection of medicine into the muscle tissue, or strenuous exercise, may increase ALT levels.

Many drugs may raise ALT levels by causing liver damage in a very small percentage of patients taking the drug. This is true of both prescription drugs and some natural health products. If your doctor finds that you have a high ALT, tell him or her about all the drugs and health products you are taking.

Aspartate Aminotransferase (AST) Test

Testing for AST is usually used to detect liver damage. Also, AST levels are often compared with levels of other liver enzymes, alkaline phosphatase (ALP) and alanine aminotransferase (ALT), to determine which form of liver disease is present. Even though AST is found in heart and other muscles, another enzyme, creatine kinase (CK), is present in much higher amounts and is usually used to detect heart or muscle injury.

When Is It Ordered?

An AST test is ordered along with several other tests to evaluate a patient who seems to have symptoms of a liver disorder. Some of these symptoms include jaundice (yellowing of the eyes and skin), dark urine, nausea, vomiting, abdominal swelling, unusual weight gain, and abdominal pain. AST can also be ordered, either by itself or with other tests, for:

- persons who might have been exposed to hepatitis viruses,
- those who drink too much alcohol,
- persons who have a history of liver disease in their family, or
- persons taking drugs that can occasionally damage the liver.

Persons who have mild symptoms, such as fatigue, may be tested for ALT to make sure they do not have chronic liver disease. ALT is often measured to monitor treatment of persons with liver disease, and may be ordered either alone or along with other tests.

What Does the Test Result Mean?

Very high levels of AST (more than 10 times the highest normal level) are usually due to acute hepatitis, often due to a virus infection.

In acute hepatitis, AST levels usually stay high for about 1–2 months, but can take as long as 3–6 months to return to normal. In chronic hepatitis, AST levels are usually not as high, often less than 4 times the highest normal level. In chronic hepatitis, AST often varies between normal and slightly increased, so doctors typically will order the test frequently to determine the pattern.

In some diseases of the liver, especially when the bile ducts are blocked, or with cirrhosis and certain cancers of the liver, AST may be close to normal, but it increases more often than ALT. When liver damage is due to alcohol, AST often increases much more than ALT (this is a pattern seen with few other liver diseases). AST is also increased after heart attacks and with muscle injury, usually to a much greater degree than is ALT.

In most cases, test results are reported as numerical values rather than as high or low, positive or negative, or normal. In these instances, it is necessary to know the reference range for the particular test. However, reference ranges may vary by the patient's age, sex, as well as the instrumentation or kit used to perform the test.

Is There Anything Else I Should Know?

Pregnancy may decrease AST levels. A shot or injection of medicine into muscle tissue, or even strenuous exercise, may increase AST levels. In rare instances, some drugs can damage the liver or muscle, increasing AST levels. This is true of both prescription drugs and some natural health products. If your doctor finds that you have high levels of AST, tell him or her about all the drugs and health products you are taking.

Bilirubin Test

When bilirubin levels are high, a condition called jaundice (a yellowing of the skin and the whites of the eyes) occurs, and further testing is needed to determine the cause. Too much bilirubin may mean that too many red cells are being destroyed, or that the liver is incapable of removing bilirubin from the blood.

It is not uncommon to see high bilirubin levels (sometimes called neonatal bilirubin) in newborns (typically 1–3 days old). Within the first 24 hours of life, up to 50% of full-term newborns, and an even greater percentage of pre-term babies, may have high a bilirubin level. At birth, the newborn lacks the intestinal bacteria that help process bilirubin. This is not abnormal and resolves itself within a few days.

In other instances, newborns' red blood cells may have been destroyed because of blood typing incompatibilities. In adults or older children, bilirubin is measured to diagnose and/or monitor liver diseases (such as cirrhosis, hepatitis, or gallstones).

What Does the Test Result Mean?

Newborns: Excessive bilirubin kills developing brain cells in infants and may cause mental retardation, physical abnormalities, or blindness. It is important that bilirubin in newborns does not get too high. When the level of bilirubin is above a critical threshold, special treatments are initiated to lower it. An excessive bilirubin level may result from the breakdown of red blood cells (RBCs) due to Rh blood typing incompatibility. For example, mother is Rh negative (Rh-), father is Rh positive (Rh+), and fetus is Rh+; mother develops antibodies against the newborn's RBCs, which are destroyed.

Adults and children: Doctors may order bilirubin tests (along with other liver enzyme tests, especially when jaundice is present) to determine if liver damage exists. Bilirubin levels can be used to monitor the progression of jaundice and to determine if it is the result of red blood cell breakdown or liver disease. This can be done by measuring two different chemical forms of bilirubin—direct (or conjugated) and indirect (or unconjugated) bilirubin. If the direct bilirubin is elevated there may be some kind of blockage of the liver or bile duct, perhaps due to gallstones, hepatitis, trauma, a drug reaction, or long-term alcohol abuse. If the indirect bilirubin is increased, hemolysis (undesirable breakdown of red blood cells) may be the cause.

In most cases, test results are reported as numerical values rather than as high or low, positive or negative, or normal. In these instances, it is necessary to know the reference range for the particular test. However, reference ranges may vary by the patient's age, sex, as well as the instrumentation or kit used to perform the test.

Is There Anything Else I Should Know?

Although bilirubin may be toxic to brain development in newborns (up to the age of about 2–4 weeks), high bilirubin in older children and adults does not pose the same threat. In older children and adults, the blood-brain barrier is more developed and prevents bilirubin from crossing this barrier to the brain cells. However, elevated bilirubin levels in children or adults strongly suggest a medical condition that must be evaluated and treated.

Jaundice results from high levels of bilirubin. Increases in bilirubin may be due to metabolic problems, obstruction of the bile duct, physical or chemical damage to the liver (cirrhosis), or an inherited abnormality (Gilbert's, Rotor's, Dubin-Johnson, or Crigler-Najjar syndromes).

Section 32.7

Protein Tests:
Albumin Test and Total Protein Test

This section includes "Albumin Test," and "Total Protein Test," © 2003 American Association for Clinical Chemistry. Reprinted with permission. For additional information on clinical lab testing, visit the Lab Tests Online website at www.labtestsonline.org.

Albumin Test

Since albumin is low in many different diseases and disorders, albumin testing is used in a variety of settings to help diagnose disease, to monitor changes in health status with treatment or with disease progression, and as a screen that may serve as an indicator for other kinds of testing.

When Is It Ordered?

A physician orders a blood albumin test (usually along with several other tests) if a person seems to have symptoms of a liver disorder or nephrotic syndrome. Doctors may also order blood albumin tests when they want to check a person's nutritional status, for example, when someone has lost a lot of weight.

What Does the Test Result Mean?

- Low albumin levels can suggest liver disease. Other liver enzyme tests are ordered to determine exactly which type of liver disease.

- Low albumin levels can reflect diseases in which the kidneys cannot prevent albumin from leaking from the blood into the urine and being lost. In this case, the amount of albumin (or protein) in the urine also may be measured.

- Low albumin levels can also be seen in inflammation, shock, and malnutrition.

- Low albumin levels may also suggest conditions in which your body does not properly absorb and digest protein (like Crohn's disease or sprue) or in which large volumes of protein are lost from the intestines.

- High albumin levels usually reflect dehydration.

In most cases, test results are reported as numerical values rather than as high or low, positive or negative, or normal. In these instances, it is necessary to know the reference range for the particular test. However, reference ranges may vary by the patient's age, sex, as well as the instrumentation or kit used to perform the test.

Is There Anything Else I Should Know?

Certain drugs increase albumin in your blood, including anabolic steroids, androgens, growth hormones, and insulin. If you are receiving large amounts of intravenous fluids, the results of this test may be inaccurate.

Total Protein Test

Total protein measurements can reflect nutritional status, kidney disease, liver disease, and many other conditions. If total protein is abnormal, further tests must be performed to identify which protein fraction is abnormal, so that a specific diagnosis can be made.

When Is It Ordered?

Total protein is ordered to provide general information about your nutritional status, such as when you have undergone a recent weight loss. It is also ordered along with several other tests to provide information if you have symptoms that suggest a liver or kidney disorder, or to investigate the cause of abnormal pooling of fluid in tissue (edema).

What Does the Test Result Mean?

Low total protein levels can suggest a liver disorder, a kidney disorder, or a disorder in which protein is not digested or absorbed properly.

More specific tests, such as albumin and liver enzyme tests, must be performed to make an accurate diagnosis. High total protein levels can indicate dehydration or some types of cancer which lead to an accumulation of an abnormal protein (such as multiple myeloma).

In most cases, test results are reported as numerical values rather than as high or low, positive or negative, or normal. In these instances, it is necessary to know the reference range for the particular test. However, reference ranges may vary by the patient's age, sex, as well as the instrumentation or kit used to perform the test.

Is There Anything Else I Should Know?

Prolonged application of a tourniquet during blood collection can increase total protein levels. Drugs that may increase protein levels include anabolic steroids, androgens, growth hormone, insulin, and progesterone. Drugs that may decrease protein levels include estrogens and oral contraceptives.

Section 32.8

Thyroid Function Tests: T3, T4, TSH

This section includes "T3," "T4," and "TSH," © 2003 American Association for Clinical Chemistry. Reprinted with permission. For additional information on clinical lab testing, visit the Lab Tests Online website at www .labtestsonline.org.

T3 Thyroid Test

A T3 test determines whether the thyroid is performing properly, and is used mainly to help diagnose hyperthyroidism, since T3 can become abnormal earlier than T4 and return to normal later than T4.

T3 is not usually helpful if your doctor thinks you have hypothyroidism.

When Is It Ordered?

A total or free T3 test may be ordered if you get an abnormal T4 test result.

What Does the Test Result Mean?

A high total or free T3 result may indicate an overactive thyroid gland (hyperthyroidism).

Low total or free T3 results may indicate an underactive thyroid gland (hypothyroidism).

In most cases, test results are reported as numerical values rather than as high or low, positive or negative, or normal. In these instances, it is necessary to know the reference range for the particular test. However, reference ranges may vary by the patient's age, sex, as well as the instrumentation or kit used to perform the test.

Is There Anything Else I Should Know?

Many medications—including estrogen, certain types of birth control pills, and large doses of aspirin—can interfere with total T3 test results, so tell your doctor about any drugs you are taking. In general, free T3 levels are not affected by these medications.

When you are sick, your body decreases production of T3 from T4. Most people who are sick enough to be in the hospital will have a low T3 or free T3 level. For this reason, doctors do not usually use T3 as a routine thyroid test for patients in hospitals.

T4 Thyroid Test

A T4 test tells whether the thyroid is performing properly. Newborns are commonly screened for T4 levels as well as TSH concentrations to check for hypothyroidism, which can cause mental retardation.

In adults, the T4 test generally aids in the diagnosis of hypothyroidism or hyperthyroidism. The test may also be used to help evaluate a patient with an enlarged thyroid gland, called a goiter. It may also aid in the diagnosis and monitoring of female infertility problems.

When Is It Ordered?

Thyroid hormone screening is commonly performed in newborns. In adults, a total T4 or free T4 test usually is ordered in response to an abnormal TSH test result.

What Does the Test Result Mean?

High free or total T4 results may indicate an overactive thyroid gland (hyperthyroidism).

Low free or total T4 results may indicate an underactive thyroid gland (hypothyroidism).

In most cases, test results are reported as numerical values rather than as high or low, positive or negative, or normal. In these instances, it is necessary to know the reference range for the particular test. However, reference ranges may vary by the patient's age, sex, as well as the instrumentation or kit used to perform the test.

Is There Anything Else I Should Know?

Many medications—including estrogen, certain types of birth control pills, and large doses of aspirin—can interfere with total T4 test results, so tell your doctor about any drugs you are taking. In general, free T4 levels are not affected by these medications.

In addition, total T4 levels may be affected by contrast material used for certain x-ray imaging tests.

TSH Thyroid Test

TSH testing is used to:

- diagnose a thyroid disorder in a person with symptoms,
- screen healthy adults for thyroid disorders as recommended by the American Thyroid Association,
- screen newborns for an underactive thyroid,
- monitor thyroid replacement therapy in people with hypothyroidism, and
- diagnose and monitor female infertility problems.

When Is It Ordered?

Your doctor orders this test if you show symptoms of a thyroid disorder. For example, symptoms of hyperthyroidism include heat intolerance, weight loss, rapid heartbeat, nervousness, insomnia, and breathlessness.

Common symptoms of hypothyroidism include fatigue, weakness, weight gain, slow heart rate, and cold intolerance.

The blood test may be ordered with other thyroid hormone tests and after a physical examination of your thyroid. TSH screening is routinely performed in newborns. The American Thyroid Association recommends that adults older than age 35 be screened for thyroid disease every five years.

What Does the Test Result Mean?

A high TSH result often means an underactive thyroid gland caused by failure of the gland (hypothyroidism). Rarely, a high TSH result can indicate a problem with the pituitary gland, such as a tumor, in what is known as secondary hyperthyroidism. A high TSH value can also occur in people with underactive thyroid glands who have been receiving too little thyroid hormone medication.

A low TSH result can indicate an overactive thyroid gland (hyperthyroidism). A low TSH result can also indicate damage to the pituitary gland that prevents it from producing TSH. A low TSH result can also occur in people with an underactive thyroid gland who are receiving too much thyroid hormone medication.

In most cases, test results are reported as numerical values rather than as high or low, positive or negative, or normal. In these instances, it is necessary to know the reference range for the particular test. However, reference ranges may vary by the patient's age, sex, as well as the instrumentation or kit used to perform the test.

Is There Anything Else I Should Know?

Many medications—including aspirin and thyroid-hormone replacement therapy—may interfere with thyroid gland function test results, so tell your doctor about any drugs you are taking.

When your doctor adjusts your dose of thyroid hormone, make sure you wait at least one to two months before you check your TSH again, so that your new dose can have its full effect.

Extreme stress and acute illness may also affect TSH test results, and results may be low during the first trimester of pregnancy.

Section 32.9

Cancer Tumor Markers

"Tumor Markers," Fact Sheet 5.18, National Cancer Institute (NCI), 1998.

Tumor markers are substances that can often be detected in higher-than-normal amounts in the blood, urine, or body tissues of some patients with certain types of cancer. Tumor markers are produced either by the tumor itself or by the body in response to the presence of cancer or certain benign (noncancerous) conditions. This section describes some tumor markers found in the blood.

Measurements of tumor marker levels can be useful—when used along with x-rays or other tests—in the detection and diagnosis of some types of cancer. However, measurements of tumor marker levels alone are not sufficient to diagnose cancer for the following reasons:

- Tumor marker levels can be elevated in people with benign conditions.

- Tumor marker levels are not elevated in every person with cancer—especially in the early stages of the disease.

- Many tumor markers are not specific to a particular type of cancer; the level of a tumor marker can be raised by more than one type of cancer.

In addition to their role in cancer diagnosis, some tumor marker levels are measured before treatment to help doctors plan appropriate therapy. In some types of cancer, tumor marker levels reflect the extent (stage) of the disease, and can be useful in predicting how well the disease will respond to treatment. Tumor marker levels may also be measured during treatment to monitor a patient's response to treatment. A decrease or return to normal in the level of a tumor marker may indicate that the cancer has responded favorably to therapy. If the tumor marker level rises, it may indicate that the cancer is growing. Finally, measurements of tumor marker levels may be used after treatment has ended as a part of follow-up care to check for recurrence.

Currently, the main use of tumor markers is to assess a cancer's response to treatment and to check for recurrence. Scientists continue to study these uses of tumor markers as well as their potential role in the early detection and diagnosis of cancer. The patient's doctor can explain the role of tumor markers in detection, diagnosis, or treatment for that person. Following are descriptions of some of the most commonly measured tumor markers.

Prostate-Specific Antigen (PSA)

Prostate-specific antigen (PSA) is present in low concentrations in the blood of all adult males. It is produced by both normal and abnormal prostate cells. Elevated PSA levels may be found in the blood of men with benign prostate conditions, such as prostatitis (inflammation of the prostate) and benign prostatic hyperplasia (BPH), or with a malignant (cancerous) growth in the prostate. While PSA does not allow doctors to distinguish between benign prostate conditions (which are very common in older men) and cancer, an elevated PSA level may indicate that other tests are necessary to determine whether cancer is present .

PSA levels have been shown to be useful in monitoring the effectiveness of prostate cancer treatment, and in checking for recurrence after treatment has ended. In checking for recurrence, a single test may show a mildly elevated PSA level, which may not be a significant change. Doctors generally look for trends, such as steadily increasing PSA levels in multiple tests over time, rather than focusing on a single elevated result.

Researchers are studying the value of PSA in screening men for prostate cancer (checking for the disease in men who have no symptoms). At this time, it is not known whether using PSA to screen for prostate cancer actually saves lives.

Researchers are also working on new ways to increase the accuracy of PSA tests. Improving the accuracy of PSA tests could help doctors distinguish BPH from prostate cancer, and thereby avoid unnecessary follow-up procedures, including biopsies.

Prostatic Acid Phosphatase (PAP)

Prostatic acid phosphatase (PAP) is normally present only in small amounts in the blood, but may be found at higher levels in some patients with prostate cancer, especially if the cancer has spread beyond the prostate. However, blood levels may also be elevated in patients who have certain benign prostate conditions or early stage cancer.

Although PAP was originally found to be produced by the prostate, elevated PAP levels have since been associated with testicular cancer, leukemia, and non-Hodgkin's lymphoma, as well as noncancerous conditions such as Gaucher's disease, Paget's disease, osteoporosis, cirrhosis of the liver, pulmonary embolism, and hyperparathyroidism.

CA 125

CA 125 is produced by a variety of cells, but particularly by ovarian cancer cells. Studies have shown that many women with ovarian cancer have elevated CA 125 levels. CA 125 is used primarily in the management of treatment for ovarian cancer. In women with ovarian cancer being treated with chemotherapy, a falling CA 125 level generally indicates that the cancer is responding to treatment. Increasing CA 125 levels during or after treatment, on the other hand, may suggest that the cancer is not responding to therapy or that some cancer cells remain in the body. Doctors may also use CA 125 levels to monitor patients for recurrence of ovarian cancer.

Not all women with elevated CA 125 levels have ovarian cancer. CA 125 levels may also be elevated by cancers of the uterus, cervix, pancreas, liver, colon, breast, lung, and digestive tract. Noncancerous conditions that can cause elevated CA 125 levels include endometriosis, pelvic inflammatory disease, peritonitis, pancreatitis, liver disease, and any condition that inflames the pleura (the tissue that surrounds the lungs and lines the chest cavity). Menstruation and pregnancy can also cause an increase in CA 125.

Carcinoembryonic Antigen (CEA)

Carcinoembryonic antigen (CEA) is normally found in small amounts in the blood of most healthy people, but may become elevated in people who have cancer or some benign conditions. The primary use of CEA is in monitoring colorectal cancer, especially when the disease has spread (metastasized). CEA is also used after treatment to check for recurrence of colorectal cancer. However, a wide variety of other cancers can produce elevated levels of this tumor marker, including melanoma; lymphoma; and cancers of the breast, lung, pancreas, stomach, cervix, bladder, kidney, thyroid, liver, and ovary.

Elevated CEA levels can also occur in patients with noncancerous conditions, including inflammatory bowel disease, pancreatitis, and liver disease. Tobacco use can also contribute to higher-than-normal levels of CEA.

Alpha-Fetoprotein (AFP)

Alpha-fetoprotein (AFP) is normally produced by a developing fetus. AFP levels begin to decrease soon after birth and are usually undetectable in the blood of healthy adults (except during pregnancy). An elevated level of AFP strongly suggests the presence of either primary liver cancer or germ cell cancer (cancer that begins in the cells that give rise to eggs or sperm) of the ovary or testicle. Only rarely do patients with other types of cancer (such as stomach cancer) have elevated levels of AFP. Noncancerous conditions that can cause elevated AFP levels include benign liver conditions such as; cirrhosis or hepatitis; ataxia telangiectasia; Wiskott-Aldrich syndrome; and pregnancy.

Human Chorionic Gonadotropin (HCG)

Human chorionic gonadotropin (HCG) is normally produced by the placenta during pregnancy. In fact, HCG is sometimes used as a pregnancy test because it increases early within the first trimester. It is also used to screen for choriocarcinoma (a rare cancer of the uterus) in women who are at high risk for the disease, and to monitor the treatment of trophoblastic disease (a rare cancer that develops from an abnormally fertilized egg). Elevated HCG levels may also indicate the presence of cancers of the testis, ovary, liver, stomach, pancreas, and lung. Pregnancy and marijuana use can also cause elevated HCG levels.

CA 19-9

Initially found in colorectal cancer patients, CA 19-9 has also been identified in patients with pancreatic, stomach, and bile duct cancer. Researchers have discovered that, in those who have pancreatic cancer, higher levels of CA 19-9 tend to be associated with more advanced disease. Noncancerous conditions that may elevate CA 19-9 levels include gallstones, pancreatitis, cirrhosis of the liver, and cholecystitis.

CA 15-3

CA 15-3 levels are most useful in following the course of treatment in women diagnosed with breast cancer, especially advanced breast cancer. CA 15-3 levels are rarely elevated in women with early stage breast cancer. Cancers of the ovary, lung, and prostate may also raise CA 15-3 levels. Elevated levels of CA 15-3 may be associated with noncancerous conditions such as benign breast or ovarian disease, endometriosis, pelvic inflammatory disease, and hepatitis. Pregnancy and lactation can also cause CA 15-3 levels to rise.

CA 27-29

Similar to the CA 15-3 antigen, CA 27-29 is found in the blood of most breast cancer patients. CA 27-29 levels may be used in conjunction with other procedures (such as mammograms and measurements of other tumor marker levels) to check for recurrence in women previously treated for stage II and stage III breast cancer.

CA 27-29 levels can also be elevated by cancers of the colon, stomach, kidney, lung, ovary, pancreas, uterus, and liver. First trimester pregnancy, endometriosis, ovarian cysts, benign breast disease, kidney disease, and liver disease are noncancerous conditions that can also elevate CA 27-29 levels.

Lactate Dehydrogenase (LDH)

Lactate dehydrogenase is a protein found throughout the body. Nearly every type of cancer, as well as many other diseases, can cause

LDH levels to be elevated. Therefore, this marker cannot be used to diagnose a particular type of cancer. LDH levels can be used to monitor treatment of some cancers, including testicular cancer, Ewing's sarcoma, non-Hodgkin's lymphoma, and some types of leukemia. Elevated LDH levels can be caused by a number of noncancerous conditions, including heart failure, hypothyroidism, anemia, and lung or liver disease.

Neuron-Specific Enolase (NSE)

Neuron-specific enolase (NSE) has been detected in patients with neuroblastoma; small cell lung cancer; Wilms' tumor; melanoma; and cancers of the thyroid, kidney, testicle, and pancreas. However, studies of NSE as a tumor marker have concentrated primarily on patients with neuroblastoma and small cell lung cancer. Measurement of NSE level in patients with these two diseases can provide information about the extent of the disease and the patient's prognosis, as well as about the patient's response to treatment.

Additional Information

Cancer Information Service
National Cancer Institute
Suite 3036A, MSC8322
6116 Executive Blvd.
Bethesda, MD 20892-8322
Toll-Free: 800-422-6237
Toll-Free TTY: 800-332-8615
Website: www.nci.nih.gov
E-mail: cancermail@icicc.nci.nih.gov

Chapter 33

Biopsy

Alternative names: Tissue sampling

Definition: A biopsy is the removal of a small piece of tissue for microscopic examination and/or culture, often to help the physician make a diagnosis.

How the Test Is Performed

The method of tissue removal varies among the type of biopsies:

- In a needle (percutaneous) biopsy, the tissue sample is simply obtained by use of a syringe. A needle is passed into the tissue to be biopsied, and cells are removed through the needle. Depending on the location of the tissue to be biopsied, needle biopsies are often performed under x-ray (usually CT scan) guidance.

- In an open biopsy, an incision is made in the skin, the organ is exposed, and a tissue sample is taken.

- Closed biopsy involves a much smaller incision than open biopsy. The small incision is made to allow insertion of a visualization device, which can guide the physician to the appropriate area to take the sample.

"Biopsy," © 2003 A.D.A.M., Inc. Reprinted with permission.

If the tissue to be sampled is in the abdomen and cannot be safely accessed with a needle or closed procedure, an open biopsy must be performed in the operating room.

How to Prepare for the Test

Check with your physician about stopping medications that can predispose to bleeding, such as aspirin, Coumadin, and nonsteroidal anti-inflammatory medications (NSAIDs). Also, mention any herbal preparations you are taking. Never change your medication regimen without first checking with your physician.

How the Test Will Feel

In a needle biopsy, you will feel a small sharp pinch at the site of the biopsy. In an open or closed biopsy, local or general anesthesia is generally used to make the procedure pain free.

Why the Test Is Performed

A biopsy may be performed to obtain healthy tissue which can be obtained for the purpose of tissue-type matching for transplants. Unhealthy tissues are more commonly biopsied to diagnose disease.

Normal Values

Normal tissue.

What Abnormal Results Mean

Abnormal biopsies mean that the material obtained differs from the usual structure or condition of the tissue. Abnormal results may indicate the presence of disease, such as cancer, depending on the particular case.

What the Risks Are

- Bleeding
- Infection

Special Considerations

The following list of biopsies indicates the many types of tissue that can be used for diagnosis and screening procedures:

- Bronchoscopy with transtracheal biopsy
- Carpal tunnel biopsy
- Bladder biopsy
- Lung needle biopsy
- Open lung biopsy
- Open pleural biopsy
- Skin lesion biopsy
- Abdominal wall fat pad biopsy
- Parathyroid biopsy
- Gum biopsy
- Nasal mucosal biopsy
- Tongue biopsy
- Oropharynx lesion biopsy
- Mediastinoscopy with biopsy
- Lymph node biopsy
- Biopsy of the biliary tract
- Small bowel biopsy
- Liver biopsy
- Adrenal biopsy
- Salivary gland biopsy
- Synovial biopsy
- Pleural needle biopsy
- Skinny-needle biopsy
- Thyroid excisional biopsy
- Muscle biopsy
- Bone marrow biopsy
- Nerve biopsy
- Renal biopsy
- Testicular biopsy
- Bone lesion biopsy
- Upper airway biopsy
- Ureteral retrograde brush biopsy cytology
- Rectal biopsy
- Myocardial biopsy
- Cervical biopsy
- Colposcopy-directed biopsy
- Breast biopsy
- Endometrial biopsy
- Cold cone biopsy
- Biopsy-polyps
- Chorionic villus biopsy

Chapter 34

Lumbar Puncture (Spinal Tap)

A lumbar puncture (LP) is a procedure in which a small amount of the fluid that surrounds the brain and spinal cord, called the cerebrospinal fluid or CSF, is removed and examined. This test is sometimes also called a spinal tap.

In infants and children, the most common reason for doing a lumbar puncture is to look for an infection of the meninges, the membrane covering the brain and spinal cord. This infection inflames the meninges, and it is called meningitis. There are other reasons to do lumbar punctures, too: sometimes they are done to remove fluid and relieve pressure with certain types of headaches, sometimes they are performed to look for bleeding in the central nervous system, and sometimes they are done to place chemotherapy medications into the spinal fluid.

What Happens during a Lumbar Puncture?

First, the child is positioned so that the spaces between the vertebrae (bones of the spine) are as wide as possible. Infants and small children lie on their sides curled up with their knees under their chin,

This information was provided by KidsHealth, one of the largest resources online for medically reviewed health information written for parents, kids, and teens. For more articles like this one, visit www.KidsHealth.org, or www.TeensHealth.org. © 2003 The Nemours Center for Children's Health Media, a division of The Nemours Foundation.

like the letter C. Teens may sit with their heads resting on a pillow placed on a table at waist level.

The skin covering the lower, or lumbar region, of the back is cleaned with an antibacterial solution and alcohol. The skin is then numbed with medication. Next, a small, hollow needle is inserted through the skin and then forward through the space between the vertebrae in the lower back until it enters the space that contains the spinal fluid. The spinal fluid drips out through the needle into a sequence of collection tubes and is sent to the lab for processing for a variety of tests. The pressure of the spinal fluid can also be measured as part of the test, which can provide important information. After the sample is collected (usually this takes a minute or so), the needle is withdrawn and a bandage is placed on the site.

The needle does not enter the spinal cord because the test is done in the lower back, below the level to which the spinal cord extends.

Understanding the Results

Fluid collected from a lumbar puncture is immediately sent to the laboratory and is processed right away in three different ways: one test looks at the chemical composition of the fluid, one test looks at the cells floating in it, and the third test searches for evidence that it's infected. Some of the results are available within 30 minutes. However, sometimes doctors may request a bacterial culture to watch for an organism growing in the sample. Culture results are usually available in 48 to 72 hours. If the doctor suspects the child has an infection, he or she may recommend starting antibiotic treatment while waiting for the results of the culture and then adjusting therapy, if needed, once the results are known.

The lab technicians look for a number of things when examining the spinal fluid sample, including:

- General appearance: spinal fluid is usually clear. Cloudy spinal fluid may indicate infection because of increased cells and proteins suspended in the fluid.

- Cell count: this includes the number of red blood cells and the number and type of white blood cells present. Spinal fluid normally does not contain significant numbers of either of these types of cells. The presence of large numbers of white cells usually indicates an infection.

- Protein: large amounts of protein in the spinal fluid also suggest an infection or other disease.

- Glucose: in bacterial infections of the spinal fluid, the glucose level of the fluid is often low.

- CSF gram stain and culture: the spinal fluid is also stained and examined under the microscope to look for bacteria. The staining technique used, called the gram stain, detects bacteria in the cerebrospinal fluid. To check for infection, it is also cultured to see if any organisms grow from the fluid.

- CSF may also be processed for other tests for which results are not available immediately.

Chapter 35

Stool Tests

Stool, also called feces, is usually thought of as nothing but waste—something to quickly flush away. But bowel movements can provide health care providers with valuable information as to what's wrong when your child has a problem in the stomach, intestines, or another part of the gastrointestinal system.

Your child's doctor may order a stool collection to test for a variety of possible conditions, including:

- allergy or inflammation in the body, such as part of the evaluation of milk protein allergy in infants;
- infection, as caused by some types of bacteria, viruses, or parasites that invade the gastrointestinal system;
- digestive problems, such as the malabsorption of certain sugars, fats, or nutrients; or
- bleeding inside of the gastrointestinal tract.

The most common reason to collect stool is to determine whether and what type of bacteria or parasite may be infecting the intestine. Many microscopic organisms live in the intestine that are necessary

This information was provided by KidsHealth, one of the largest resources online for medically reviewed health information written for parents, kids, and teens. For more articles like this one, visit www.KidsHealth.org, or www.TeensHealth.org. © 2003 The Nemours Center for Children's Health Media, a division of The Nemours Foundation.

for normal digestion. Sometimes, however, the intestine may become infected with harmful bacteria or parasites that cause a variety of conditions, such as certain types of bloody diarrhea. It may then be necessary to examine the stool under a microscope, culture the stool, and perform other tests to help find the cause of the problem.

Stools are also sometimes analyzed for the substances they contain. An example of stool analysis includes examining the fat content of stools. Normally, fat is completely absorbed from the intestine, and the stool contains virtually no fat. In certain types of digestive disorders, however, fat is incompletely absorbed and remains in the stool.

Collecting a Stool Specimen

Unlike most other lab tests, stool is sometimes collected by the child's family at home, not by a health care professional. Here are some tips for collecting a stool specimen from your child:

- Collecting stool can be messy, so be sure to wear latex gloves and wash your hands and your child's hands well afterward.

- Many children with diarrhea, especially young children, can't always let a parent know in advance when a bowel movement is coming. Sometimes a hat-shaped plastic lid is used to collect the stool specimen. This catching device can be quickly placed over the toilet bowl or your child's rear end to collect the specimen. Using a catching device can prevent contamination of the stool by water and dirt. If urine contaminates the stool sample, it will be necessary to take another sample. Also, if you're unable to catch your child's stool sample before it touches the inside of the toilet, the sample will need to be repeated.

- Another way to collect a stool sample is to loosely place plastic wrap over the lid of the toilet. Then place the stool sample in a clean, sealable container before taking to the laboratory. Plastic wrap can also be used to line the diaper of an infant or toddler who is not yet using the toilet.

Fishing a bowel movement out of the toilet does not provide a clean specimen for the laboratory to analyze.

The stool should be collected into clean, dry plastic jars with screw cap lids. These containers can be obtained from your health care provider or through hospital laboratories or pharmacies, although any clean, sealable container could do the job. For best results, the stool should then be brought to the laboratory immediately.

If it is impossible to get the sample to the laboratory right away, the stool should be refrigerated, then taken to the laboratory to be cultured as soon as possible after collection. When the sample arrives at the laboratory, it is either examined and cultured immediately or placed in a special liquid medium that attempts to preserve potential bacteria or parasites.

Your child's doctor or the hospital laboratory will usually provide written instructions on how to successfully collect a stool sample; if written instructions are not provided, take notes on how to collect the sample and what to do once you've collected it. If you have any questions about how to collect the specimen, be sure to ask. The doctor or the laboratory will also let you know if a fresh stool sample is needed for a particular test, and if it will need to be brought to the laboratory right away.

Most of the time, disease-causing bacteria or parasites can be identified from a single stool specimen. Sometimes, however, up to three samples from different bowel movements must be taken. Your child's provider will let you know if this is the case.

Testing the Stool Sample

In general, the results of stool tests are usually reported back within 3 to 4 days, although it often takes longer for parasite testing to be completed.

Examining the Stool for Blood

Your health care provider will sometimes check your child's stool for blood, which may be caused by certain kinds of infectious diarrhea, bleeding within the gastrointestinal tract, and other conditions. However, most of the time, blood streaking in the stool of an infant or toddler is from a slight rectal tear, called a fissure, which is caused by straining against a hard stool (this is fairly common in infants and children with ongoing constipation).

Testing for blood in the stool is often performed with a quick test in the office that can provide the results immediately. First, stool is smeared on a card, then a few drops of a developing solution are placed on the card. An instant color change shows that blood is present in the stool. Sometimes, stool is sent to a laboratory to test for blood, and the result will be reported within hours.

Culturing the Stool

Stool can be cultured for disease-causing bacteria. In a culture, a sample of the stool is placed in an incubator for at least 48 to 72 hours and any disease-causing bacteria in the stool are identified and isolated. Remember that not all bacteria in the stool cause problems; in fact, over 80% of stool is bacteria, most of which live there normally and are necessary for digestion. In a stool culture, lab technicians are most concerned with identifying bacteria that cause disease.

For a stool culture, the lab will need a fresh or refrigerated sample of stool. The best samples are of loose, fresh stool; well-formed stool is rarely positive for disease-causing bacteria. Sometimes, more than one stool will be collected for a culture.

Swabs from a child's rectum can also be tested for viruses. Although this procedure is not done routinely, it can sometimes give clues in the case of certain illnesses, especially in newborns or very ill children. Viral cultures can take a week or longer to grow, depending on the virus.

Testing the Stool for Ova and Parasites

Stool may be tested for the presence of parasites and ova (the egg stage of a parasite) if a child has prolonged diarrhea or other intestinal symptoms. Sometimes, the doctor will collect 2 or more samples of stool to successfully identify parasites. If parasites—or their eggs—are seen when a smear of stool is examined under the microscope, the child will be treated for a parasitic infestation. Your child's doctor may give you special collection containers that contain chemical preservatives for parasites.

Chapter 36

Strep Screen/Throat Culture

A child's throat can be sore for many reasons. When a sore throat is caused by an infection, the most common cause is a virus. In most cases, the soreness goes away as the infection does and almost always causes no further problems.

But about 15% of sore throats are caused by a more serious bacterial infection from germs known as group A streptococci, or strep. These germs cause strep throat, an infection that affects school-age children who develop a sore throat.

"Strep throat is more serious than the other 85% of sore throats, because if not treated with antibiotics, it sometimes can cause more serious pus-forming infections," says Frederick Meier, MD, a pathologist. In fact, the scientific name for the strep that causes sore throats is pyogenes, or pus-maker. Group A streptococci also produce toxins that can cause circulatory collapse (shock) in streptococcal toxic shock syndrome or fever and a rash in scarlet fever. Furthermore, strep-caused glomerulonephritis can damage the kidneys. Rheumatic fever can damage the heart, joints, and sometimes the brain. Damage from these poststreptococcal diseases can be life-threatening and even permanent.

This information was provided by KidsHealth, one of the largest resources online for medically reviewed health information written for parents, kids, and teens. For more articles like this one, visit www.KidsHealth.org, or www.TeensHealth.org. © 2003 The Nemours Center for Children's Health Media, a division of The Nemours Foundation.

Timely antibiotic treatment can dramatically decrease a child's chance of developing rheumatic fever and many of the other possible complications of a strep infection. Although a strep infection may come to a doctor's attention because of a skin infection, such as impetigo, the most common complaint is a sore throat. To determine whether a sore throat is caused by strep, either a strep screen or throat culture can be performed.

How Is a Strep Screen/Throat Culture Done?

In a strep screen or throat culture, the doctor or medical assistant wipes the back of your child's throat with a long cotton swab. In the laboratory, the swab is placed in a test tube with a chemical mix that extracts part of the strep germ from the swab. This extract is then combined with antibodies to the group A strep. (Antibodies are natural substances that attach to the group A strep bacteria's surface— just as they would in the body.) When a third substance is added to the tube, the liquid changes color if strep germs are present.

A positive test means your child would benefit from taking antibiotics to kill the strep germs. The test is 95% sensitive, meaning that it will detect the bacteria in 95 of 100 people with strep throat.

How Long Does It Take to Get the Results?

A rapid strep screen can offer results in minutes, whereas a throat culture takes 2 to 3 days. It's important to find out whether strep is the cause of the sore throat since early treatment for strep throat reduces symptoms and decreases the risk of rheumatic fever. Waiting for results will allow enough time to treat the strep and avoid the serious, preventable complications. Sometimes, depending on the severity of the illness and other specific circumstances, your child's doctor may begin antibiotic treatment while waiting for the culture results.

Chapter 37

Sweat Testing for Cystic Fibrosis

Sweat Testing Procedure and Commonly Asked Questions

The sweat test has been the gold standard for diagnosing cystic fibrosis (CF) for more than 40 years. When it is performed by trained technicians, and evaluated in an experienced, reliable laboratory, the sweat test is still the best test to diagnose CF. It is recommended that the sweat test be performed in a Cystic Fibrosis Foundation-accredited care center where strict guidelines are followed to ensure the accuracy of the results. The test can be performed on individuals of any age. However, some infants may not make enough sweat for the laboratory to analyze. If an infant does not produce enough sweat on the first sweat test, it should be repeated to collect more.

What Happens during a Sweat Test?

The sweat test determines the amount of chloride in the sweat. There are no needles involved in the procedure. In the first part of the test, a colorless, odorless chemical, known to cause sweating, is applied to a small area on an arm or leg. An electrode is then attached to the arm or leg, which allows the technician to apply a weak electrical current to the area to stimulate sweating. Individuals may feel a tingling sensation in the area, or a feeling of warmth. This part of

"Sweat Testing," © 2001 Cystic Fibrosis Foundation. Reprinted by permission. For further information about cystic fibrosis, visit www.cff.org.

the procedure lasts approximately five minutes. The second part of the test consists of cleaning the stimulated area and collecting the sweat on a piece of filter paper or gauze or in a plastic coil. Thirty minutes later, the collected sweat is sent to a hospital laboratory for analysis. The entire collection procedure takes approximately one hour.

What Does the Sweat Test Reveal?

Your physician has asked that this test be performed to rule out the presence of CF, an inherited disorder of the lungs, intestines, and sweat glands. Children and adults with CF have an increased amount of sodium and chloride (salt) in their sweat. In general, sweat chloride concentrations less than 40 mmol/L are normal (does not have CF); values between 40 to 60 mmol/L are borderline, and sweat chloride concentrations greater than 60 mmol/L are consistent with the diagnosis of CF. For individuals who have CF, the sweat chloride test will be positive from birth. Once a test result is positive, it is always positive. Sweat test values do not change from positive to negative or negative to positive as a person grows older. Sweat test values also do not vary when individuals have colds or other temporary illnesses.

Is There Any Preparation for the Sweat Test?

There are no restrictions on activity or diet or special preparations before the test. However, one should not apply creams or lotions to the skin 24 hours before the test. All regular medications may be continued and will have no effect on the test results.

When Are Sweat Test Results Made Available?

Sweat test results are usually available to your physician on the next working day after the test is performed. In a small number of cases, the quantity of sweat obtained is not sufficient to give an accurate result, and the test may need to be repeated.

Can the Test Results Be Inconclusive?

Yes. In a small number of cases, the test results fall into borderline range between not having CF and indicative of CF. In these situations, repeat sweat tests, as well as other diagnostic procedures, may need to be carried out. These will only be done after consultation with a physician.

Chapter 38

Urine Tests

Chapter Contents

Section 38.1

Urinalysis

This information was provided by KidsHealth, one of the largest resources online for medically reviewed health information written for parents, kids, and teens. For more articles like this one, visit www.KidsHealth.org. or www.TeensHealth.org. © 2003 The Nemours Center for Children's Health Media, a division of The Nemours Foundation. Also in this section, "24-Hour Urine Collection," Warren Grant Magnuson Clinical Center, National Institutes of Health, 1999.

Urinalysis

Examining urine for signs of disease has been recommended since at least the time of Hippocrates, the father of Western medicine, who told his followers to check urine color in those who were sick.

Kidneys act as filters for the bloodstream, purifying all the blood as it passes through them. The kidneys filter the equivalent of about 150 quarts of blood that recycles daily. The kidneys remove wastes and ensure that needed substances are left in the blood. Urine is produced by the kidneys when they remove soluble waste products from the body. Kidneys, like most of the organs of the body, perform a number of functions. Among their biological roles, kidneys help control blood pressure and synthesize an active form of vitamin D.

A urinalysis is most often ordered if a urinary tract infection is suspected, although there are other reasons why such a test could be useful. Like the complete blood count, a urinalysis can check on several different things:

- The number and kind of cells from the lining of the kidneys and bladder that have appeared in the urine;

- The number and variety of both red (RBCs) and white blood cells (WBCs);

- The presence of bacteria or other organisms;

- A variety of chemicals that the kidneys filter (when healthy or sick), such as glucose;

- The pH, measuring how acidic or basic the urine is;

- The concentration of the urine.

Sometimes results that may seem abnormal, such as the presence of white or red cells in the urine, may be the result of how or when the urine was collected rather than disease. For example, a dehydrated, crying child may have a few RBCs or WBCs in the urine. Once she is rehydrated, these "abnormal" results may disappear.

How Is a Urinalysis Done?

Urine is collected in a clean container. The first part of the test is the urine dipstick. Here, a plastic stick that has patches of chemical indicators on it (the dipstick) is placed in the urine. Depending on the color changes of the patches, various things will be revealed. These include the presence or absence of hemoglobin (found in red blood cells), white blood cells, sugar, and pH (whether the urine is acid or base).

The urine also is examined under a microscope. In addition to looking for red and white cells, the doctor or laboratory technologist can check for crystals, measure how concentrated the urine is, and perform other useful measures. In order to be accurate, the urine must be "fresh" when tested, and there needs to be enough collected.

How Long Will It Take to Get Results?

Some of the tests can be done rapidly. Some of the tests may take minutes to hours. As with all tests, it also depends on how busy the laboratory is. Most urinalyses are reported back within a few days.

Urine Culture

If a urinalysis shows white blood cells and bacteria, which may indicate infection in the kidneys or bladder, the doctor may decide to culture the urine. This will identify the kind of bacteria present.

"It is hard to get a good urine sample from children," says Dr. Fred Meier, a clinical laboratory expert, and it's easy to understand why. The skin around the urinary opening normally is home to the same bacteria that cause infection inside the body. Contamination with these bacteria can make the sample inaccurate or unusable. To avoid this, the skin surrounding the urinary opening must either be cleaned and rinsed immediately before the urine is collected, or bypassed through use of a catheter—a narrow, soft tube inserted gently through the urinary tract opening (urethra) into the bladder.

How Is a Urine Culture Done?

In the "clean-catch" method, the patient (or parent) cleans the skin around the urethra, urinates, stops urination, and then urinates again into the collection container. Catching urine in "midstream" is the goal. "Understandably, this is difficult for young children to do," said Dr. Meier. The "clean-catch" method may be difficult for girls under four or five, who have most of the urinary infections. Very young children who are not yet toilet trained and need a urine culture may be catheterized to obtain an accurate specimen.

How Long Does It Take until the Culture Is Done?

About 48–72 hours.

24-Hour Urine Collection

You have been asked to collect a 24-hour urine sample. This procedure checks the function of your kidneys or measures certain products in your urine. For accurate results, it is important to collect all your urine for exactly 24 hours.

Preparation

1. Before you begin the collection, you will be given a urine collection container (a urinal for males, a "hat" for females), a urine storage container, and a name tag. You may need more than one storage container to contain all of your urine for the 24-hour period.

2. Make sure each storage container has a name tag with your full name and hospital number written on it. If your container is not labeled properly, you may be asked to repeat the 24-hour collection.

3. Keep your storage container refrigerated throughout the 24-hour collection period until you bring it back to the clinical center. If you do not have access to a refrigerator, your collection should be kept on ice or in a cooler.

4. Some tests require using a double storage container or adding a preservative to the storage container. If you need a double

container, preservative, or if there are special instructions to follow, your doctor or nurse will tell you.

5. If you are staying on an inpatient unit during your 24-hour urine collection, your nurse will make sure your container is labeled correctly and show you where to keep your storage container.

Procedure

1. Start the 24-hour urine test by urinating directly into the toilet. Do not save this urine. After you urinate, write the date and time on your storage container. For the next 24 hours, urinate first into your collection container, then pour the urine into your storage container.

2. If you need to use more than one container during the 24-hour period, use one container at a time. When it is full, collect your urine in the next container.

3. Exactly 24 hours after you started the test, urinate one last time and place the urine in your storage container. This is the end of your test. Write the date and time the test ended on your storage container.

4. Take the urine to the clinical center as soon as possible. To prevent leaks, make sure the lid is on tightly, and that the container is transported upright inside a plastic bag. If the weather is warm and you must travel a long distance, transport your urine container on ice or in a cooler.

5. If you are an inpatient, your nurse will tell you what time to begin and end the collection and will set up more containers, as needed.

If you have questions about the procedure, please ask. Your nurse and doctor are ready to assist you at all times.

Section 38.2

Urodynamic Testing

"Urodynamic Testing," National Institute of Diabetes and Digestive and Kidney Diseases (NIDDK), NIH Publication No. 02-5106, May 2002.

If you have a problem with urine leakage or blocked urine flow, your doctor or nurse can help. One of the first steps may be urodynamic testing to find precisely what the problem is.

Several muscles, organs, and nerves are involved in collecting, storing, and releasing urine. The kidneys form urine by filtering wastes and extra water from the bloodstream. The ureters are tubes that carry urine from the kidneys to the bladder. Normal urine flow is one way. If urine backs up toward the kidneys, infections are more likely.

The bladder, a hollow muscular organ shaped like a balloon, sits in the pelvis and is held in place by ligaments attached to other organs and to the pelvic bones. The bladder stores urine until you are ready to empty it. It swells into a round shape when it is full and gets smaller as it empties. A healthy bladder can hold up to 16 ounces (2 cups) of urine comfortably for 2 to 5 hours.

The bladder opens into the urethra, the tube that allows urine to pass outside the body. Circular muscles called sphincters close tightly to keep urine from leaking. The involuntary leakage of urine is called incontinence.

Nerves in the bladder tell you when it is time to empty your bladder. When the bladder begins to fill with urine, you may notice a feeling that you need to urinate. The sensation becomes stronger as the bladder continues to fill and reaches its limit. At that point, nerves in the bladder send a message to the brain, and your urge to urinate intensifies.

When you are ready to urinate, the brain signals the sphincter muscles to relax. At the same time, the brain signals the bladder muscles to tighten, squeezing urine out. Urine can then leave the bladder through the urethra. When these signals occur in the correct order, normal urination occurs.

Problems in the urinary system can be caused by aging, illness, or injury. The muscles in your ureters, bladder, and urethra tend to become weaker with age. You may have more urinary infections because your bladder muscles have weakened and cannot empty your bladder completely. Also, weakening of the muscles of the sphincters and the pelvis can cause incontinence because the sphincter cannot remain tight enough to hold urine in the bladder or does not have enough support from the pelvic muscles.

Urodynamics is the study of how the body stores and releases urine. Urodynamic tests help your doctor or nurse see how well your bladder and sphincter muscles work and can help explain symptoms such as:

- incontinence
- frequent urination
- sudden, strong urges to urinate
- problems starting a urine stream
- painful urination
- problems emptying your bladder completely
- recurrent urinary tract infections

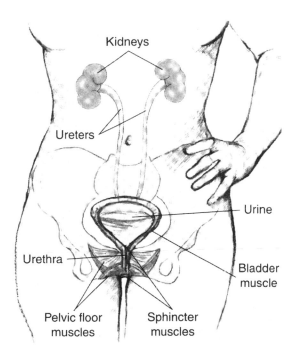

Figure 38.1. *Urinary Tract*

These tests may involve imaging equipment that films urination or may be as simple as urinating behind a curtain while a doctor or nurse listens.

Seeing Your Doctor or Nurse

The first step in solving a urinary problem is to talk to your doctor or nurse. He or she should ask you about your general medical history, including any major illnesses or surgeries. You should talk about the medicines you take, both prescription and nonprescription, because they might be part of the problem. You should talk about how much fluid you drink a day and whether you use alcohol or caffeine. Give as many details as you can about the problem and when it started. The doctor or nurse may ask you to keep a voiding diary, which is a record of fluid intake and trips to the bathroom, plus any episodes of leakage.

If leakage is the problem, a pad test is a simple way to measure how much urine seeps out. You will be given a number of absorbent pads and plastic bags of a standard weight. You will be told to wear the pad for 1 or 2 hours and then seal it in a bag. Your health care team will then weigh the bags to see how much urine has been caught in the pad. A simpler but less precise method is to change pads as often as you need to and keep track of how many pads you use in a day.

A physical exam will also be performed to rule out other causes of urinary problems, such as weakening pelvic muscles or prostate enlargement.

Preparing for the Test

If the doctor or nurse recommends bladder testing, usually no special preparations are needed, but make sure you understand any instructions you do receive. Depending on the test, you may be asked to come with a full bladder or an empty one. Also, ask whether you should change your diet or skip your regular medicines and for how long.

Taking the Test

Any procedure designed to provide information about a bladder problem can be called a urodynamic test. The type of test you take depends on your problem.

Most urodynamic testing focuses on the bladder's ability to empty steadily and completely. It can also show whether the bladder is having abnormal contractions that cause leakage. Your doctor will want to know whether you have difficulty starting a urine stream, how hard you have to strain to maintain it, whether the stream is interrupted, and whether any urine is left in your bladder when you are done (postvoid residual). Urodynamic tests can range from simple observation to precise measurement using sophisticated instruments.

Uroflowmetry: Measurement of Urine Speed and Volume

A uroflowmeter automatically measures the amount of urine and the flow rate (how fast the urine comes out). You may be asked to urinate privately into a toilet that contains a collection device and scale. This equipment creates a graph that shows changes in flow rate from second to second so the doctor or nurse can see the peak flow rate and how many seconds it took to get there. This test will be abnormal if the bladder muscle is weak or urine flow is obstructed.

Your doctor or nurse can also get some idea of your bladder function by using a stopwatch to time you as you urinate into a graduated container. The volume of urine is divided by the time to see what your average flow rate is. For example, 330 milliliters (mL) of urine in 30 seconds means that your average flow rate is 11 mL per second.

Measurement of Postvoid Residual

After you have finished, you may still have some urine, usually only an ounce or two, remaining in your bladder. To measure this postvoid residual, the doctor or nurse may remove it with a catheter, a thin tube that can be gently glided into the urethra. Ultrasound equipment that uses harmless sound waves to create a picture of the bladder can also be used. A postvoid residual of more than 200 mL, about half a pint, is a clear sign of a problem. Even 100 mL, about half a cup, requires further evaluation. However, the amount of postvoid residual can be different each time you urinate.

Cystometry: Measurement of Bladder Pressure

A cystometrogram (CMG) measures how much your bladder can hold, how much pressure builds up inside your bladder as it stores urine, and how full it is when you feel the urge to urinate. The doctor or nurse will use a catheter to empty your bladder completely. Then a special, smaller catheter with a pressure-measuring tube called a cystometer will be used to fill your bladder slowly with warm water. Another catheter may be placed in the rectum to record pressure there as well. You will be asked how your bladder feels and when you feel the need to urinate. The volume of water and the bladder pressure will be recorded. You may be asked to cough or strain during this procedure. Involuntary bladder contractions can be identified.

Measurement of Leak Point Pressure

While your bladder is being filled for the CMG, it may suddenly contract and squeeze some water out without warning. The cystometer will record the pressure at the point when the leakage occurred. This reading may provide information about the kind of bladder problem you have. You may also be asked to try to exhale while holding your nose and mouth to apply abdominal pressure to the bladder, cough, or shift positions. These actions help the doctor or nurse evaluate your sphincter muscles.

Pressure Flow Study

After the CMG, you will be asked to empty your bladder so that the catheter can measure the pressures required to urinate. This pressure

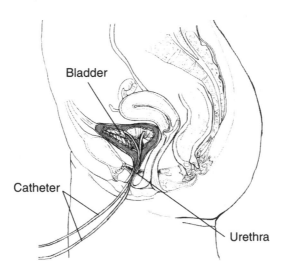

Figure 38.2. *Cystometry in a Female Patient*

flow study helps to identify bladder outlet obstruction that men may experience with prostate enlargement. Bladder outlet obstruction is less common in women, but can occur with a fallen bladder or rarely after a surgical procedure for urinary incontinence. Some catheters can be used for both CMG and pressure flow studies.

Electromyography: Measurement of Nerve Impulses

If your doctor or nurse thinks that your urinary problem is related to nerve damage, you may be given an electromyography test. This test measures the muscle activity in the urethral sphincter using sensors placed on the skin near the urethra and rectum. Sometimes the sensors are on the urethral or rectal catheter. Muscle activity is recorded on a machine. The patterns of these impulses will show whether the messages sent to the bladder and urethra are coordinated correctly.

Video Urodynamics

Urodynamic tests may be performed with or without equipment to take pictures of the bladder during filling and emptying. The imaging equipment may use x-rays or sound waves. If x-ray equipment is used, the liquid used to fill the bladder may be a contrast medium that will show up on the x-ray. The pictures and videos show the size and shape of the urinary tract and help your doctor or nurse understand your problem.

After the Test

You may have mild discomfort for a few hours after these tests. Drinking two 8-ounce glasses of water each hour for 2 hours should help. Ask your doctor whether you can take a warm bath. If not, you may be able to hold a warm, damp washcloth over the urethral opening to relieve the discomfort.

Your doctor may give you an antibiotic to take for 1 or 2 days to prevent an infection. If you have signs of infection—including pain, chills, or fever—call your doctor at once.

Getting the Results

Results for simple tests can be discussed with your doctor or nurse immediately after the test. Other tests may take a few days. You will have the chance to ask questions about the results and possible treatments for your problem.

Additional Information

American Foundation for Urologic Disease
1128 North Charles Street
Baltimore, MD 21201
Toll-Free: 800-828-7866
Phone: 410-468-1800
Website: www.afud.org
E-mail: admin@afud.org

Interstitial Cystitis Association of America, Inc.
110 N. Washington St., Suite 340
Rockville, MD 20850
Toll-Free: 800-HELP-ICA
Phone: 301-610-5300
Fax: 301-610-5308
Website: www.ichelp.org
E-mail: icamail@ichelp.org

National Kidney and Urologic Diseases Information Clearinghouse
3 Information Way
Bethesda, MD 20892-3580
Toll-Free: 800-891-5390
Phone: 301-654-4415
Fax: 301-907-8906
Website: http://kidney.niddk.nih.gov
E-mail: nkudic@info.niddk.nih.gov

Section 38.3

Bladder Cancer Test Approved for General Screening

Reprinted with permission from "A Kinder, Gentler Bladder Cancer Test" by Mark Moran, MPH, WebMD Medical News Archive, January 16, 2001. © 2001 WebMD Corporation. All rights reserved.

A simple, painless urine test may soon help doctors tell which patients with bladder cancer are at risk for having the disease recur. That's important because such cancer reappears about 80% of the time, say researchers from Yale University, and the current method used to test for it—which involves inserting a scope through the urethra into the bladder—is quite uncomfortable for patients.

That method, called a cystoscopy, might become just an unpleasant memory if the Yale team's urine test continues to prove effective. The new test looks for the presence of something called survivin in the urine, says Dario Altieri, MD, professor of pathology at the Yale School of Medicine in New Haven, Connecticut.

Altieri explains that survivin is a natural substance that hinders apoptosis, the body's built-in system of killing off unnecessary cells. "For this reason, survivin is very important during fetal development," Altieri says. "By inhibiting apoptosis, it helps keep cells alive."

In the case of cancer cells, which are multiplying out of control, it is not surprising that there is an excess of survivin. "The molecule helps preserve the viability of cancer cells and makes them more resistant to chemotherapy," Altieri says.

In collaboration with physicians from Yale's department of surgery, Altieri devised a strategy for exploiting this phenomenon to determine if a patient with a history of bladder cancer is at risk for having the cancer come back."

The assumption is that if there were a tumor in the bladder, the tumor cells, which would be released in the urine, would contain the survivin molecule," he says. "We reasoned that we might be able to detect it with a simple urine test." Their hunch appears to be borne out.

Altieri and colleagues surveyed urine samples from various groups of individuals: healthy volunteers, patients with noncancerous urinary tract disease, patients with genitourinary cancer, and patients with bladder cancer. They found that survivin was detected in the urine samples of all of the patients with new or recurrent bladder cancer, but was not found in healthy volunteers or in patients with prostate, kidney, vaginal, or cervical cancer.

The results indicate a high degree of test sensitivity, Altieri says, meaning the presence of the molecule is a strong signal a tumor is present. At the same time, however, he notes that three of the patients with noncancerous urinary tract disease, and one patient with increased prostate specific-antigen, also tested positive for survivin. This indicates the test may not be perfectly specific for bladder cancer and could therefore lead to false-positive results.

"Clearly, this study needs to be expanded in a much larger population," Altieri cautions. "We are following the three individuals who had a false-positive test and have found after six months had elapsed, that one of them did develop bladder cancer."

While more research is necessary, and approval by the FDA is required before the test can become routinely available, Altieri says the technology for performing the test already is available and could be performed by doctors at low cost. Ultimately, if proven successful in future research, the test may be best used in combination with other diagnostic tests.

The survivin study is particularly promising because of the invasive and uncomfortable nature of cystoscopy, says Sudhir Srivastava, PhD, MPH, chief of the cancer biomarkers research group at the National Cancer Institute. He says the effort to use survivin to detect bladder cancer recurrence is part of a broad scientific effort to develop biomarkers for a variety of diseases. But the problem of false-positives is one that plagues many of these efforts, some of which have been highly touted by commercial companies without appropriate scientific validation. "For many years, we have been discovering biomarkers and leaving it there, without taking it further along to prove whether they are clinically applicable," Srivastava says. "Validation studies are not very glamorous and do not get the same kind of funding and attention that discovery does."

For that reason, the NCI has developed an Early Detection Research Network to shepherd research on biomarkers from discovery to validation. And Srivastava says that the NCI is likely to instigate large-scale trials of survivin to validate the results found by Altieri and colleagues. "Anyone who has a cancer is looking for the light at the end of the tunnel," he says. "Naturally, they hope to be the first one to use it. We owe it to them to have something that has been proven." The study by Altieri and colleagues appeared in the Jan. 17, 2001 edition of the *Journal of the American Medical Association.*

Part Six

Imaging Tests

Chapter 39

X-Rays

Chapter Contents

Section 39.1

Bone Radiography

This section includes "Diagnostic X-Rays," reprinted with permission from the Beth Israel Deaconess Medical Center, Department of Radiology, © 2003 Beth Israel Deaconess Medical Center. All Rights Reserved. For additional information, visit http://radiology.bidmc.harvard.edu/. Also, "We Want You to Know about X-Rays: Get the Picture on Protection," Center for Devices and Radiological Health (CDRH), U.S. Food and Drug Administration (FDA), 1999.

Diagnostic X-Rays

This is the original field from which radiology developed, and is probably still the most commonly employed form of radiology. X-rays can be either still images or movies, and can often be done quickly. They are frequently used to complement other kinds of radiology as well. The films created by x-rays show different features of the body in various shades of gray. The gray is darkest in those areas that do not absorb x-rays well; the grays are lighter in dense areas (like bones) that absorb more of the x-rays. Some x-ray exams improve visibility by using contrast, a range of substances which may be introduced into the patient by swallowing, injection, or enema.

Types of Diagnostic X-Ray Exams

There are many kinds of x-rays. Most of them (for example, chest x-rays) don't require any special preparation by the patient. The following list includes some of the x-ray tests that do require special preparation on your part.

- Barium enema
- Gall bladder exam
- GI (gastrointestinal) series
- Hysterosalpingogram
- IVP (intravenous pyelogram)
- Lumbar puncture myelogram

398

We Want You to Know about X-Rays: Get the Picture on Protection

Will you be one of the 7 out of 10 Americans who will get a medical or dental x-ray picture this year? Most of the time that's fine because the x-ray will help your doctor find out what's wrong and decide how you should be treated The information from diagnostic x-rays can even save your life.

But sometimes x-rays are taken when they're not medically needed. And even when there is a good medical reason for an x-ray, if proper care is not taken, the patient can get more radiation than necessary. Like many things, x-rays may do harm as well as good. X-rays may add slightly to the chance of getting cancer in later life. And if the sex organs are in or near the x-ray beam, changes could be produced in the reproductive cells. Those changes might be passed on and could cause harm in future children and grandchildren.

Because of the amount of radiation used in x-ray examinations is small, the chance that x-rays will cause these problems is very low. Still, it makes sense to avoid unnecessary risks, no matter how small. By avoiding x-rays that aren't medically needed, you avoid the risks, and you can also avoid unnecessary medical costs. You may now be asking, "How many x-ray exams are safe?" There's really no answer to this question. There is no number that is definitely safe, just as there is no number that is definitely dangerous. Every x-ray can involve some tiny risk. If the x-ray is needed to find out about a medical problem, then that small risk is certainly worth taking.

Here's what you can do:

Ask how it will help to find out what's wrong. How will it help determine your treatment? Feel free to talk with your doctor; you have a right to understand why an x-ray is suggested.

Don't refuse an x-ray if the doctor explains why it is medically needed. Remember, the risk of not having a needed x-ray is greater than the tiny risk from the radiation.

Don't insist on an x-ray. Sometimes doctors give in to people who ask for an x-ray, even if it isn't medically needed.

Tell the doctor if you are, or think you might be pregnant before having an x-ray of your abdomen or lower back. Because the unborn baby is growing so quickly, it can be more easily affected by radiation than a grownup. If you need an abdominal x-ray during your pregnancy, remember that the chance of harm to the unborn baby is very tiny. But be sure to talk with your doctor.

Keep up on new mammography information. There is agreement that mammography (breast x-rays) is important in the fight against breast cancer. But scientific information is still growing on the proper role of mammography. Right now it is believed that women more likely to need mammography are those with symptoms, those past menopause, or those with a personal or family history of breast cancer. Talk with your doctor about the value of breast x-rays in your particular case.

Ask if a gonad shield can be used if you or your children are to have x-rays of the lower back, abdomen, or near the sex organs. A lead shield over the sex organs can keep x-rays from reaching your reproductive cells, thereby protecting future generations. Gonad shielding should be considered if the patient might have children in the future. But remember, a shield can't always be used, particularly over the female ovaries, because it may hide what the doctor needs to see on the x-ray.

Keep an x-ray record card. When an x-ray is taken, have the date, the type of exam, and where the x-ray is kept, filled out on the card. Then, if another doctor suggests an x-ray of the same part of your body, you can tell him or her about the previous x-ray. Sometimes the doctor can use the previous x-ray instead of taking a new one. Or, if a new x-ray is needed, the previous one might help show any change in your medical problem. Keep a record card for everyone in your family.

Section 39.2

Hysterosalpingogram

Reprinted with permission from the Beth Israel Deaconess Medical Center, Department of Radiology. © 2003 Beth Israel Deaconess Medical Center. All Rights Reserved. For additional information, visit http://radiology.bidmc.harvard.edu.

What is a hysterosalpingogram?

A hysterosalpingogram is an x-ray exam of the uterus and the fallopian tubes.

How do I prepare for this exam?

It is important that this exam be scheduled seven to ten days after the first day of your last menstrual period. There are no dietary restrictions. For maximum comfort, your doctor may recommend that you take 400 mg Motrin one hour before the exam. Motrin (ibuprofen) is available from your local pharmacy.

Can I take my usual medication?

You may take medications.

What will happen in the x-ray room?

A radiologist and a technologist will administer the exam. You will be placed in a position similar to a routine pelvic exam. The radiologist will clean off your skin with a sterile iodine solution to prevent infection, cover you with a sterile towel, and insert a speculum. The radiologist will place a small catheter into the cervical canal and inject an x-ray dye to visualize the uterus and fallopian tubes. The radiologist will watch on a special x-ray television screen. At intervals, the radiologist will ask you to hold your breath, to breathe out, or to change your position so that snapshots or spot films may be taken.

Special note: For your comfort, a companion may accompany you. Also, for 24 hours after the test do not douche, use tampons, or have intercourse. You may take Tylenol or Motrin as needed for minor cramps. It is normal to have some spotting or light bleeding, but if you have heavy bleeding or a fever at any time following this procedure, call your doctor immediately.

Will the exam hurt?

There may be some cramping associated with the injection of the x-ray dye.

How long will the exam take?

The exam will take about 30 to 45 minutes.

How will I learn the results?

Your primary-care physician will discuss the results with you.

Section 39.3

Intravenous Pyelogram

"IVP X-Ray," reprinted with permission from the Beth Israel Deaconess Medical Center, Department of Radiology. © 2003 Beth Israel Deaconess Medical Center. All Rights Reserved. For additional information, visit http://radiology.bidmc.harvard.edu.

Intravenous Pyelogram

An IVP is a special x-ray exam of your kidneys and other parts of your urinary system. This includes your ureters (the tubes leading from the kidneys) and your bladder. Another name for this test it IV urogram.

How do I prepare for this exam?

In order to see the kidneys well on x-ray, the bowel needs to be cleaned out. This is done by following a simple diet.

- On the day before your exam, eat a light lunch and dinner. An example of a light meal would be: clear soup, plain chicken or turkey, broiled meat, mashed potatoes, and Jell-O. Do not eat heavy food or roughage.

- At your drug store, buy a ten ounce bottle of magnesium citrate. You do not need a prescription.

- Drink it at 8 p.m. on the night before your test. Drink as much clear fluid as you can during the evening. Clear fluid includes: water, apple juice, and tea/coffee without milk or cream. But stop eating solid food after 8 p.m. On the day of the exam, do not eat solid food. You may continue to drink clear liquids up until 3 hours before your appointment.

- If you have a history of severe allergies or asthma, you may be asked to take some medicine called prednisone before your scan. Please ask your doctor for more information.

Special note: If you are scheduled for any other test on the same day, please be sure to ask if there are any dietary requirements. If there are, please consult your doctor or call the radiology department.

If you have asthma or any allergies to foods or medications, be sure to inform the technologist and the radiologist before the test.

What about my medications?

If you need regular medications on the morning of your test, take them with water.

I have diabetes. Are there special instructions for me?

- If you are a diabetic and take insulin or another medicine for diabetes, please check with you doctor to see if your medicine will have to be adjusted while you are not eating.

- If you are taking Glucophage (metformin), for diabetes, please be sure to tell the person doing your exam. You will be given special instructions about your medication.

What else do I need to know?

- If you have asthma or any allergies to foods or medications, be sure to tell the people who are doing your exam. Also, be sure to tell them about any reactions to x-ray dye you've had in the past. Tell them even if you think the information is on your record, or you think they already know about it. This is for your safety. You will be getting a dye for this test, and some people who have allergies are also allergic to the dye.

- If you have been scheduled for any other x-ray test on the same day as your IVP, call the radiology department to make sure one test will not interfere with the other.

What will happen during the test?

First, a technologist will take a test x-ray to see if your bowel is empty enough for the test. If there is a lot of gas or bowel contents over the kidneys, your test may need to be rescheduled. If not, an IV (intravenous) line will be started in your arm.

You will be given a special x-ray dye through the IV. This dye will outline the kidneys and urinary system so they can be seen on x-ray. This will show the radiologist (the doctor who reads the x-rays) how well your kidneys are working, and the structure of your urinary system. After the injection, a number of x-rays will be taken. Each time, you will be asked to hold your breath for a brief period.

After the radiologist has seen your bladder fill with dye, you will be asked to go to the bathroom to urinate. Then, an x-ray of your empty bladder will be taken.

Will it hurt?

No. However, some people experience a mild feeling of warmth or coolness with the injection. Others experience a metallic taste. If you experience nausea or breathing difficulties, please inform the technologist.

How long will the exam take?

The exam takes about one hour. Occasionally, more time is necessary when delayed films need to be taken.

When may I eat?

In most cases, you may eat as soon as the exam is over.

How will I learn the results?

Your doctor will discuss the results with you.

Section 39.4

Lower Gastrointestinal (GI) Series

"Lower GI Series," National Institute of Diabetes and Digestive and Kidney Diseases (NIDDK), NIH Publication No. 02-4331, February 2002.

A lower gastrointestinal (GI) series uses x-rays to diagnose problems in the large intestine, which includes the colon and rectum. The lower GI series may show problems like abnormal growths, ulcers, polyps and diverticuli, and colon cancer.

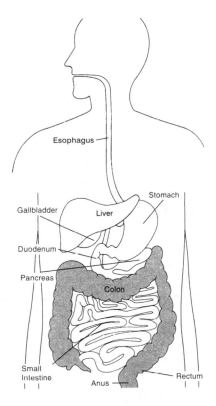

Figure 39.1. The Digestive System: Lower GI Series

Before taking x-rays of your colon and rectum, the radiologist will put a thick liquid called barium into your colon. This is why a lower GI series is sometimes called a barium enema. The barium coats the lining of the colon and rectum and makes these organs, and any signs of disease in them, show up more clearly on x-rays. It also helps the radiologist see the size and shape of the colon and rectum.

You may be uncomfortable during the lower GI series. The barium will cause fullness and pressure in your abdomen and will make you feel the urge to have a bowel movement. However, that rarely happens because the tube used to inject the barium has a balloon on the end of it that prevents the liquid from coming back out.

You may be asked to change positions while x-rays are taken. Different positions give different views of the intestines. After the radiologist is finished taking x-rays, you will be able to go to the bathroom. The radiologist may also take an x-ray of the empty colon afterwards.

A lower GI series takes about 1 to 2 hours. The barium may cause constipation and make your stool turn gray or white for a few days after the procedure.

Preparation

Your colon must be empty for the procedure to be accurate. To prepare for the procedure you will have to restrict your diet for a few days beforehand. For example, you might be able to drink only liquids and eat only foods that do not contain sugar or dairy products for 2 days before the procedure; only clear liquids the day before; and nothing after midnight the night before. A liquid diet means fat-free bouillon or broth, gelatin, strained fruit juice, water, plain coffee, plain tea, or diet soda. To make sure your colon is empty, you will be given a laxative or an enema before the procedure. Your physician may give you other special instructions.

Additional Information

National Digestive Diseases Information Clearinghouse
2 Information Way
Bethesda, MD 20892-3570
Toll-Free: 800-891-5389
Phone: 301-654-3810
Fax: 301-907-8906
Website: http://digestive.niddk.nih.gov
E-mail: nddic@info.niddk.nih.gov

Section 39.5

Mammography

This section is excerpted from PDQ® Cancer Information Summary. National Cancer Institute; Bethesda, MD. Screening for Breast Cancer (PDQ®): Health Professional. Updated 06/19/2002. Available at: http://cancer.gov. Accessed October, 28, 2003.

Mammography utilizes ionizing radiation to image breast tissue. The examination is performed by compressing the breast firmly between a plastic plate and an x-ray cassette which contains special x-ray film. For routine screening, examination films are taken in mediolateral oblique and craniocaudal projections. Both views should include breast tissue from the nipple to the pectoral muscle. Studies have shown that two-view examinations decrease the recall rate for suspicious findings found at screening mammography, compared to single view examinations. A retrospective analysis of 61,273 screening mammograms showed that 3.3% of studies had false positives due to superimposition of normal breast structures. About half of these false positives could be eliminated by performance of two-view studies and 29% by additional diagnostic imaging.[1]

Under the Mammography Quality Standards Act (MQSA) enacted by Congress in 1992, all facilities that perform mammography must be certified by the U.S. Food and Drug Administration (FDA). This mandate has resulted in improved mammography technique, lower radiation dose, and better training of personnel. Image contrast has improved with the use of lower voltage, specialized aluminum grids, and higher film optical density. The 1998 MQSA Reauthorization Act requires that patients receive a written lay-language summary of mammography results.

Mammography can identify breast cancers too small to palpate on physical examination, and can also find ductal carcinoma in situ (DCIS), a noninvasive condition. Since all cancers develop as a consequence of a series of mutations, it is theoretically beneficial to diagnose these noninvasive lesions. A large increase in the frequency of DCIS diagnosis occurred in the United States beginning in the early 1980s[2] due to the increased use of screening mammography. Appropriate management of DCIS is not well understood, because its natural history is incompletely defined.

Numerous uncontrolled trials and retrospective series have documented the capacity of mammography to diagnose small, early-stage breast cancers, including those that have a favorable clinical course.[3] These trials also show that cancer-related survival is better in screened compared to nonscreened women. These comparisons are susceptible, however, to a number of important biases:

1. Lead-time bias: Survival time for a cancer found mammographically includes the time between detection and when it would have become detected because of clinical symptoms, but this time is not included in the survival time of those found because of symptoms.

2. Length bias: Mammography detects a cancer while it is preclinical and preclinical durations vary; cancers with longer preclinical durations are more likely to be detected by screening and these cancers tend to be slow growing and to have good prognoses.

3. Overdiagnosis bias, which is an extreme form of length bias: Screening may find cancers that are very slow growing and that would never have become manifest clinically.

4. Healthy volunteer bias: The screened population may be healthier or more health conscious than the general population. Since the extent of these biases is never clear in a particular study, one must rely on randomized controlled trials to assess the benefits of screening.

The sensitivity of mammography is the proportion of breast cancer detected when breast cancer is present. Sensitivity depends on several factors, including lesion size, lesion conspicuity, breast tissue density, patient age, the hormone status of the tumor, overall image quality, and interpretive skill of the radiologist. Sensitivity is of great importance to patients and physicians alike; failure to diagnose breast cancer is the most common cause of medical malpractice litigation. Half of the cases resulting in payment to the claimant had negative mammograms.[4]

Retrospective correlations of mammographic findings with population-based cancer registries show that sensitivity ranges from 54% to 58% in women under age 40 to 81% to 94% in those over 65.[5,6] Using data from screened women in the Group Health Cooperative of Puget Sound health maintenance organization, characteristics of 150 cancers not detected at screening, but diagnosed within 24 months of a normal screening examination (interval cancers), were compared with those of 279 screen-detected cancers. Interval cancers were much more likely to occur in women under 50, and to be of mucinous or lobular histology, high histologic grade, and high proliferative activity. Screen-detected cancers were more likely to have tubular histology, and to be smaller, of low stage, hormone sensitive, and to have a major component of in situ cancer.[7]

A critical factor determining mammographic sensitivity is the radiologist's interpretation. One study, using the Breast Imaging Reporting and Data System (BI-RADS) reporting terminology, correlated 2 radiologists' interpretations of 2,616 mammograms with each other and with patient outcome. There were 302 breast cancers diagnosed within 1 year of the mammogram. The 2 radiologists had recommended additional testing in 73.8% and 78.1% of the patients with cancer.[8] Other studies have shown more inter-observer variability. In one, 150 mammograms (123 without and 27 with pathologically proven breast cancer) were read by 10 radiologists, with a median weighted agreement of 78%. For the women without cancer, an immediate work-up was recommended in 11% to 65%, and for those with cancer, work-up was recommended in 74% to 96%.[9] In another study, 10 radiologists read the same 100 mammograms twice, with a 5-month interval between readings, and with the addition of a sham history in one or the other reading. Their recommendations for further testing varied by +/-20%, having been influenced by the sham history.[10] Sensitivity and specificity are also associated with the volume of mammograms read by a radiologist.[11] Radiologists from low-, medium-, and high-volume mammography practices were enrolled in a study to assess the sensitivity and specificity of mammography using a standardized 60-film teaching set of mammograms. Sensitivity and specificity were associated with the volume of mammograms read in the practices. The average sensitivity ranged from 70.3% for low-volume radiologists to 78.6% among high-volume radiologists. Specificity ranged from 83.6% to 88% for low- to high-volume radiologists, respectively. Affixing specificity at 90%, sensitivity ranged from 64.8% to 75.6% from low-volume radiologists to high-volume radiologists.[11]

High breast density is associated with low sensitivity. At all ages, regardless of hormone replacement therapy (HRT), also called hormone therapy (HT), high breast density is associated with 10% to 29%

lower sensitivity.[5] High breast density is an inherent trait, which can be familial,[12] but also may be affected by age, endogenous[13] and exogenous[14,15] hormones,[16] selective estrogen receptor modulators (SERMs) such as tamoxifen,[17] and diet.[18] Strategies have been proposed to improve mammographic sensitivity by altering diet, by timing mammograms with menstrual cycles, or by interrupting HRT/HT use prior to the examination.

The specificity of mammography is the likelihood of the test being normal when cancer is absent. One minus specificity is the false-positive rate. If specificity is low, there are many false positive examinations which result in unnecessary follow-up examinations and procedures. An improvement in reporting mammography results has been the adoption of BI-RADS categories, which standardizes the terminology used in assessing the significance of the findings and recommending future action. A study correlating needle localization biopsies with BI-RADS categories showed that categories 0 and 2 yielded benign tissue in 87% and 100% of 65 cases. Category 3 (probably benign) yielded benign tissue in 98% of 141 cases, category 4 (suspicious) yielded benign tissue in 70% of 936 cases, and category 5 (highly suspicious) yielded benign tissue in only 3% of 170 cases. The authors' recommendation is that BI-RADS category 3 cases might be safely observed, without biopsy.[19] One concern about false positive tests is that women will be dissuaded from future examinations; however, two studies show the opposite to be true.[20,21]

The optimal interval between screening mammograms is unknown, and practice varies widely. A prospective trial that was undertaken in the United Kingdom randomized women aged 50 to 62 to annual versus the standard 3-year interval for screening mammograms. More cancers, of slightly smaller size, were detected in the annual screening group with a lead time of 7 months. However, the grade and node status were similar in both groups.[22] As a general rule, cancers which arise between screening examinations (interval cancers) have characteristics of rapid growth [7,23] and are frequently of advanced stage.[24] The likelihood of diagnosing cancer is highest with the prevalent (first) screening examination, ranging from 9 to 26 cancers per 1000 screens, depending on age. That likelihood decreases for follow-up examinations, ranging from only 1 to 3 cancers per 1000 screens.[25]

One study examined the usefulness of mammography in evaluating breast complaints in 1,908 women aged 35 years or younger. Although 23 were found to have palpable cancers, none of the 1,908 mammograms contributed any information that affected patient management.[26]

410

References

1. Sickles EA: Findings at mammographic screening on only one standard projection: outcomes analysis. *Radiology* 208 (2): 471-5, 1998.

2. Ernster VL, Barclay J, Kerlikowske K, et al.: Incidence of and treatment for ductal carcinoma in situ of the breast. *JAMA* 275 (12): 913-8, 1996.

3. Moody-Ayers SY, Wells CK, Feinstein AR: "Benign" tumors and "early detection" in mammography-screened patients of a natural cohort with breast cancer. *Arch Intern Med* 160 (8): 1109-15, 2000.

4. *Physician Insurers Association of America: Breast Cancer Study*. Washington, DC: Physician Insurers Association of America, 1995.

5. Rosenberg RD, Hunt WC, Williamson MR, et al.: Effects of age, breast density, ethnicity, and estrogen replacement therapy on screening mammographic sensitivity and cancer stage at diagnosis: review of 183,134 screening mammograms in Albuquerque, New Mexico. *Radiology* 209 (2): 511-8, 1998.

6. Kerlikowske K, Grady D, Barclay J, et al.: Likelihood ratios for modern screening mammography. Risk of breast cancer based on age and mammographic interpretation. *JAMA* 276 (1): 39-43, 1996.

7. Porter PL, El-Bastawissi AY, Mandelson MT, et al.: Breast tumor characteristics as predictors of mammographic detection: comparison of interval- and screen-detected cancers. *J Natl Cancer Inst* 91 (23): 2020-8, 1999.

8. Kerlikowske K, Grady D, Barclay J, et al.: Variability and accuracy in mammographic interpretation using the American College of Radiology Breast Imaging Reporting and Data System. *J Natl Cancer Inst* 90 (23): 1801-9, 1998.

9. Elmore JG, Wells CK, Lee CH, et al.: Variability in radiologists' interpretations of mammograms. *N Engl J Med* 331 (22): 1493-9, 1994.

10. Elmore JG, Wells CK, Howard DH, et al.: The impact of clinical history on mammographic interpretations. *JAMA* 277 (1): 49-52, 1997.

11. Esserman L, Cowley H, Eberle C, et al.: Improving the accuracy of mammography: volume and outcome relationships. *J Natl Cancer Inst* 94 (5): 369-75, 2002.

12. Pankow JS, Vachon CM, Kuni CC, et al.: Genetic analysis of mammographic breast density in adult women: evidence of a gene effect. *J Natl Cancer Inst* 89 (8): 549-56, 1997.

13. White E, Velentgas P, Mandelson MT, et al.: Variation in mammographic breast density by time in menstrual cycle among women aged 40-49 years. *J Natl Cancer Inst* 90 (12): 906-10, 1998.

14. Harvey JA, Pinkerton JV, Herman CR: Short-term cessation of hormone replacement therapy and improvement of mammographic specificity. *J Natl Cancer Inst* 89 (21): 1623-5, 1997.

15. Laya MB, Larson EB, Taplin SH, et al.: Effect of estrogen replacement therapy on the specificity and sensitivity of screening mammography. *J Natl Cancer* Inst 88 (10): 643-9, 1996.

16. Baines CJ, Dayan R: A tangled web: factors likely to affect the efficacy of screening mammography. *J Natl Cancer Inst* 91 (10): 833-8, 1999.

17. Brisson J, Brisson B, Coté G, et al.: Tamoxifen and mammographic breast densities. *Cancer Epidemiol Biomarkers Prev* 9 (9): 911-5, 2000.

18. Boyd NF, Greenberg C, Lockwood G, et al.: Effects at two years of a low-fat, high-carbohydrate diet on radiologic features of the breast: results from a randomized trial. Canadian Diet and Breast Cancer Prevention Study Group. *J Natl Cancer Inst* 89 (7): 488-96, 1997.

19. Orel SG, Kay N, Reynolds C, et al.: BI-RADS categorization as a predictor of malignancy. *Radiology* 211 (3): 845-50, 1999.

20. Burman ML, Taplin SH, Herta DF, et al.: Effect of false-positive mammograms on interval breast cancer screening in a health maintenance organization. *Ann Intern Med* 131 (1): 1-6, 1999.

21. Pisano ED, Earp J, Schell M, et al.: Screening behavior of women after a false-positive mammogram. *Radiology* 208 (1): 245-9, 1998.

22. The Breast Screening Frequency Trial Group: The frequency of breast cancer screening: results from the UKCCCR

Randomised Trial. United Kingdom Co-ordinating Committee on Cancer Research. *Eur J Cancer* 38 (11): 1458-64, 2002.

23. Hakama M, Holli K, Isola J, et al.: Aggressiveness of screen-detected breast cancers. *Lancet* 345 (8944): 221-4, 1995.

24. Tabár L, Faberberg G, Day NE, et al.: What is the optimum interval between mammographic screening examinations? An analysis based on the latest results of the Swedish two-county breast cancer screening trial. *Br J Cancer* 55 (5): 547-51, 1987.

25. Kerlikowske K, Grady D, Barclay J, et al.: Positive predictive value of screening mammography by age and family history of breast cancer. *JAMA* 270 (20): 2444-50, 1993.

26. Hindle WH, Davis L, Wright D: Clinical value of mammography for symptomatic women 35 years of age and younger. *Am J Obstet Gynecol* 180 (6 Pt 1): 1484-90, 1999.

Section 39.6

Upper Gastrointestinal (GI) Series

"Upper GI Series," National Institute of Diabetes and Digestive and Kidney Diseases (NIDDK), NIH Publication No. 02-4335, February 2002.

The upper gastrointestinal (GI) series uses x-rays to diagnose problems in the esophagus, stomach, and duodenum (first part of the small intestine). It may also be used to examine the small intestine. The upper GI series can show a blockage, abnormal growth, ulcer, or a problem with the way an organ is working. During the procedure, you will drink barium, a thick, white, milkshake-like liquid. Barium coats the inside lining of the esophagus, stomach, and duodenum and makes them show up more clearly on x-rays. The radiologist can also see ulcers, scar tissue, abnormal growths, hernias, or areas where something is blocking the normal path of food through the digestive system. Using a machine called a fluoroscope, the radiologist is also able to watch your digestive system work as the barium moves through it.

This part of the procedure shows any problems in how the digestive system functions, for example, whether the muscles that control swallowing are working properly. As the barium moves into the small intestine, the radiologist can take x-rays of it as well.

An upper GI series takes 1 to 2 hours. X-rays of the small intestine may take 3 to 5 hours. It is not uncomfortable. The barium may cause constipation and white-colored stool for a few days after the procedure.

Preparation

Your stomach and small intestine must be empty for the procedure to be accurate, so the night before you will not be able to eat or drink anything after midnight. Your physician may give you other specific instructions.

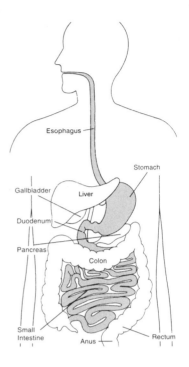

Figure 39.2. *The Digestive System: Upper GI Series*

Additional Information

National Digestive Diseases Information Clearinghouse
2 Information Way
Bethesda, MD 20892-3570
Toll-Free: 800-891-5389
Phone: 301-654-3810
Fax: 301-907-8906
Website: http://digestive.niddk.nih.gov
E-mail: nddic@info.niddk.nih.gov

Chapter 40

Ultrasound

Chapter Contents

Section 40.1

Ultrasound Exams Overview

"Ultrasound Exams," reprinted with permission from the website of the Society of Radiologists in Ultrasound, www.sru.org. © 2003 Society of Radiologists in Ultrasound. All rights reserved.

This section describes what an ultrasound procedure is like. You or a loved one may have had an ultrasound procedure prescribed by your physician. When you call to schedule your procedure, the radiologist, an M.D. specializing in diagnosis, or one of his co-workers may talk to you on the telephone to answer any questions.

Because there are many different types of ultrasound tests, there are different ways to prepare. The radiologist probably has your previous x-ray and imaging studies to review with your ultrasound examination, but sometimes the radiologist will call your doctor to find out more clinical information about you. The examination itself may be performed by a trained ultrasound technologist, by the radiologist, or both. Because interpreting images is their medical specialty, unlike most other specialists, radiologists have special training in the technology and techniques of ultrasound to get the best examinations. They also can bring together all the available clinical and radiological information to come to a quick and correct diagnosis.

The different types of ultrasound and the kinds of things they are used for are described in Table 41.1.

Table 40.1. Ultrasound Examinations (continued on next page)

Types of Ultrasound Examinations	Some Reasons for Having an Ultrasound
Vascular ultrasound, carotid ultrasound, peripheral arterial ultrasound, lower extremity venous ultrasound	**Carotid:** Symptoms of stroke, bruit in neck, dizziness. **Peripheral arterial ultrasound:** Symptoms of poor arterial circulation, follow-up after arterial graft. **Lower extremity venous ultrasound:** Signs of blood clot in leg vein, deep venous thrombosis, DVT, leg swelling.

Table 40.1. Ultrasound Examinations (continued on next page)

Echocardiogram, cardiac echo, cardiac ultrasound	Diseases of the heart valves, effectiveness of heart's pumping ability, newly diagnosed murmur, diagnosis and follow-up of congenital heart disease, blood clot in chamber of the heart.
Abdominal ultrasound, gallbladder ultrasound, liver ultrasound, liver Doppler	Abdominal pain, suspected gallstones, abdominal mass felt by physician, enlarged spleen, abnormal liver blood test, jaundice, fluid in abdomen (ascites), abdominal infection, cirrhosis of liver to check blood flow toward liver and to rule out cancers of the liver, screening for cirrhosis in patients diagnosed with hepatitis B or C.
Renal ultrasound, ultrasound of the kidneys, kidney ultrasound, renal echography, renal Doppler	Flank (side) pain, blockage of urinary tract (hydronephrosis), severe kidney infection, blood in urine, history of kidney stones, unexplained kidney failure, to follow growth of kidneys in children with infections or reflux, possible cyst of kidney seen on IVP or CT scan.
Obstetrical ultrasound, OB ultrasound, level I or level II OB ultrasound, pregnancy ultrasound or echography, high risk pregnancy ultrasound	Initial ultrasound of pregnancy to estimate fetal age, number of fetuses, abnormal bleeding during pregnancy, abnormal fetal heartbeat, large for dates, high risk pregnancy, diabetes, history of birth defects, follow-up scan for possible fetal abnormality.
Pelvic ultrasound, endovaginal ultrasound	Pelvic pain, mass felt by doctor or nurse during pelvic examination, ectopic pregnancy, abnormal bleeding, women taking certain medications, pelvic infection (PID or TOA), fibroid uterus, family history of ovarian cancer (screening), infertility work-up, fertility drug effects on woman.
Breast ultrasound	Evaluation of mass seen by radiologist on mammogram, drainage of breast cysts, biopsy of breast masses, placement of marker-wire in breast mass prior to surgery to guide surgeon to mass.
Thyroid ultrasound	Mass in neck over thyroid gland, abnormal thyroid blood tests, history of neck irradiation, abnormality on nuclear medicine imaging of thyroid, incidental thyroid mass seen on carotid ultrasound, CT scan or neck MRI.
Scrotal ultrasound, testicular ultrasound, ultrasound of testicles, scrotal echography	Pain in testicle, mass felt in testicle by patient or doctor, infertility, abnormal swelling of testicles, trauma to testicles, suspected torsion of testicle, mass suspected after specific abnormality seen on imaging study (CT scan, MRI, chest CT, or chest x-ray).

Table 40.1. Ultrasound Examinations (continued from previous page)

Prostate ultrasound, transrectal ultrasound of the prostate, TRUS	Elevated blood test (PSA), nodule felt by doctor during rectal exam (during routine physical exam or prostate cancer screening examination).
Musculoskeletal ultrasound	Rotator cuff tear, shoulder pain, muscle tear, doctor or patient feels mass in soft tissues, unable to have MRI of problem area, tendonitis, acute sports injuries.
Interventional ultrasound, intraoperative ultrasound	Placement of biopsy needles, drainage of infections (abscesses), assisting the surgeon during operations that require looking where the surgeon can't see or feel, or exact placement of special cancer destroying devices during operation.

Section 40.2

Abdominal Ultrasound

Reprinted with permission from the website of the Society of Radiologists in Ultrasound, www.sru.org. © 2003 Society of Radiologists in Ultrasound. All rights reserved.

Some reasons your doctor ordered your abdominal ultrasound:

- Abdominal pain.
- Unexplained weight loss.
- Your doctor felt a lump or mass.
- Abnormal laboratory test result.

Common diseases the radiologist/sonologist might discover:

- Gallstones.
- Abdominal aortic aneurysm (ballooning of aorta).
- Dilated bile ducts.
- Enlarged pancreas or pancreatitis.
- Tumor or mass in liver.
- Enlarged spleen or liver.

How Do You Prepare for an Abdominal Ultrasound Examination?

- Nothing by mouth past midnight (except a small amount of water for medications). This prevents you from swallowing air (bad for ultrasound images) or increasing bowel activity. Any food could cause your gallbladder to contract. The radiologist wants your gallbladder full and in its resting state.

What Happens in the Ultrasound Laboratory?

- You will probably change into a patient gown to prevent the ultrasound gel from staining your clothes.

- You will meet your sonographer, the person that will perform most of your scan. This trained technologist is an expert in ultrasound scanning. Most have been certified by the American Registry of Diagnostic Medical Sonographers (ARDMS).

- You will lie comfortably on an examination table. You may be asked to roll to either side.

- The sonographer squirts a special pre-warmed gel onto your skin that helps the sound penetrate into your body. This gel is harmless and easily wipes off after your examination.

- The transducer, or ultrasound scan head, emits a very high frequency sound. The sound waves bounce off structures inside your body and are detected by the same ultrasound transducer. The ultrasound machine is a sophisticated computer that converts these reflected sound waves into images that are recorded by the sonographer and interpreted by the radiologist.

- Often, before you leave the examination room, the radiologist will come in to meet you and may also scan you in order to answer questions not fully answered on the initial ultrasound images.

Section 40.3

Echocardiogram

Reprinted with permission from www.heartsite.com. © 2003 A.S.M. Systems, Inc. All rights reserved. For additional information, visit www .heartsite.com.

What Is an Echocardiogram?

An echocardiogram is a test in which ultrasound is used to examine the heart. The equipment is far superior to that used by fishermen. In addition to providing single-dimension images, known as M-mode echo that allows accurate measurement of the heart chambers, the echocardiogram also offers far more sophisticated and advanced imaging. This is known as two-dimensional (2-D) Echo and is capable of displaying a cross-sectional slice of the beating heart, including the chambers, valves, and the major blood vessels that exit from the left and right ventricle.

An echocardiogram can be obtained in a physician's office or in the hospital. For a resting echocardiogram (in contrast to a stress echo or TEE) no special preparation is necessary. Clothing from the upper body is removed and covered by a gown or sheet to keep you comfortable and maintain the privacy of females. The patient then lies on an examination table or a hospital bed.

Sticky patches or electrodes are attached to the chest and shoulders and connected to electrodes or wires. These help to record the electrocardiogram (EKG or ECG) during the echocardiography test. The EKG helps in the timing of various cardiac events (filling and emptying of chambers). A colorless gel is then applied to the chest and the echo transducer is placed on top of it. The echo technologist then makes recordings from different parts of the chest to obtain several views of the heart. You may be asked to move from your back and to the side. Instructions may also be given for you to breathe slowly or to hold your breath. This helps in obtaining higher quality pictures. The images are constantly viewed on the monitor. It is also recorded on photographic paper and on videotape. The tape offers a permanent record of the examination and is reviewed by the physician prior to completion of the final report.

What Is a Doppler Examination?

Doppler is a special part of the ultrasound examination that assesses blood flow (direction and velocity). In contrast, the M-mode and 2-D Echo evaluates the size, thickness, and movement of heart structures (chambers, valves, etc.). During the Doppler examination, the ultrasound beams will evaluate the flow of blood as it makes its way through and out of the heart. This information is presented visually on the monitor (as color images or grayscale tracings and also as a series of audible signals with a swishing or pulsating sound).

What Information Does Echocardiography and Doppler Provide?

Echocardiography is an invaluable tool in providing the doctor with important information about the heart's function and status.

Size of the chambers of the heart, including the dimension or volume of the cavity and the thickness of the walls. The appearance of the walls may also help identify certain types of heart disease that predominantly involve the heart muscle. In patients with long standing hypertension or high blood pressure, the test can determine the thickness and stiffness of the left ventricle (LV) walls. When the LV pump function is reduced in patients with heart failure, the LV and right ventricle (RV) tends to dilate or enlarge. Echocardiography can measure the severity of this enlargement. Serial studies performed on an annual basis can gauge the response of treatment.

Pumping function of the heart can be assessed by echocardiography. One can tell if the pumping power of the heart is normal or reduced to a mild or severe degree. This measure is known as an ejection fraction (EF). A normal EF is around 55% to 65%. Numbers below 45% usually represent some decrease in the pumping strength of the heart, while numbers below 30% to 35% are representative of an important decrease.

Echocardiography can also identify if the heart is pumping poorly due to a condition known as cardiomyopathy (pronounced cardio-myo-puth-e), or if one or more isolated areas have depressed movement (due to prior heart attacks). Thus, echocardiography can assess the pumping ability of each chamber of the heart and also the movement of each visualized wall. The decreased movement, in turn, can be graded from mild to severe. In extreme cases, an area affected by a heart attack may have no movement (akinesia, pronounced a-kine-neez-ya), or may even bulge in the opposite direction (dyskinesia, pronounced dis-kine-neez-ya). The latter is seen in patients with aneurysm (pronounced an-new-riz-um) of the left ventricle. It must be remembered that LV aneurysm due to an old heart attack does not usually rupture or burst.

Valve Function: Echocardiography identifies the structure, thickness, and movement of each heart valve. It can help determine if the valve is normal, scarred from an infection or rheumatic fever, thickened, calcified (loaded with calcium), or torn. It can also assess the function of prosthetic or artificial heart valves.

The additional use of Doppler helps to identify abnormal leakage across heart valves and determine their severity. Doppler is also very useful in diagnosing the presence and severity of valve stenosis (pronounced stee-no-sis) or narrowing. Remember, unlike echocardiography, Doppler follows the direction and velocity of blood flow rather than the movement of the valve leaflets or components. Thus, reversed blood direction is seen with leakages while increased forward velocity of flow with a characteristic pattern is noted with valve stenosis.

Echocardiography is used to diagnose mitral valve prolapse (MVP), while Doppler identifies whether it is associated with leakage or regurgitation of the mitral valve (MR). The presence of MVP frequently prompts the use of antibiotics prior to any dental or non-sterile surgical procedure. Such action helps reduce the rare complication of valve infection.

Volume status: Low blood pressure can occur in the setting of poor heart function, but may also be seen when patients have a reduced volume of circulating blood (as seen with dehydration, blood loss, or use of diuretics or water pills). In many cases, the diagnosis can be made on the basis of history, physical examination, and blood tests. However, confusion may be caused when patients have a combination of problems. Echocardiography may help clarify the confusion. The inferior vena cava (the major vein that returns blood from the lower half of the body to the right atrium) is distended or increased in size in patients with heart failure and reduced in caliber when the blood volume is reduced.

Other Uses: Echocardiography is useful in the diagnosis of fluid in the pericardium (the sac that surrounds the heart). It also determines when the problem is severe and potentially life-threatening.

Other diagnoses (plural for diagnosis) made by Doppler or echocardiography include congenital heart diseases, blood clots or tumors within the heart, active infection of the heart valves, and abnormal elevation of pressure within the lungs.

How Safe Is Echocardiography?

Echocardiography is extremely safe. There are no known risks from the clinical use of ultrasound during this type of testing.

How Long Does It Take?

A brief examination in an uncomplicated case may be done within 15 to 20 minutes. The additional use of Doppler may add 10 to 20 minutes. However, it may take up to an hour when there are multiple problems or when there are technical problems (for example, patients with lung disease, obesity, restlessness, or significant shortness of breath, may be more difficult to image).

When Can I Expect to Receive the Results?

If a doctor is present during the test or reviews it while you are still in the office, you may be able to get the results before you leave. However, the doctor is not routinely present during the test and you may have to wait from one to several days before the images have been reviewed by a physician and the results are sent to you by phone or mail. Some physicians will discuss your case before the study is performed and will contact you if there are significant unexpected findings. For example, if you are expected to have a finding or known to have a given disease, your physician may indicate that he or she will call you only if there are significant unexpected findings. You may also be contacted if echocardiography reveals a finding that influences a change in treatment. For example, the presence of a distended inferior vena cava may result in increasing the dose of your diuretic or water pill, if it is indicated by other aspects of your condition. If you are anxious or confused about the results, feel free to contact the physician's office staff. They can usually clarify a question for you.

Section 40.4

Vascular Ultrasound

Reprinted with permission from the website of the Society of Radiologists in Ultrasound, www.sru.org. © 2003 Society of Radiologists in Ultrasound. All rights reserved.

Some reasons your doctor ordered your vascular ultrasound:

- Symptoms of stroke can sometimes be explained by the discovery of a narrowing of one or more of the carotid arteries in your neck.

- The doctor heard a whooshing sound over the neck with a stethoscope. Frequently a narrowing of more than 50% will cause the flowing blood to make a sound audible to your doctor. If the bruit (pronounced brew-ee) is due to a narrowing of the arteries directly leading to the brain ultrasound may spot this narrowing and determine the degree of narrowing (or stenosis).

- Other arteries can be evaluated in the ultrasound laboratory. These include superficial blood vessels in the arms and legs.

- After an arterial bypass procedure, the openness, or patency of an arterial bypass graft can be directly or indirectly assessed with ultrasound.

- Some ultrasound laboratories attempt to detect narrowing of deeper vessels in the abdomen. Two examples are the renal arteries (arteries supplying the kidneys) and superior mesenteric artery (supplying the gut).

- Ultrasound is a very sensitive and non-invasive way to check the veins in the legs, to rule out the possibility of clots. Clots in leg veins can migrate centrally and lodge in the lungs (pulmonary embolism). They need to be treated.

How Do I Prepare for a Vascular Ultrasound?

- Studies of peripheral veins and arteries require no special preparation. Because cigarette smoking can cause blood vessels to constrict, smoking prior to an arterial study may be discouraged.

- Studies of the vessels deep in the abdomen are adversely affected by bowel activity and gas. For this reason, restriction of food and liquid intake is recommended for at least 6–8 hours prior to the vascular ultrasound.

- There is no special preparation for vascular ultrasound of the neck arteries (carotid ultrasound).

What Will Happen to Me during My Vascular Ultrasound?

- You will meet a sonographer who will perform the examination. In many cases the sonographer will have special training and be called an RVT, or Registered Vascular Technologist.

- The sonographer will place the transducer, or ultrasound probe, over the artery or vein to be studied. To help the ultrasound beam penetrate the skin, a special gel is placed on the skin.

- The ultrasound image is formed on a screen, and the sonographer will occasionally stop to take a picture of the image. The sonographer may videotape the entire procedure.

- In many instances the sonographer may leave the room to show the pictures to the radiologist. The radiologist may even come into the examination room, perform additional scans, and discuss the findings with you.

- During the procedure, depending on the type of study, the sonographer may ask you to hold your breath, stop swallowing, or even elevate or compress a different part of the extremity (called augmentation of flow in the study of the deep venous system).

Section 40.5

Transrectal Ultrasound

The information in this section has been provided by UPMC Cancer Centers. Illustration by Linda Rowley. For additional information, visit http://www.upmccancercenters.com/cancer/prostate/what.html. © 2003 University of Pittsburgh Medical Center. Reprinted with permission.

The digital rectal examination (DRE) and the prostate-specific antigen (PSA) blood test are two important ways to detect changes in the prostate gland.

However, they cannot determine if the changes are due to prostate cancer or to a non-cancerous condition. In the event of a significantly elevated PSA test and/or abnormal DRE, a prostate needle biopsy—the surgical removal of tissue for examination under a microscope—must be performed in order to make a definitive diagnosis of prostate cancer. The biopsy is taken with the guidance of transrectal ultrasound.

Transrectal ultrasound (TRUS) is a 5–15-minute outpatient procedure that uses sound waves to create a video image of the prostate gland. A small, lubricated probe placed into the rectum releases sound waves, which create echoes as they enter the prostate. Prostate tumors sometimes create echoes that are different from normal prostate tissue. The echoes that bounce back are sent to a computer that translates the pattern of echoes into a picture of the prostate. While the probe may be temporarily uncomfortable, TRUS is essentially a painless procedure. Although TRUS alone cannot detect every tumor, it has been shown to detect some tumors that cannot be felt by a DRE. In addition, TRUS is used to estimate the size of the prostate gland, helping doctors get a better idea of PSA density, which helps distinguish benign prostatic hyperplasia (BPH) from prostate cancer. Finally, it plays a vital role in a prostate needle biopsy, guiding the needle to just the right part of the prostate gland.

Preparation for TRUS

Prior to TRUS, the patient may be instructed to have an enema to remove feces and gas from the rectum, which might impede the progress of the rectal probe.

TRUS Technique

The patient traditionally lies on his left side, which is considered a more relaxing position as well as allowing for easier insertion of the rectal probe. After the probe is inserted into the rectum, the tester adjusts the console on the ultrasound machine to a baseline for the echoes of normal prostate tissue, which will serve as the standard by which other tissue will be classified. Imaging is usually begun at the base of the bladder, as the probe is rotated to provide a full picture of the prostate.

Images

The rectal probe sends sound waves to the prostate gland; normal and abnormal tissue bounce back different kinds of echoes that are relayed to the computer, which translates their pattern into a video picture of the prostate.

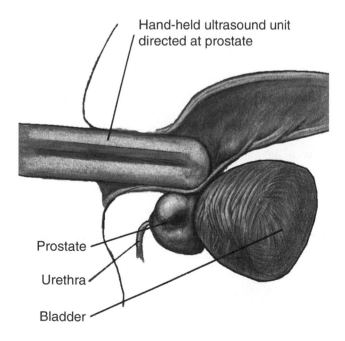

Hand-held ultrasound unit directed at prostate

Prostate

Urethra

Bladder

Figure 40.1. Transrectal Ultrasound

- *Isoechoic areas*, which represent normal tissue, bounce back, or echo, the same amount of sound waves as they received.

- *Hypoechoic areas* send back significantly fewer echoes than they received and often indicate the presence of cancer.

- *Hyperechoic areas* send back significantly more echoes than they received and often indicate the presence of prostatic calcifications, or tiny stones, in the prostate. The stones are usually harmless unless they become infected.

PSA Density (PSAD)

Most men in the age group for prostate cancer usually have some BPH as well, which can elevate PSA levels and make prostate cancer diagnosis more difficult. PSA density—the blood PSA level divided by the size of the prostate, as determined by TRUS—can help distinguish between BPH and prostate cancer. Basically, with BPH, the PSA level should not be more than 15 percent of the size of the prostate. PSA levels exceeding 15 percent of the size of the prostate are more likely to indicate the presence of prostate cancer and the need for a biopsy.

Additional Information

UPMC Cancer Centers Administration
5150 Centre Avenue
Pittsburgh, PA 15232
Toll-Free: 800-237-4724
Phone: 412-647-2811
Website: www.upmccancercenters.com
E-mail: PCI-INFO@msx.upmc.edu

Section 40.6

Transesophageal Echocardiogram (TEE)

"TEE or Transesophageal Echo," reprinted with permission from www .heartsite.com. © 2003 A.S.M. Systems, Inc. All rights reserved. For additional information, visit www.heartsite.com.

How Does TEE Differ from a Standard ECHO?

A standard echocardiogram or echo is obtained by applying a transducer to the front of the chest. The ultrasound beam travels through the chest wall (skin, muscle, bone, tissue) and lungs to reach the heart. Because it travels through the front of the chest or thorax (pronounced thow-racks) a standard echocardiogram is also known as a transthoracic (pronounced trans-thow-rassic) echo.

At times, closely positioned ribs, obesity, and emphysema may create technical difficulties by limiting the transmission of the ultrasound beams to and from the heart. In such cases, your physician may select to get a transesophageal (pronounced trans-esoff-a-gee-ul) echo, where the echo transducer is placed in the esophagus (pronounced esoff-a-gus) or food pipe that connects the mouth to the stomach. Since the esophagus sits behind the heart, the echo beam does not have to travel through the front of the chest, avoiding many of the obstacles described. In other words, it offers a much clearer image of the heart, particularly, the back structures, such as the left atrium, which may not be seen as well by a standard echo taken from the front of the heart.

How Is a TEE Performed?

The patient is made to lie on the left side. A sedative is given through an intravenous (IV) line to help in relaxation and the throat is sprayed with an anesthetic to numb it. The TEE echo transducer is much smaller than the standard echo equipment and is positioned at the end of a flexible tube (similar to the tube used to examine the stomach during endoscopy). The tube transfers the images from the transducer to the echo monitor. The patient begins to swallow the tube and the procedure begins. The use of anesthesia and the sedative minimizes discomfort and there is usually no pain. The tube goes down the esophagus the same way as swallowed food. Therefore, it is important that the patient swallow the tube rather than gag on it.

The transducer at the end of the tube is positioned in the esophagus, directly behind the heart. By rotating and moving the tip of the transducer, the physician can examine the heart from several different angles. The heart rate, blood pressure, and breathing are monitored during the procedure. Oxygen is given as a preventive measure and suction is used, as needed. After the procedure, driving is not allowed for 12 hours (because of the use of sedatives). Eating and drinking should be avoided for at least two hours because the throat will still be numb and the food or drink could be aspirated into the lungs. Hot food and drinks should not be used for about 24 hours. The throat may be sore and throat lozenges can be used two hours after the procedure. It is unusual to experience bleeding, persistent pain, or fever. These should be reported to the physician.

Preparing for the TEE

- Do not eat or drink for six hours. This will minimize the risk of vomiting and aspirating during the procedure.
- Medications prescribed by your doctor may be taken with sips of water, if you are not instructed to hold them.
- Arrange for a drive home if the procedure is performed on an outpatient basis.
- Be sure to notify the doctor or nurse if you have any allergies, if you have any difficulty in swallowing, or problems with your mouth, esophagus, or stomach.
- Dentures should be removed.

How Long Does a TEE Procedure Take?

You should plan to be in the cardiac lab for about two hours. The actual procedure usually lasts 10 to 30 minutes. The remainder of the time is spent in preparation and observation.

How Safe Is TEE?

TEE is a relatively common procedure and considered to be fairly safe. However, it does require entrance into your esophagus and stomach.

On occasions, patients may experience breathing problems, abnormal or slow heart rhythm, reaction to the sedative, and minor bleeding. In extremely rare cases TEE may cause perforation or tearing of the esophagus.

How Soon Will I Get the Results?

The physician can usually provide the results immediately after the procedure. However, the doctor may prefer to review the tape again before giving a final report. Also, if the patient appears drowsy from the sedative, a conference may be set up for a later time.

What Information Is Provided by TEE?

A TEE is extremely useful in detecting blood clots, masses, and tumors that are located inside the heart. It can also gauge the severity of certain valve problems and help detect infection of heart valves, certain congenital heart diseases (like a hole between the upper chambers of the heart, known as an ASD or atrial septal defect), and a tear (dissection) of the aorta (major artery of the body). TEE is also very useful in evaluating patients who have had mini or major stokes as a result of blood clots. The procedure may detect the responsible clot inside the left atrium.

Section 40.7

Endoscopic Ultrasound (EUS)

Reprinted with permission from Dr. Peter B. Cotton, Director of the Digestive Disease Center of the Medical University of South Carolina, http://www.ddc.musc.edu. © 2003 Medical University of South Carolina. All rights reserved.

Endoscopic ultrasound combines the techniques of endoscopy and ultrasound examination to obtain images and information about various parts of the digestive tract. Endoscopes are thin, flexible telescopes that allow trained specialists to examine most areas of the gut. At the end of the endoscope is a tiny television camera which allows the doctor to see the lining of the gut on a television monitor. Traditionally, ultrasound examinations of the abdomen have been performed using a probe which the radiologist moves over the surface of the abdomen to obtain pictures which resemble sonar images. In EUS, a small ultrasound transducer is mounted on the tip of a modified endoscope. By passing this endoscope into the upper or lower digestive tract, it is possible to obtain high quality ultrasound images internally.

The use of sound waves allows your doctor to obtain unique information about the different layers of the gut wall. The ultrasound waves also penetrate through the gut wall and allow doctors to obtain pictures of important organs adjacent to the gut such as blood vessels, lymph nodes, pancreas, liver, gallbladder, and bile ducts. In this way it is sometimes, but not always, possible to obtain images and information which cannot be obtained from other investigations, for example CT scan.

Several different types of instruments are currently used and these allow doctors to obtain ultrasound pictures in different planes in order to obtain the maximum amount of information. Sometimes it is possible to study the flow of blood in vessels by Doppler ultrasound, or pass a fine needle down the endoscope and direct it, under ultrasound guidance, into enlarged lymph nodes or suspicious masses. In this way tissue can be aspirated for analysis by a pathologist. This technique is known as fine needle aspiration biopsy (FNA).

In another type of study doctors pass a thin (2 mm) flexible plastic catheter, containing a tiny ultrasound miniprobe, down through an ordinary endoscope to obtain ultrasound images. These miniprobes use higher frequency sound waves (12–30 mega Hertz) and are used to examine the fine structure of small lesions, such as nodules arising in the wall of the gut.

When Is EUS Performed?

Because it is a relatively new technique, the indications for performing EUS are still being developed, but it is useful in the following situations:

- **Staging of cancers of the esophagus, stomach, pancreas, and rectum.** During the diagnostic work up of a patient with cancer, it is important to find out how early or advanced the tumor is, in order to select the most appropriate therapy and to give information about prognosis. This is called staging and is carried out according to standardized criteria which include assessing the depth of the penetration of the tumor through the gut wall, the involvement of adjacent lymph nodes, and spread of the tumor to distant organs such as the liver. Because ultrasound waves do not penetrate deeply through tissues, EUS cannot give information about tumor spread to distant organs, but it is highly accurate in evaluating involvement of the different gut wall layers and the surrounding lymph nodes. It can, for example, provide detailed information about whether the tumor has spread into nearby blood vessels or organs, and this helps the surgeon decide whether the tumor can be removed or not.

- **Staging of lung cancer.** Lung cancer often spreads to involve lymph nodes in the center of the chest (mediastinum). These lymph nodes may or may not be visible on CT scans, but are usually well seen and easily visualized at EUS. Sampling of these nodes by EUS guided fine needle aspiration is valuable in determining the most appropriate treatment in patients with this condition.

- **Submucosal lesions.** Sometimes patients are found at routine upper gastrointestinal endoscopy to have small nodules or lumps bulging from the wall of the esophagus or stomach. The overlying lining (mucosa) may appear normal because the nodule is coming from deeper in the gut wall. There are many different types of nodule, most of which are benign, but it can be difficult to distinguish them on their appearances at endoscopy alone. Ultrasound scanning over these submucosal nodules is often helpful in determining their nature and subsequent therapy.

- **Chronic pancreatitis.** Chronic inflammation and damage to the pancreas may be difficult to diagnose. EUS can provide detailed information about the pancreas gland and the pancreatic duct which carries digestive juices to the small bowel. This information complements that obtained at ERCP. In patients with severe, chronic, intractable abdominal pain resulting from chronic pancreatitis, it is sometimes possible to perform a nerve block (neurolysis) under EUS guidance.

- **Disorders of the bile duct** (the tube which carries bile from the liver to the small bowel). EUS is capable of detecting stones in the gallbladder and bile duct, but so can other tests such as ERCP and ordinary transabdominal ultrasound. It is not yet known if EUS is superior to these other tests.

- **Fecal incontinence.** This distressing condition is often the result of damage to the muscles lining the lower rectum and anal canal (sphincters). EUS is very accurate at detecting damage to these muscles. It has proven valuable in helping surgeons decide whether an operation will be helpful or not for patients with this disorder.

There are many other situations where EUS may be useful, some of which are still being developed. These are not yet fully established and are performed only at specialist centers with appropriate expertise.

How Is the Procedure Performed?

When you arrive for your EUS, the nurse and doctor will talk to you again about the procedure and answer your questions. Only then should you be asked to sign a consent form, signaling your understanding and agreement to proceed. You will put on a hospital gown and you will need to remove any eye glasses, contact lenses, or dentures. An IV needle will be placed into a vein, normally on the back of your hand or arm. Fluids will drip through the IV to stop you from getting thirsty. During EUS the IV line will be used to administer sedative medicines and to make you relaxed and sleepy. Complete anesthesia is rarely necessary.

You will be taken into a specially equipped room and the EUS procedure will be carried out while you lie on your left side. Local anesthetic throat spray will be given to make your throat numb, a plastic guard will be placed in your mouth to protect your teeth, and small monitoring devices will be placed on your skin so that the nurses can measure your pulse, blood pressure, and blood oxygen as necessary. When you are sleepy the doctor will place the thin flexible endoscope through the mouth guard and when you swallow the doctor will gently move the endoscope down the esophagus. The doctor can see with a small video camera on the end of the endoscope. Initially you may feel like gagging, but this will settle quickly and the endoscope will not interfere with your breathing. You will not feel the doctor doing the diagnostic maneuvers and any treatments. The procedure generally takes between thirty and ninety minutes at the end of which the doctor will remove the endoscope without any discomfort.

After EUS, you will be sleepy for up to one hour and will not be able eat or drink during that time. Once you are awake the doctor will discuss the results of the procedure with you and the person accompanying you (since your memory may be dulled by the sedative medication). They can take you home if the procedure has been straightforward. At home you should rest quietly until the next day, having only light meals with plenty of fluids. You may feel slightly bloated because of air inserted into your stomach during the examination. This is normal and will pass spontaneously. Your throat may be slightly sore for a day or two. You should call the clinic and your doctor if you have concerns about progress during the next few days, and especially if you have severe pain, vomiting, passage or vomiting of blood, or chills and fever. If EUS has involved treatment or been difficult, you may be admitted to the hospital overnight. This will be discussed with you by the doctors when you wake up.

What Are the Risks of EUS?

Like all other types of endoscopy, EUS is generally safe and well tolerated, but it is not without risk and you must understand what can happen. Firstly, you could have a reaction to the medicines, which can cause nausea and skin reactions such as reddening and hives. A tender lump may form in the vein where the IV was placed. This will usually settle spontaneously, but you should call your doctor if redness or swelling develops or persists.

For patients undergoing diagnostic EUS without fine needle aspiration or other intervention, specific complications occur in approximately one in two thousand (0.05%) cases. This is similar to the complication rate of routine upper gastrointestinal endoscopy or sigmoidoscopy. The main complication of serious concern is perforation of the esophagus or stomach (making a hole in the wall) which can occur during manipulation of the tip of the endoscope. All possible precautions are taken to minimize this risk. Perforation usually requires prolonged admission. Some cases can be treated medically (with IV fluids, antibiotics, etc.), but other cases require surgery. Perforation is extremely rare except in patients with large tumors of the esophagus which require stretching (dilation) before or during the EUS procedure.

When FNA sampling of tumors or lymph nodes is performed; complications occur more often but are still uncommon (0.5-1%). Passing the needle through the gut wall into the target tissue may cause bleeding, but this is usually minor and not serious. Occasionally, it is necessary for patients to be admitted for observation, but rarely are blood transfusions or surgery required for bleeding. Infection is another rare complication of FNA carried out during EUS. This is more likely to occur in patients undergoing aspiration of cystic (fluid filled) masses or lumps, and, in this setting, antibiotics are usually given before the procedure. Very rarely patients may develop acute pancreatitis following biopsy of the pancreas. This will require admission to hospital for observation, rest, IV fluids, and pain relief, but usually settles spontaneously over a few days.

Thus, EUS is a safe procedure and complications are uncommon. Most of these involve only a day or two of hospital treatment and death is extremely rare.

Chapter 41

Computed Tomography (CT) Scan

Chapter Contents

Section 41.1

What Is Computed Tomography?

"Computed Tomography (CT): Questions and Answers," Fact Sheet 5.2,
National Cancer Institute (NCI), reviewed 9/2003.

Computed tomography (CT) is a diagnostic procedure that uses special x-ray equipment to obtain cross-sectional pictures of the body. The CT computer displays these pictures as detailed images of organs, bones, and other tissues. This procedure is also called CT scanning, computerized tomography, or computerized axial tomography (CAT).

What Can a Person Expect during the CT Procedure?

During a CT scan, the person lies very still on a table. The table slowly passes through the center of a large x-ray machine. The person might hear whirring sounds during the procedure. People may be asked to hold their breath at times, to prevent blurring of the pictures.

Often, a contrast agent, or dye, may be given by mouth, injected into a vein, given by enema, or given in all three ways before the CT scan is done. The contrast dye can highlight specific areas inside the body, resulting in a clearer picture.

Computed tomography scans do not cause any pain. However, lying in one position during the procedure may be slightly uncomfortable. The length of the procedure depends on the size of the area being x-rayed; CT scans take from 15 minutes to 1 hour to complete. For most people, the CT scan is performed on an outpatient basis at a hospital or a doctor's office, without an overnight hospital stay.

Are There Risks Associated with a CT Scan?

Some people may be concerned about the amount of radiation they receive during a CT scan. It is true that the radiation exposure from a CT scan can be higher than from a regular x-ray. However, not having the procedure can be more risky than having it, especially if cancer is suspected. People considering CT must weigh the risks and benefits.

In very rare cases, contrast agents can cause allergic reactions. Some people experience mild itching or hives (small bumps on the skin). Symptoms of a more serious allergic reaction include shortness of breath and swelling of the throat or other parts of the body. People should tell the technologist immediately if they experience any of these symptoms, so they can be treated promptly.

What Is Spiral CT?

A spiral (or helical) CT scan is a new kind of CT. During a spiral CT, the x-ray machine rotates continuously around the body, following a spiral path to make cross-sectional pictures of the body. Benefits of spiral CT include:

- It can be used to make 3-dimensional pictures of areas inside the body;
- It may detect small abnormal areas better than conventional CT; and
- It is faster, so the test takes less time than a conventional CT.

What Is Total or Whole Body CT? Should a Person Have One?

A total or whole body CT scan creates images of nearly the entire body—from the chin to below the hips. This test has not been shown to have any value as a screening tool. (Screening means checking for signs of a disease when a person has no symptoms.)

The American College of Radiology (as well as most doctors) does not recommend scanning a person's body on the chance of finding signs of any sort of disease. In most cases abnormal findings do not indicate a serious health problem; however, a person must often undergo more tests to find this out. The additional tests can be expensive, inconvenient, and uncomfortable. The disadvantages of total body CT almost always outweigh the benefits.

What Is Virtual Endoscopy?

Virtual endoscopy is a new technique that uses spiral CT. It allows doctors to see inside organs and other structures without surgery or special instruments. One type of virtual endoscopy, known as CT colonography or virtual colonoscopy, is under study as a screening technique for colon cancer.

439

What Is Combined PET/CT Scanning?

Combined positron emission tomography (PET)/CT scanning joins two imaging tests, CT and PET, into one procedure. A PET scan creates colored pictures of chemical changes (metabolic activity) in tissues. Because cancerous tumors usually are more active than normal tissue, they appear different on a PET scan.

Combining CT with PET scanning may provide a more complete picture of a tumor's location and growth or spread than either test alone. Researchers hope that the combined procedure will improve health care professionals' ability to diagnose cancer, determine how far it has spread, and follow patients' responses to treatment. The combined PET/CT scan may also reduce the number of additional imaging tests and other procedures a patient needs. However, this new technology is currently only available at some facilities.

Additional Information

American College of Radiology
CT Accreditation Department
1891 Preston White Drive
Reston, VA 20191-4397
Toll-Free: 800-347-7748
Phone: 703-648-8900
Fax: 703-264-2093
Website: www.acr.org
E-mail: ctaccred@acr.org

Radiological Society of North America, Inc.
820 Jorie Blvd.
Oak Brook, IL 60523-2251
Toll-Free: 800-381-6660
Phone: 630-571-2670
Fax: 630-571-7837
Website: www.rsna.org or www.radiologyinfo.org

Section 41.2

Radiation Risks from Computed Tomography (CT)

"What Are the Radiation Risks from CT?" Center for Devices and Radiological Health (CDRH), U. S. Food and Drug Administration (FDA), updated 4/2002.

What Are the Radiation Risks from Computed Tomography (CT)?

As in many aspects of medicine, there are both benefits and risks associated with the use of CT. The main risks are those associated with:

1. abnormal test results, for a benign or incidental finding, leading to unneeded, possibly invasive, follow-up tests that may present additional risks; and

2. the increased possibility of cancer induction from x-ray radiation exposure.

The probability for absorbed x-rays to induce cancer is thought to be very small for radiation doses of the magnitude that are associated with CT procedures. Such estimates of the cancer risk from x-ray exposure have a broad range of statistical uncertainty, and there is some scientific controversy regarding the effects from very low doses and dose rates as discussed later. Under some rare circumstances of prolonged, high-dose exposure, x-rays can cause other adverse health effects, such as skin erythema (reddening), skin tissue injury, genetic effects, and birth defects. But at the exposure levels associated with most medical imaging procedures, including CT, these other adverse effects would not occur.

Risk Estimates

In the field of radiation protection, it is commonly assumed that the risk for adverse health effects from cancer is proportional to the

441

amount of radiation dose absorbed, and the amount of dose depends on the type of x-ray examination. A CT examination with an effective dose of 10 millisieverts (abbreviated mSv; 1 mSv = 1 mGy in the case of x-rays.) may be associated with an increase in the possibility of fatal cancer of approximately 1 chance in 2000. This increase in the possibility of a fatal cancer from radiation can be compared to the natural incidence of fatal cancer in the U.S. population, about 1 chance in 5. In other words, for any one person, the risk of radiation-induced cancer is much smaller than the natural risk of cancer. Nevertheless, this small increase in radiation-associated cancer risk for an individual can become a public health concern if large numbers of the population undergo increased numbers of CT screening procedures of uncertain benefit.

It must be noted that there is uncertainty regarding the risk estimates for low levels of radiation exposure as commonly experienced in diagnostic radiology procedures. There are some that question whether there is adequate evidence for a risk of cancer induction at low doses. However, this position has not been adopted by most authoritative bodies in the radiation protection and medical arenas.

Radiation Dose

The effective doses from diagnostic CT procedures are typically estimated to be in the range of 1 to 10 mSv. This range is not much less than the lowest doses of 5 to 20 mSv received by some of the Japanese survivors of the atomic bombs. These survivors, who are estimated to have experienced doses only slightly larger than those encountered in CT, have demonstrated a small but increased radiation-related excess relative risk for cancer mortality.

Radiation dose from CT procedures varies from patient to patient. A particular radiation dose will depend on the size of the body part examined, the type of procedure, and the type of CT equipment and its operation. Typical values cited for radiation dose should be considered as estimates that cannot be precisely associated with any individual patient, examination, or type of CT system. The actual dose from a procedure could be two or three times larger or smaller than the estimates. Facilities performing screening procedures may adjust the radiation dose used to levels less (by factors such as 1/2 to 1/5 for so called low dose CT scans) than those typically used for diagnostic CT procedures. However, no comprehensive data is available to permit estimation of the extent of this practice and reducing the dose can have an adverse impact on the image quality produced. Such reduced image quality may be acceptable in certain imaging applications.

The quantity most relevant for assessing the risk of cancer detriment from a CT procedure is the effective dose. Effective dose is evaluated in units of millisieverts (abbreviated mSv; 1 mSv = 1 mGy in the case of x-rays.) Using the concept of effective dose allows comparison of the risk estimates associated with partial or whole-body radiation exposures. This quantity also incorporates the different radiation sensitivities of the various organs in the body.

Estimates of the effective dose from a diagnostic CT procedure can vary by a factor of 10 or more depending on the type of CT procedure, patient size, and the CT system and its operating technique. A list of representative diagnostic procedures and associated doses are given in Table 41.1 that is adapted from the European Commission, Radiation Protection Report 118, "Referral guidelines for imaging." Directorate-General for the Environment of the European Commission, 2000.

Table 41.1. Radiation Dose Comparison

Diagnostic Procedure	Typical Effective Dose (mSv)[1]	Number of Chest X-Rays (PA film) for Equivalent Effective Dose[2]	Time Period for Equivalent Effective Dose from Natural Background Radiation[3]
Chest x-ray (PA film)	0.02	1	2.4 days
Skull x-ray	0.07	4	8.5 days
Lumbar spine	1.3	65	158 days
I.V. urogram	2.5	125	304 days
Upper G.I. exam	3.0	150	1.0 year
Barium enema	7.0	350	2.3 years
CT head	2.0	100	243 days
CT abdomen	10.0	500	3.3 years

1. Effective dose in millisieverts (mSv).

2. Based on the assumption of an average effective dose from chest x-ray (PA film) of 0.02 mSv.

3. Based on the assumption of an average effective dose from natural background radiation of 3 mSv per year in the United States.

Section 41.3

Computed Tomography (CT) of the Brain

"Cranial CT Scan," © 2003 A.D.A.M., Inc. Reprinted with permission.

Alternative names: Head CT; CT scan-skull; CT scan-head; CT scan-orbits; CT scan-sinuses

Definition: A CT scan (computed tomography) of the head, including the skull, brain, orbits (eyes), and sinuses.

How the Test Is Performed

A head CT will image from the upper neck to the top of the head. If the patient cannot keep his/her head still, immobilization may be necessary. All jewelry, glasses, dentures, and other metal should be removed from the head and neck to prevent artifact. Intravenous contrast media may be administered to further evaluate for vascular masses, determine whether masses enhance (become brighter) with contrast, or allow for visualization of the vessels of the head and/or brain.

The total amount of time in the CT scanner should be a few minutes.

How to Prepare for the Test

There is no preparation necessary.

Infants and children:

The physical and psychological preparation you can provide for this or any test or procedure depends on your child's age, interests, previous experiences, and level of trust.

How the Test Will Feel

As with any intravenous iodinated contrast injection, there may be a slight temporary burning sensation in the arm, metallic taste in the mouth, or whole body warmth. This is a normal occurrence and will subside in a few seconds. Otherwise, the CT is painless.

Why the Test Is Performed

A CT scan is recommended to help:

- evaluate acute cranial-facial trauma
- determine acute stroke
- evaluate suspected subarachnoid or intracranial hemorrhage
- evaluate headache
- evaluate loss of sensory or motor function
- determine if there abnormal development of the head and neck

CT scans are also used to view the facial bones, jaw, and sinus cavities.

What Abnormal Results Mean

There may be signs of:

- trauma
- bleeding (for example, chronic subdural hematoma, subarachnoid or intracranial hemorrhage)
- stroke
- masses or tumors
- abnormal sinus drainage
- sensorineural hearing loss
- malformed bone or other tissues
- brain abscess
- cerebral atrophy (loss of brain tissue)
- cerebral edema (brain tissue swelling)
- hydrocephalus (fluid collecting in the skull)

Additional conditions under which the test may be performed:

- acoustic neuroma
- acoustic trauma
- acromegaly
- acute (subacute) subdural hematoma
- amyotrophic lateral sclerosis
- arteriovenous malformation (cerebral)

445

- benign positional vertigo
- cancer of the throat
- central pontine myelinolysis
- cerebral aneurysm
- Cushing's syndrome
- deep intracerebral hemorrhage
- delirium
- dementia
- dementia due to metabolic causes
- drug-induced tremor
- encephalitis
- epilepsy
- essential tremor
- extradural hemorrhage
- familial tremor
- general paresis
- generalized tonic-clonic seizure
- hemorrhagic stroke
- hepatic encephalopathy
- Huntington's disease
- hypertensive intracerebral hemorrhage
- hypopituitarism
- intracerebral hemorrhage
- juvenile angiofibroma
- labyrinthitis
- lobar intracerebral hemorrhage
- Ludwig's angina
- mastoiditis
- melanoma of the eye
- Ménière's disease
- meningitis
- metastatic brain tumor
- multi-infarct dementia
- multiple endocrine neoplasia (MEN) I
- neurosyphilis

- normal pressure hydrocephalus (NPH)
- occupational hearing loss
- optic glioma
- orbital cellulitis
- otitis media; chronic
- otosclerosis
- partial (focal) seizure
- partial complex seizure
- petit mal seizure
- pituitary tumor
- primary brain tumor
- primary lymphoma of the brain
- prolactinoma
- retinoblastoma
- Reye syndrome
- schizophrenia
- senile dementia/Alzheimer's type
- acute sinusitis
- stroke secondary to atherosclerosis
- stroke secondary to cardiogenic embolism
- stroke secondary to FMD (fibromuscular dysplasia)
- stroke secondary to syphilis
- subarachnoid hemorrhage
- syphilitic aseptic meningitis
- temporal lobe seizure
- toxoplasmosis
- transient ischemic attack (TIA)
- Wilson's disease

What the Risks Are

Iodine is the usual contrast media (dye). Some patients are allergic to iodine and may experience a reaction that may include hives, itching, nausea, breathing difficulty, or other symptoms.

As with any x-ray examination, radiation is potentially harmful. Consult your health care provider about the risks if multiple CT scans are needed over a period of time.

Special Considerations

A CT scan can decrease or eliminate the need for invasive procedures to diagnose problems in the skull. This is one of the safest means of studying the head and neck.

Chapter 42

Magnetic Resonance Imaging (MRI)

Chapter Contents

Section 42.1

MRI: X-Ray Vision without the X-Rays

"Stories of Discovery: MRI: X-Ray Vision without the X-Rays," National Center for Research Resources (NCRR), National Institutes of Health, 4/2002.

Ever since the discovery of x-rays in 1895, scientists have been developing techniques to see inside the body without using surgery. One of today's most ubiquitous imaging tools is magnetic resonance imaging (MRI), which provides clear pictures of the body's interior—including tissues, organs, and blood vessels—without the use of hazardous radiation. Through its support of advanced technologies and instruments, NCRR helped to usher MRI from its obscure beginnings nearly three decades ago into the widely used diagnostic tool now found in hospitals and research centers nationwide.

MRI is based on a phenomenon known as nuclear magnetic resonance (NMR), first observed more than 50 years ago. When placed in strong magnetic fields, the nuclei of certain atoms resonate—that is, absorb specific radiofrequencies beamed at them and then emit their own radiofrequency signals. Because these signals are influenced by the chemical environment surrounding the resonating nuclei, scientists can identify a sample's constituent chemicals by their NMR frequencies. In the early 1970s, NCRR established some of the first national NMR centers devoted to biomedical research.

A critical breakthrough came in the mid-1970s, when Dr. Paul Lauterbur showed that NMR frequencies could be used to produce two-dimensional (2-D) images of samples, ranging from vials of water to a pecan nut to a live clam, as long as the samples contained resonating nuclei, such as hydrogen. The basic principles behind these early MRI scans underlie even today's most sophisticated MRI instruments. Dr. Lauterbur's investigations of MRI and NMR tools and technologies, from the late 1970s through the 1990s, depended in part on the technology-based infrastructure that NCRR funding provided.

Since its debut, MRI has become the primary imaging technique for analyzing internal structures to diagnose disorders of the brain and spinal cord, major blood vessels, other organs, and systems. With

2-D or 3-D MRI, clinicians can detect structural abnormalities caused by tumors, trauma, or tissue degeneration, possibly even before symptoms appear. A recent MRI study conducted in part at the NCRR-supported Neuroimaging Analysis Center at Brigham and Women's Hospital found that individuals in the early stages of Alzheimer's disease show distinctive changes in three brain regions.

Other researchers at the NCRR-supported Laboratory of Neuro Imaging (LONI) Resource at the University of California, Los Angeles, observed a wave of nerve cell loss that spread through the brains of schizophrenic patients in their late teens or early 20s, as the disease progressed. These same researchers, headed by LONI Director Dr. Arthur Toga, have identified periods of rapid growth of certain brain regions in normal children. Brain systems involved in learning languages grow swiftly between the age of 6 and puberty, a period in which children most easily grasp new languages.

Besides studying structure, MRI also can be used to study the physiology of the body through techniques such as functional MRI (fMRI), which was pioneered with NCRR support. Using fMRI, researchers can determine which parts of the brain are functioning during various activities.

The first published fMRI studies were conducted by separate teams of NCRR-supported investigators. With equipment purchased through NCRR Shared Instrumentation Grants, Dr. Bruce Rosen and his colleagues in 1991 used fMRI to see increased activity in a brain region associated with visual perception when people watched flashing visual patterns. The technique involved infusing a volunteer's bloodstream with a chemical contrast agent, which enabled imaging of increased blood flow to activated brain regions. Today, Dr. Rosen heads the NCRR-supported Center for Functional Neuroimaging Technologies at Massachusetts General Hospital.

Then in 1992, three scientific teams reported an additional breakthrough—the ability to acquire fMRI images without the use of a contrast agent. Instead, the new method relied on the increased radio-frequency signal produced by oxygen-rich blood in the vicinity of active brain regions. Being completely noninvasive, this technique soon became the standard for fMRI. The three research teams, who published their findings within one month of each other, were headed by Dr. Kamil Ugurbil, director of the NCRR-supported NMR Imaging and Localized Spectroscopy resource at the University of Minnesota; Dr. James Hyde, then-director of an NCRR-supported Paramagnetic Resonance Resource at the Medical College of Wisconsin; and Dr. Rosen at Massachusetts General Hospital.

More recent fMRI studies, conducted with NCRR support, have identified brain regions involved in responding to a visual cue with appropriate movements, and the regions involved in recognizing human faces or common objects. This technique also facilitates the study of mental processes such as memory formation. NCRR-supported scientists have identified patterns of brain activity associated with transforming short-term memories into long-term memories and other patterns that indicate whether an experience will be remembered well, remembered poorly, or totally forgotten.

The standard MRI scanner used in human studies contains a 1.5 tesla magnet. However, researchers are finding that higher magnetic power provides higher levels of resolution. In structural MRI, stronger magnets make the images more distinct, and in fMRI they allow researchers to observe brain responses to rapid events. Several NCRR-funded biomedical technology resource centers are conducting clinical MRI studies with magnets that range from 2.0 to 4.1 tesla.

Besides functional imaging, other physiology-based MRI techniques include MR angiography, which produces images of blood flow, and MR spectroscopy, which reveals the biochemistry of specific organs or tissues. Recently, Dr. Warren Manning and his colleagues at Beth Israel Deaconess Medical Center in Boston showed that MR angiography could detect impaired blood flow to the heart muscle, which could lead to a heart attack.

In operating rooms, surgeons are beginning to use another type of MRI technology known as interventional MRI, in which they watch 3-D images in real time to observe details of tissues during surgery. Dr. Ron Kikinis, director of the Neuroimaging Analysis Center, and his colleagues developed rapid computational methods that combine structural MRI, fMRI, and MR angiography into a single image. This technique has allowed neurosurgeons to determine the exact boundaries of brain tumors and their proximity to vital brain regions and major blood vessels.

Interventional MRI, with its integration of three different types of MR images, exemplifies the increasing sophistication of both MRI instruments and computers. These integrated technologies now allow scientists to conduct entirely new types of studies. For example, 3-D brain images of many patients with a disease (such as Alzheimer's disease or schizophrenia) can now be integrated into a composite image of a typical brain of someone with that disease. However, to produce these composite images requires thousands of patients and trillions of bytes of computer memory, both of which are beyond the capacities of the average laboratory. To address this problem, NCRR is funding the new Biomedical Informatics Research Network (BIRN), a high-performance computer network that allows laboratories around the country to share data. The network also connects various computers around the country into one large supercomputer, which can rapidly analyze the shared data. Through BIRN, researchers in different disciplines will be able to collaborate on projects and make discoveries that previously would have been impossible. BIRN is just one example of how NCRR serves as a catalyst for discovery, by creating and providing critical research technologies and shared resources.

—*Steven Stocker*

Section 42.2

Magnetic Resonance Imaging: Body

"NIH Licenses New MRI Technology That Produces Detailed Images of Nerves, Other Soft Tissues," NIH News Release, National Institutes of Health (NIH), July 29, 2002.

NIH Licenses New MRI Technology That Produces Detailed Images of Nerves and Other Soft Tissues

A new technology that allows physicians and researchers to make detailed, three-dimensional maps of nerve pathways in the brain, heart muscle fibers, and other soft tissues has been licensed by the National Institutes of Health (NIH).

The new imaging technology, called Diffusion Tensor Magnetic Resonance Imaging (DT-MRI) was invented by researchers now at the National Institute of Child Health and Human Development (NICHD). DT-MRI may allow physicians and researchers to better understand and diagnose a wide range of medical conditions such as stroke, amyotrophic lateral sclerosis (Lou Gehrig's disease), multiple sclerosis (MS), autism, attention deficit disorder (ADD), and schizophrenia. NIH has signed an agreement with GE Medical Systems, licensing them to produce and market the product.

"NIH's mission is to support research that improves the health of the public," said Duane Alexander, M.D., Director of NICHD. "The recent licensing of DT-MRI ensures that the technology produced as a result of NIH research is further developed and marketed to medical institutions where patients can benefit from its use."

Like conventional MRI, DT-MRI is a technology that produces high quality 3-D images of the inside of the body, painlessly, non-invasively, and without using contrast agents or dyes. In addition, DT-MRI produces sophisticated images of soft tissues by measuring the three-dimensional random motion of water molecules (diffusion) within the tissues.

Although water may appear placid in a jar or cup, individual water molecules are constantly in motion, colliding with each other at extremely high speeds. These high-speed collisions cause the water molecules to spread out, or diffuse, similar to the way a drop of dye placed in a jar of water spreads in a spherical pattern. In some tissues, such as gray matter in the brain, water also diffuses in an approximately spherical pattern. In contrast, in tissues containing a large number of parallel fibers, such as skeletal muscle, cardiac muscle, and white matter in the brain, water diffuses fastest along the direction in which the fibers are pointing, and slowest at right angles to it. DT-MRI uses this information to produce intricate three-dimensional images of the tissue's architectural organization and local structure.

Changes in tissue properties that can be measured with DT-MRI can often be correlated with processes that occur in development, degeneration, disease, and aging. As a result, doctors and scientists can use DT-MRI to diagnose and assess a growing number of diseases and better understand how tissues in the body function.

Since its invention, DT-MRI has had a wide range of applications. Scientists and clinicians have used it to map nerve pathways in the brain, diagnose acute stroke, and determine the effectiveness of new stroke prevention medications. DT-MRI has also been used to map subtle changes in white matter in diseases such as Lou Gehrig's Disease (Amyotrophic Lateral Sclerosis–ALS), adrenoleukodystrophy (ALD), MS, and epilepsy. This information has helped scientists and clinicians better understand the development of these disorders, an important first step in eventually devising new methods to treat them.

Others are using DT-MRI to assess the type and severity of brain tumors and to plan the surgical procedure to remove them. For example, brain surgeons planning tumor removal surgeries are beginning to use DT-MRI images to help them better distinguish between healthy brain tissue and tumors. Other researchers are investigating DT-MRI's use in diagnosing and determining the stage of certain cancers, such as prostate cancer.

DT-MRI has also been used to study cognitive and behavioral disorders, such as schizophrenia, ADD, and dyslexia. Presently, scientists are using the new technology to associate these conditions with specific anomalies in brain anatomy.

"If we could establish a strong connection between an anatomical deficit and a particular disorder, it might be possible to one day use DT-MRI as a screening tool," said Peter Basser, Ph.D., principal inventor of DT-MRI and Chief of the NICHD Section on Tissue Biophysics and Biomimetics.

Pediatric researchers are using DT-MRI to learn more about normal brain development in infants and children. Other researchers are investigating DT-MRI's use in assessing head trauma and cardiac abnormalities.

"Licensing technology like DT-MRI benefits the NIH, the private sector, and the public at large," said Krishna Balakrishnan, Ph.D., MBA, Marketing Group Leader of NIH's Office of Technology Transfer, "It motivates the business world to further develop the product invented at NIH and get it to the public. It also benefits further NIH research by validating its societal applications."

In addition to Peter Basser, Dennis LeBihan and James Mattiello also contributed to the development of this invention.

Section 42.3

Magnetic Resonance Imaging: Heart

This section includes "Cardiac Magnetic Resonance Imaging Examination," reproduced with permission from the American Heart Association World Wide Web Site, www.americanheart.org © 2003, Copyright American Heart Association; and "NIH Study Shows MRI Provides Faster, More Accurate Way to Diagnose Heart Attacks," NIH News Release, National Heart, Lung, and Blood Institute (NHLBI), January 29, 2003.

Cardiac Magnetic Resonance Imaging Examination

What Is the MRI Test?

Magnetic resonance imaging (referred to as MRI or NMR) is a way to examine the heart. The human body is made up of many atoms, and when it's placed in a magnet, these atoms produce very weak signals. By using electronics and a computer, these signals can be magnified, recorded, and used to make pictures of the body.

Why Is It Done?

MRI pictures can give very clear images of the size of the heart chambers and the thickness of the heart muscle. The images also can show the large blood vessels leading to and from the heart. With special methods, the test can show the heart's pumping action and obtain information about blood flow.

How Is It Done?

MRI scanners or magnets usually look like very large, thick-walled pipes or tubes. You will lie down on a mobile examination table, which is then moved into the center of the tube. Using a computer and TV system, the technologist will watch you from a room next to the magnet room. You should not move during the examination, which will take 45 minutes to one hour. Ideally, the only movement should be normal breathing during the exam period.

When you are brought to the magnet, the technologist will put you on the examination table. Most parents stay in the magnet room with their child during the examination. An intercom will let you or your child talk with the doctor and technologist during the examination. Sometimes children become uncomfortable from holding still for long periods of time. Let the technologist know if this happens. The technologist can reposition your child before the study begins. Besides lying still, a patient doesn't have to do anything during an MRI imaging examination. Occasionally, additional information is obtained by having an intravenous (IV) placed and injecting a contrast agent to show the blood vessels (MRA).

Younger patients usually require sedation. Then a child usually falls asleep within 30 minutes and sleeps for about one hour. Upon awakening after sedation, your child may have poor balance for more than an hour. During this time he or she must be carefully attended and not allowed to sit, stand, or walk alone.

Does It Hurt?

An MRI examination is painless and cannot be felt. During the period when the test is being run, you will hear thumping and buzzing noises. Don't be afraid. These noises are a normal part of the test.

Is It Harmful?

There are no known harmful effects. No x-rays or other types of radiation are used in the MRI test.

Specific Concerns

The MRI tube contains a strong magnet that attracts metal. These special precautions should be noted:

- No person with a pacemaker should enter the magnet room.

- Watches and credit cards should be removed before entering the MRI room. The magnet can affect watches and can erase the magnetic strips on credit cards.

- Jewelry and other metal objects such as hairpins and clips should be taken off before going into the magnet room. Clothing should contain as little metal as possible. No large or sharp metal objects should be brought into the MRI room.

- Your doctor and the MRI technologist should be aware of any metal implants that you or your child have (bone pins, plates, or rods). You don't have to worry about dental fillings, or metal clips, or wires from various types of heart surgery.

- Your doctor and the MRI technologist should be aware if you or your child had accidents in which metal pieces (welding chips, shrapnel) have entered the eyes.

- If your child is afraid of confinement, discuss this with the doctor ahead of time.

- If you or your daughter might be pregnant, you should tell the doctor or technologist before the examination.

Prepared by the Committee on Congenital Cardiac Defects of the Council on Cardiovascular Disease in the Young.

NIH Study Shows MRI Provides Faster, More Accurate Way to Diagnose Heart Attacks

Advanced magnetic resonance imaging (MRI) technology can detect heart attack in emergency room patients with chest pain more accurately and faster than traditional methods, according to a new study supported by the National Heart, Lung, and Blood Institute (NHLBI).

Published in the February 4, 2003 issue of *Circulation: Journal of the American Heart Association*, the findings suggest that more patients who are suffering a heart attack or who otherwise have severe blockages in their coronary arteries could receive treatment to reduce or prevent permanent damage to the heart if they are assessed with MRI.

Researchers evaluated the ability of high-resolution MRI to detect acute coronary syndrome (heart attack or unstable angina) in emergency department patients with chest pain. MRI results were compared with three standard diagnostic tests: an electrocardiogram (ECG or EKG), blood enzyme test, and the TIMI risk score, which assesses the risk of complications or death in patients with chest pain based on a combination of several clinical characteristics. MRI detected all of the patients' heart attacks, including three in patients who had normal EKGs. In addition, MRI detected more patients with unstable angina than the other tests.

Of the more than 5 million patients who visit emergency departments with chest pain each year, only about 40 percent can be immediately diagnosed with heart attack using standard tests. The majority of patients must undergo a number of tests and further hospitalization for a conclusive diagnosis to be reached.

"This study lays the groundwork for what could mean a dramatic change in how heart attacks are diagnosed—and how rapidly patients receive treatment once they arrive at the hospital," said NHLBI Director Dr. Claude Lenfant. "Using MRI to detect heart problems in the emergency department will ultimately save lives. Because patients will be diagnosed and treated more quickly, cardiac MRIs might save costs, as well."

The study is part of a collaborative program among the NHLBI, the Warren Grant Magnuson Clinical Center—both components of the National Institutes of Health (NIH), the Federal Government's primary agency for biomedical and behavioral research—and Suburban Hospital in Bethesda, Maryland. Another area of the program, supported by NIH's National Institute of Neurological Disorders and Stroke, is studying the use of MRI to diagnose and treat stroke. NIH is part of the U.S. Department of Health and Human Services.

In the chest pain study, 161 patients whose initial EKG did not indicate a heart attack were evaluated with traditional diagnostic tests and a cardiac MRI after their condition was stabilized. The MRI lasted around 38 minutes. All patients were followed up 6 to 8 weeks after the initial visit to the emergency department.

Researchers studied the ability of each test to detect acute coronary syndrome (sensitivity) as well as how often an abnormal test result correctly identified a patient with acute coronary syndrome (specificity). MRI accurately diagnosed 21 of the 25 patients (84 percent) determined to have acute coronary syndrome—a significantly higher level of sensitivity than EKG criteria for ischemia (restricted blood flow), blood enzyme levels, and TIMI risk score. MRI was also more specific than abnormal EKG.

"MRI was the strongest predictor of acute coronary syndrome—for both heart attacks and unstable angina," said Dr. Andrew Arai, principal investigator of the study, who leads the cardiovascular imaging section of the NHLBI Laboratory of Cardiac Energetics. "MRI allows us to look at how well the heart is pumping, how good the supply of blood to the heart is in specific areas, and whether there is evidence of permanent damage to the heart."

MRI addresses another critical issue in assessing patients with acute coronary syndrome: time. Patients can be scanned in under 40 minutes; if severe blockages are found, they could receive vital treatment to restore blood flow, such as clot-busting drugs, angioplasty, or coronary artery bypass surgery. Current recommendations are for such therapies to begin within one hour from the start of a heart attack for optimal effectiveness.

EKG records the electrical activity of the heart to detect abnormal heart rhythms, some areas of damage, inadequate blood flow, and heart enlargement. Like MRI, EKG is noninvasive. Because of its low degree of sensitivity, however, EKG immediately diagnoses only about 10 percent of patients with acute coronary syndrome. It is not uncommon for an EKG to appear normal during a heart attack or an episode of unstable angina.

Patients suspected of having a heart attack that is not confirmed by an EKG typically have their blood tested for enzymes or other substances (markers) that indicate permanent damage to the heart tissue. Because the markers are not evident in the blood until several hours after a heart attack, patients whose EKG appears normal may need to stay in the hospital for 12 to 24 hours to ensure the blood test is accurate. Furthermore, because the blood test detects only permanently damaged tissue, it does not detect unstable angina.

Unstable angina can be considered an impending heart attack. Heart attacks are caused by a blood clot from a tear or break in fatty deposits (plaque) that have built up inside a coronary artery; when the blood clot suddenly cuts off most or all blood supply to the heart, heart tissue is permanently damaged. In unstable angina, the coronary artery has many or all of the same characteristics as a heart attack, except that the problems are not quite severe enough to cause permanent heart damage. Because no heart cells die in unstable angina, the condition is harder to detect with standard tests.

Approximately two percent of patients with a heart attack are discharged home from the emergency department without the heart attack being detected and treated. In addition, many patients with unstable angina are sent home without diagnosis; they may progress to a heart attack after discharge or require urgent medical therapy soon thereafter. Patients with undetected acute coronary syndrome are twice as likely to die as those whose condition is detected and treated. In the study, three of the patients were not characterized as having acute coronary syndrome until their follow-up visit.

"MRI provides us with additional and more precise information than is currently accessible from other imaging methods, such as echocardiography, coronary angiography, and positron emission tomography," added Dr. Robert S. Balaban, scientific director of the NHLBI Laboratory Research Program, and a co-author of the paper. "MRI technology could help us get another 20 percent of patients with acute coronary syndrome to life-saving treatment more quickly, and reduce the number of patients spending hours in the hospital for long-term EKG and enzyme monitoring."

Balaban estimates that MRI to detect acute coronary syndrome in the emergency department could be used in hospitals nationwide within a few years. Many U.S. hospitals currently have equipment that could be upgraded for this use.

"This study represents a shift of moving technology directly from the basic science laboratory to the clinical setting," added Balaban. "Working with physicists and engineers, we hope to further develop MRI to provide even more precise imaging and quantifiable ways to measure coronary blockages."

"MRI is a noninvasive imaging tool that we can now interact with in real time allowing us to see soft tissues, such as the wall of a diseased artery or the heart muscle itself while measuring physiological functions such as contraction, blood flow, and viability," Balaban noted. "The future of MRI is to go from diagnostic uses, as described in this study, to therapeutic applications. MRI can be used to guide minimally invasive procedures, including cardiac catheterization to open blocked arteries, direct the injection of therapeutic agents such as gene vectors or stem cells into damaged areas of the heart, replace heart valves, or remove cells that are causing arrhythmias."

Chapter 43

Angiography

Chapter Contents

Section 43.1

Catheter Angiography

This section includes "Angiography," Reprinted with permission from the Beth Israel Deaconess Medical Center, Department of Radiology © 2003 Beth Israel Deaconess Medical Center. All Rights Reserved. For additional information, visit http://radiology.bidmc.harvard.edu/. Also, "Coronary Angiography and Cardiac Catheterization," © 2003 Florida Cardiovascular Institute. All rights reserved. Reprinted with permission. For additional information on cardiac procedures, visit http://www.fciheart.com.

Angiography

Angiography is a special x-ray procedure that takes pictures (angiograms) of your blood vessels. It is usually done by inserting a catheter into an artery or vein in your groin. In some cases another site is selected; if so, the radiologist will discuss this with you.

The catheter is a small, flexible, hollow tube about the size of a thin strand of spaghetti. The radiologist carefully threads it into your blood vessel and guides it to the area to be studied. He watches the catheter moving through your blood vessels on a special x-ray television screen. When the catheter reaches the site under investigation, x-ray dye is injected through the catheter. This clearly outlines the blood vessels and enables the radiologist to see any irregularities or blockages.

A day or two before the exam, you may be asked to go in for a pretest appointment. At that time you will be seen by a radiologist and/or a nurse, who will give you more information about your procedure and answer any questions you may have. They will give you written instructions telling you what to do before the test and where to go on the day of the test. They will also ask you to sign a form giving your consent for the procedure. You will then be sent to have blood tests.

What Will Happen during My Procedure?

After you arrive at the hospital you will change into a gown. You do not need to remove your dentures, eyeglasses, or hearing aids. You'll proceed to a special procedures area, where you'll meet your team, and then be taken into the x-ray room. If you have not already been set up with one, your nurse will start an intravenous in order to give you fluids. She will check your vital signs—your heart rate and blood pressure. These vital signs will be checked frequently throughout your procedure. Your nurse will also check the pulses in your feet. The x-ray technologist will also be preparing you for this exam. This involves shaving the hair on your groin and washing the area with a special soap. Finally, sterile sheets will be placed over you. It is important to keep your hands at your sides under these sterile sheets.

What Will I Feel during My Angiogram?

The radiologist will numb your groin with a local anesthetic such as Xylocaine. This will sting a bit, but only for a few seconds. After this, you should feel only pressure where the doctor is working.

The nurse will also give you some intravenous medications to help relax you and make you more comfortable. As the doctor places the catheter, you may notice that the lights go on and off in the room. This allows the doctor to see the TV screen more clearly, to follow the catheter's progress. Just as you cannot feel blood flowing in your body, you will not feel the catheter moving inside your blood vessels. When x-ray dye is injected, you may feel a warm or hot flushed feeling. This is a normal response and passes in a few seconds.

While the x-ray pictures are being taken, you will be given breathing instructions from time to time. Also, you will be told before the x-rays are taken what you can expect to feel and hear. Once all the necessary pictures are taken, the doctor will remove the catheter, and apply pressure to the puncture site for ten to twenty minutes. This allows the blood vessel to seal over so it does not bleed (stitches are not necessary). A bandage will be placed on the site.

What Can I Expect after My Angiogram?

After your angiogram you will rest in bed for six to eight hours in a recovery area. You must keep your leg straight to keep the puncture site from bleeding, since movement could dislodge the seal in your blood vessel. Your nurses can carefully turn you onto your side for back comfort. You may resume your normal diet. The x-ray dye that was used will cause you to urinate more than usual after your procedure, and you will need to drink more fluids. The intravenous fluids will also help keep you hydrated. You may use a bedpan or urinal.

Your nurse will check on you frequently. She'll take your vital signs, check the puncture site, and check your foot pulses. You should let her know if you have any discomfort such as nausea, headache, a cold feeling, or numbness/tingling in your foot. Please call her immediately if you feel a warm wet sensation or swelling in your groin.

Before you leave the hospital, you will be given written information about caring for yourself at home.

How Will I Learn the Results?

Your doctor will discuss the results of the angiogram with you.

Coronary Angiography and Cardiac Catheterization

Cardiac catheterization is the insertion of a catheter (a long, narrow, flexible tube) through a blood vessel into the heart. This technique makes it possible to explore within the heart to find out precisely how the heart and coronary arteries are working, and, in some cases, to treat disease. One of the most important tests that can be done along with the catheterization is coronary angiography, or the injection of a substance through the tube that causes the coronary arteries to show up on x-rays. Although cardiac catheterization is a highly specialized diagnostic technique, and is performed only in a specially equipped hospital laboratory by a carefully trained staff, it is an extremely common procedure. In fact, about three-quarters of a million cardiac catheterizations are conducted each year in this country.

Why Is Catheterization Done?

You may go to your doctor for symptoms that could indicate heart trouble—such as shortness of breath, chest pain, palpitations, dizziness, or blackouts. Or your doctor may have picked up signs of heart or coronary artery disease during the course of a physical examination. In either case, you have probably been through a sequence of diagnostic steps: personal history, electrocardiogram (EKG), x-rays, treadmill stress tests, blood tests, and even nuclear tests or dobutamine stress echocardiography. At this point, your doctor may recommend cardiac catheterization to more precisely identify the problem.

Be sure to tell your doctor if:

- You suspect that you are pregnant. Cardiac catheterization will usually be delayed until after the birth of your baby.

- You have had allergic reactions. An infrequent complication of angiography is a reaction to the contrast medium injected.

To better understand why your doctor considers cardiac catheterization necessary, you may find it useful to review some basic facts about the heart and how it works. For additional information, consult your physician.

Basically, the heart is a tough muscle that contracts rhythmically to pump blood on its course throughout the body. Each contraction of a healthy heart is strong enough to pump out at least 55% of the heart's blood contents. These contractions, which we feel as heartbeats, are kept steady by a natural electrical pacemaker cell in the heart muscle. A system of valves inside the heart chambers prevents the blood from flowing backwards. Blood is pumped from the left side of the heart through the aorta to the rest of the body which uses oxygen. Oxygen-rich blood returns from lungs to left side of heart.

Blood is pumped from the right side of the heart to the lungs, where it picks up oxygen. Because the heart itself is a muscle doing hard work, it needs its own direct supply of oxygen-rich blood. This blood is supplied by the coronary arteries which branch off from the aorta, the great artery leaving the left side of the heart. The coronary arteries, in turn, branch into smaller and smaller arteries over the entire heart muscle.

One or more catheters are inserted into an artery or vein, or both, located in the arm or upper thigh. As the catheter is gently advanced toward the heart, its progress is watched on an x-ray screen. When the catheter enters the heart, its specially shaped tip helps your doctor guide it into its proper position. Because your cooperation is required from time to time, you will be awake, although mildly sedated, during the entire procedure.

Different catheters may be used for various diagnostic tests. These tests include measuring the heart's electrical activity, drawing blood samples, and taking pressure readings in the heart chambers and in the arteries. A substance called a contrast medium can be injected to reveal pumping action of the heart chambers, leaks in valves, or obstructions in the coronary arteries.

The tests done during cardiac catheterization can provide your doctor with a wealth of detail about the condition of your heart.

One of the most important reasons for cardiac catheterization is the need to see the blood flowing through the heart and coronary arteries. Contrast medium is injected through the catheter and the resulting x-ray pictures or cinefilms show the heart's blood flow clearly. In the heart itself, angiography can reveal faulty motion of the heart wall, leakage of blood back through diseased valves, or shunting (the pushing of blood back and forth through a hole between the heart's

465

right and left sides). In the coronary arteries, angiography can help locate blockages due to fatty deposits on the inner arterial walls. These deposits may prevent blood from reaching the heart muscle. Delicate sensors in the tip of or connected to the catheter can measure the volume of blood pumped by the heart, and can show if this flow is less than normal. Measurements taken in more than one place help to locate any blockage or any leaking in the valves. If it appears that catheterization itself may upset the heart's electrical system, a temporary artificial pacemaker will be introduced through the catheter to keep the heartbeat regular. This pacemaker is removed at the end of the test. Blood samples drawn through the catheter are measured for their oxygen content. Before cardiac catheterization can be performed, your doctor will discuss the procedure and any possible risks with you, and have you sign a legal consent form.

Before the Procedure

You may enter the hospital the afternoon before or possibly the day of the catheterization. After midnight you won't be allowed to have anything to eat or drink, but you may rinse your mouth out with water. In the morning, you will be given a mild sedative, and the area where the catheter is to be inserted (either the upper thigh or arm) will be shaved. Then you will be taken to the catheterization laboratory.

In the Laboratory

At first the laboratory may feel cool, but it will warm up as the machinery starts to run. Because the lab must be absolutely sterile, you will be draped just as if you are going to have an operation. Your doctor, and the nurses and technicians, will be wearing gowns and gloves. Only the patch of skin where the catheter is to be inserted is exposed. The preparations for catheterization are extensive, and they often take as long as half an hour. However, not all of the lab's various cameras, monitors, and instruments will necessarily be used— they are set up simply to take care of all possible needs. First, you will be given a local anesthetic where the catheter is to go in. This injection feels like a bee sting and will probably be the most uncomfortable part of the entire examination. Once the anesthetic has taken effect, the catheter is inserted, which may cause a sensation of slight pressure. If the catheter is going in through your arm, a tiny incision is made to expose a blood vessel; then, having made a hole in the vein or artery, your doctor inserts the catheter directly into the pathway to the heart. If the catheter is going in through your thigh, no incision is made. Instead, a needle is inserted into a blood vessel. Then a wire is put in, the needle removed, and the catheter slipped over the wire and advanced toward the heart. X-ray cameras allow accurate positioning of the catheter within the heart. After it is in place, you may be asked to cooperate in some simple tests: for example, you may breathe into an airbag for a measurement of your oxygen consumption. During these tests, the personnel in the lab are recording measurements and continually monitoring your condition. When the contrast medium for angiography is administered through the catheter, you will feel a hot flush all over your body that lasts about 15 to 30 seconds. This is a normal reaction to the contrast medium and is not cause for concern. There may be several injections of the contrast medium, and the catheter may be advanced or new ones inserted to get different views of your heart and coronary arteries. During the angiography procedure, you may be asked to cough a few times to help move the contrast medium through your heart. Test results are recorded through x-ray cameras.

After the catheters are removed, your doctor will close the point of insertion with stitches if the insertion was in your arm. If the catheter was inserted into your thigh, one of the staff will press down with a firm hand for about 15 minutes. A sandbag will then be put on the spot before you're taken back to your room. The entire procedure, including about half an hour of preparation, takes about an hour.

After the Procedure

Once you are back in your hospital room, you will be watched carefully. If you have a sandbag on your thigh, you will have to remain lying down for four to six hours. Your nurse will bring a bedpan if you need one, but even then try to move as little as possible. Your blood pressure will be checked every 15 minutes for several hours. A nurse will also keep checking the point where the catheter was inserted to be sure there is no bleeding. Your doctor may come in to check you as well.

The risks involved in cardiac catheterization are very low. There is less than a 1% chance that the procedure could cause a heart attack, a stroke, bleeding or clotting, or perforation of the heart. In rare instances, a rapid increase in heart rate might require electrical stimulation to return it to normal. Fatalities are extremely rare. It is important to keep in mind that the risks involved in cardiac catheterization are far outweighed by the benefit of knowing the exact state of your heart. The more your doctor knows about the condition of your heart, the greater the chance that treatment will be successful. The contrast material may cause you to pass more urine than usual. For this reason, and because you won't have drunk anything since midnight, you may be advised to drink a lot of fluid.

Although most people have no pain at all following catheterization, your doctor will prescribe a pain medication if you need it. A small black and blue spot or a lump under the skin at the point of insertion is common, and will disappear in about a week.

Your doctor should have all the information from your tests later in the day and will probably discuss the results with you some time during the evening. You will probably be discharged from the hospital the evening of the procedure or, in some cases, the next morning.

If you have symptoms of heart or coronary artery disease, your doctor will want to use every available method to find out precisely what the trouble is. The techniques of cardiac catheterization and coronary angiography can give exact information that will help your doctor to make a more accurate diagnosis of your condition.

The knowledge gained from cardiac catheterization enables your doctor to make a much more informed decision about the kind of treatment you may need. It is possible that you may be told to stop taking medication because your symptoms are not caused by heart disease. Your medication or dosage may be changed, or a new medication prescribed. You may be advised to have surgery—possibly coronary bypass surgery, or a repair to the heart's walls or its valves. You may be recommended for coronary angioplasty to treat your coronary artery disease.

Section 43.2

Computed Tomography (CT) Angiography

"CT Angiography," Copyright © 2002 Mater Imaging. All rights reserved. Additional information about imaging procedures is available at www.mater-imaging.com.au.

What Is the Test Used For?

Computerized tomography (or CT) angiography is used to look at the blood vessels (arteries and veins) of the body. CT images are cross-sections of the body, but the CT computer can generate a reconstruction where the blood vessels are shown in three dimensions, just like conventional angiography. The main advantage over conventional angiography is that there is no need to perform an injection into a main artery. With CT angiography, injection is made into an arm vein, which is much safer and more comfortable. Also, less contrast is used.

What Is the Preparation for the Test?

This depends on the area of the body being examined. You may be asked to fast (no solid food, and only clear liquids) for 2–3 hours before the procedure. When you go into the CT room, you may also be asked about any history of allergy, or what medications you are taking.

Will I Have to Undress?

For a scan of the head, arms, or legs, you are generally not required to undress, but may be asked to remove jewelry, hairclips, dentures, etc. These items show up too well on x-ray and can be confusing to interpret or hide abnormalities.

For most other scans, you will be asked to remove most of your clothes, but may keep wearing your underpants. You will be asked to change into a cotton gown.

Where Will I Be for the Test?

You will be asked to lie on the CT table, which as the name implies, is fairly hard. Pillows and foam pads can be used to make things more comfortable for you, and pads or Velcro straps may be used to help keep an area of the body still for the scan. The CT table will move during the scan, but nothing will touch you. The table moves into or out of the scanner, which is a very short tunnel. The tunnel is not enclosed, and only a small part of your body will be in it at any time.

Most examinations are performed with you lying on your back, although occasionally you may be asked to lie face down.

How Is the Test Done?

CT scanners are very specialized x-ray machines. As you move through the scanner, x-rays are taken and a powerful computer builds a very detailed image of the internal structure of the part of the body being examined.

To perform CT angiography, you will be given an injection of x-ray contrast, just before or during the scan. This injection highlights the blood supply to the organs of the body. The contrast is given via a small needle in the arm or hand. The needle is about the size of that used when blood tests are taken. The injection contains an iodine compound. It is important to tell the CT staff if you have any allergy to x-ray contrast. The injection may make you feel warm for a few minutes, and also give you a metallic taste in the mouth. These feelings are quite normal, although many people experience nothing at all. You may be asked to hold your breath during the scan, but only for 15 or 20 seconds. This is because breathing will blur the images.

How Long Will It All Take?

Most CT appointments are for 20 minutes, although for many scans, you will only be on the table for 5 to 10 minutes. The rest of the time is for explaining the procedure, getting you changed, and getting you off the table.

And after the Test?

If you have had barium, drink plenty of clear fluids over the next day to wash it through. You may eat and drink as normal. If you have had an x-ray contrast injection, there should be no lasting effects, although if you do experience anything unusual following the scan, contact your doctor.

Section 43.3

Magnetic Resonance Angiography (MRA)

"MR Angiography Can See Heart Bypass Grafts, Look for Blockage," Reproduced with permission from the American Heart Association World Wide Web Site, www.americanheart.org. © 2003, Copyright American Heart Association.

MR Angiography Can See Heart Bypass Grafts, Look for Blockage

High-resolution magnetic resonance angiography (MRA) may offer a risk-free way to identify narrowed vein grafts after bypass surgery, according to a report in the January 22, 2002 *Circulation: Journal of the American Heart Association*.

High-resolution MRA provides clear 3-dimensional images of blood vessels. MRA accurately identifies blockage in vein grafts, as well as the extent of narrowing, researchers say.

"The high-resolution images were comparable to images obtained with x-ray angiography, which is the gold standard test for diagnosing blocked arteries and veins," says Ernst E. van der Wall, M.D., an author of the study and professor of cardiology at Leiden University Medical Center, Leiden, Netherlands.

In bypass surgery, surgeons take a blood vessel from another part of the body and create a detour around the blocked part of a coronary artery. In the procedure, an artery may be detached from the chest wall and the open end attached to the coronary artery below the blocked area. Or, a piece of a long vein in the leg may be used. One end is sewn onto the large artery leaving the heart—the aorta. The other end of the vein is attached or grafted to the coronary artery below the blocked area.

The MRA technique in this study was used to look only at bypasses that had used the patient's leg vein.

"Recurrent chest pain after coronary artery bypass surgery is alarming for the patient and can pose a clinical dilemma for the physician: Should the patient undergo an invasive test, such as an angiography, to determine the cause of the pain, or is it better to follow a course of watchful waiting?" says van der Wall. MRA may provide the needed answers without the risk of invasive testing or the anxiety associated with waiting, he says.

Narrowed or blocked arteries and veins are caused by the buildup of a hard, fatty substance called plaque. This buildup of deposits on the inner surface of arteries and veins is called atherosclerosis. When blocked arteries are bypassed, the disease may progress to the new vein grafts and can cause recurrent chest pain called angina.

"The beauty of MRA is that it is a non-invasive test," says van der Wall, whereas the traditional diagnostic test, coronary angiography, is invasive. He says coronary angiography is an excellent tool for diagnosing disease in coronary arteries and grafts, but it can be risky after surgery.

Patients who undergo coronary angiography have a thin catheter (tube) inserted in the groin, which is then carefully guided into the heart. Dye is released through this catheter and makes the arteries and grafts visible on an x-ray. While most patients undergo angiography with no ill effects, sometimes the catheter can tear a blood vessel or cause other complications. With MRA there are no such risks, he says.

In the study, van der Wall's team used high-resolution MRA to assess the condition of 56 vein grafts in 38 patients who complained of recurrent chest pain after bypass surgery. The patients, whose mean age was 67, were already scheduled for standard angiography to determine the cause of the pain, but agreed to have MRA in addition to the standard treatment. Nineteen of the patients had MRA before x-ray angiography and 19 patients underwent MRA following standard angiography.

Eighteen grafts were found to be narrowed by 50 percent or more, while 11 grafts were at least 70 percent narrowed and six were completely blocked.

Two observers who were blinded to the findings of the standard angiogram or the report of the other observer assessed the MRA scans.

When the graft was at least 50 percent narrowed, the diagnostic accuracy of high-resolution MRA compared to traditional angiography was 65 percent to 88 percent. When the vessel was narrowed by 70 percent or more, accuracy was 73 percent to 87 percent, and when the vein graft was completely blocked, the accuracy was 83 percent to 100 percent.

Since MRA technology is still developing, van der Wall says it is too soon to suggest that it can replace standard angiography, but he says it could be considered as a useful diagnostic adjunct. "Also, the technique costs about $500, which is about half the cost of standard angiography."

According to the American Heart Association's latest statistics, about 12.6 million Americans have coronary heart disease. In 1999 more than 570,000 heart bypass surgeries were performed in the United States.

Chapter 44

Nuclear Medicine Procedures

What Patients Should Know about Nuclear Medicine Procedures

Your doctor has referred you or a family member for a test in the nuclear medicine department because the information obtained from the test will be important in determining the diagnosis and treatment of the medical problem you may have. You probably have a number of questions such as:

- What is a nuclear medicine test?
- What preparation is needed for the test?
- What will happen during the test?

This chapter provides information on some of the more commonly performed diagnostic and therapeutic nuclear medicine procedures. First, an overview of nuclear medicine is discussed; answers to frequently asked questions as well as key points to know are provided. Lastly, procedures for specific tests are outlined.

However, the material presented here is for informational purposes only and is not intended as a substitute for discussion between you

---

This chapter includes "What Patients Should Know about Nuclear Medicine Procedures," "Frequently Asked Questions about Nuclear Medicine," "Bone Imaging," "Renal Imaging in Children," "Liver and Hepatobiliary Imaging," and "Brain Imaging," all reprinted by permission of the Society of Nuclear Medicine, www.snm.org. © 2003 Society of Nuclear Medicine.

and your physician. If you require more information about a nuclear medicine procedure, please consult your physician or the nuclear medicine department of the institution where the test will be performed.

What Is Nuclear Medicine?

Nuclear medicine involves the use of small amounts of radioactive materials (or tracers) to help diagnose and treat a variety of diseases. Nuclear medicine determines the cause of the medical problem based on the function of the organ, tissue, or bone. This is how nuclear medicine differs from an x-ray, ultrasound, or other diagnostic tests that determine the presence of disease based on structural appearance.

Millions of nuclear medicine tests are performed each year in the United States. Nuclear medicine tests (also known as scans, examinations, or procedures) are safe and painless. In a nuclear medicine test, the radioactive material is introduced into the body by injection, swallowing, or inhalation. Different tracers are used to study different parts of the body. The amount of tracer used is carefully selected to provide the least amount of radiation exposure to the patient, but ensure an accurate test. A special camera (scintillation or gamma camera) is used to take pictures of your body. The camera does this by detecting the tracer in the organ, bone, or tissue being imaged, and then records this information on a computer screen or on film. Generally, nuclear medicine tests are not recommended for pregnant women because unborn babies have a greater sensitivity to radiation than children or adults. If you are pregnant or think that you are pregnant, your doctor may order a different type of diagnostic test.

Frequently Asked Questions

Why May Several Different Tests Be Needed?

Sometimes a variety of diagnostic tests are performed to determine the nature of a medical problem and the most appropriate treatment. Although a diagnosis is usually made with one nuclear medicine test, it may be necessary to confirm the test results with another test or study.

Are Nuclear Medicine Procedures Safe?

Nuclear medicine procedures are very safe. A patient only receives an extremely small amount of tracer, just enough to provide accurate diagnostic information. The amount of radiation in a nuclear medicine test is no more than that received during an x-ray.

Who Performs Nuclear Medicine Tests?

- A nuclear medicine technologist, a health care professional trained and experienced in the theory and practice of nuclear medicine procedures, performs the test by administering the tracer, positioning the patient under the camera, and operating the equipment used in the test.

- A nuclear medicine physician, who is specially trained in physics and chemistry and is licensed to use tracers, interprets the images.

How Should I Prepare for the Test?

Generally, no special preparation is required, but if preparation is needed, you will be notified before the test. Certain tests may require some slight preparation. For example, if you are having a cardiac stress-rest test, you may be asked not to eat three to four hours before the test because the pictures of your heart will be easier to interpret if the stomach is empty. Or, if you are having a prostate, ovarian, or colorectal cancer scan, it is important to let the technologist know if you have had a nuclear medicine test recently, have had previous surgery, or are allergic or sensitive to any substances or drugs.

You need not worry about stopping your regular, daily activities or stop taking previously prescribed medications. Although you should check with your doctor, most medications generally do not affect the accuracy of the test results.

The key to having a successful nuclear medicine test is to remain as still as possible. Any movement may distort the image results, making them difficult to interpret and increasing the possibility of redoing the test. Be sure to dress comfortably so that you are relaxed during the test. You should dress warmly since some imaging rooms may be cold. Also, if lying on your back for long periods of time causes discomfort, you may take a pain reliever before the test is performed.

What Should I Tell My Doctor before the Test Is Scheduled?

You should tell your doctor if you are pregnant or think that you are pregnant. You should also tell your doctor if you are breastfeeding.

Why Do Nuclear Medicine Tests Take a Long Time to Perform?

The amount of time needed for a procedure depends on the type of test. Nuclear medicine tests are performed in three parts: tracer administration, taking the pictures, and analyzing the images. For many tests, a certain amount of time is needed (from a few hours to a few days) for the tracer to accumulate in the part of the body being studied before the pictures can be taken. During the imaging session, the time needed to obtain the pictures (from minutes to hours) will vary depending on the test.

Does the Tracer Cause Side Effects?

Adverse reactions, or side effects, are rare, but do let the technologist know if you experience any symptoms during or after the tracer injection.

What Happens after the Test?

When the exam is completed, the nuclear medicine physician reviews your images, prepares a report, and discusses the results with your doctor. Your doctor will explain the test results to you and discuss what further procedures, if any are needed.

After the test, should I avoid physical contact with others? No. However, if you have had radioiodine treatment, there are guidelines that your doctor may recommend that you follow to reduce the chance of radiation exposure to others. In general, the tracer you are given will remain in your body for a short period of time, and is cleared from the body through natural bodily functions. Drinking fluids will help eliminate the tracer more quickly.

Can I Resume My Daily Activities after the Test?

You should be able to resume your daily activities after a nuclear medicine test. If you were temporarily asked to stop taking any medication prior to the test or if your doctor changed your usual dosage because of the test, be sure to ask when and if you should resume taking your medication(s).

Are Nuclear Medicine Tests Performed on Children?

Yes, scans are performed on children. The tests are usually done to evaluate bone pain, injuries, infection, or kidney or bladder functions.

The amount of tracer is carefully adjusted based on the child's size. Sedation is sometimes required, depending on the child and type of test being given.

What You Should Know

- Remember to remain still while the pictures are being taken. Movement may distort the images and make the test results difficult to interpret.

- Do not worry about the amount of radiation you will receive during the test. It is no more than what you would receive from similar x-ray procedures.

- Be sure to tell your doctor if you are pregnant, think you are pregnant, or are a nursing mother.

- Let the technologist know if you experience any symptoms during or after the tracer is administered.

- The radioactive tracer remains in your body for a short time, and it is cleared from the body through natural bodily functions. Drinking plenty of fluids will help the tracer clear through your body more quickly.

- Ask the technologist to explain any part of the procedure that you do not understand.

Nuclear Medicine Procedures

Scans may be used to diagnose a host of medical problems. Some of the more frequently performed tests include:

- Bone scans to examine orthopedic injuries, fractures, tumors, or unexplained bone pain.

- Heart scans to identify normal or abnormal blood flow to the heart muscle, measure heart function, or determine the existence or extent of damage to the heart muscle after a heart attack.

- Breast scans which are used in conjunction with mammograms to more accurately detect and locate cancerous tissue in the breasts.

- Liver and gallbladder scans to evaluate liver and gallbladder function.

- Ovarian and colorectal cancer imaging to detect tumors and determine the severity (staging) of various types of cancer.

- Prostate cancer imaging to detect tumors and to determine the extent and spread of various types of cancers.
- Brain imaging to investigate problems within the brain itself or in blood circulation to the brain.
- Renal imaging in children to examine kidney function.

Other commonly performed procedures include thyroid uptake scans to analyze the overall function of the thyroid and show the structure of the gland; lung scans to evaluate the flow of blood and movement of air into and out of the lung as well as determine the presence of blood clots; gallium scans to evaluate infection and certain types of tumors; and gastrointestinal bleeding scans.

Nuclear medicine can also be used for treatment (therapy). Radioiodine treatment for the thyroid is a common therapeutic procedure.

The material presented here is for informational purposes only and is not intended as a substitute for discussion between you and your physician. Be sure to consult with your physician or the nuclear medicine department where the test will be performed if you require more information about specific nuclear medicine procedures.

Bone Imaging

Bone scans are used to detect arthritis, osteoporosis, fractures, sports injuries, tumors, and even cases of child abuse. Bone scans may also be used to evaluate unexplained bone pain; malignancies in the breast; prostate, thyroid, and certain types of heart or brain damage.

Test Preparation

For most bone studies, you will be asked to drink as many fluids as possible, both before and after the procedure.

Exam Procedure

During the first part of the test, the tracer is injected. It generally takes about two hours for the tracer to be absorbed by the bones. The technologist will let you know if it is okay to eat during this waiting period. During the waiting period, you should try to urinate as often as possible because it will help eliminate the tracer from your body that is not going to the bones.

Depending on the study, the technologist may take pictures of your bones as the tracer is moving through your bloodstream before it reaches your bones. It takes about 30 minutes to complete the images. In most bone studies, however, the imaging portion takes much longer, from two to four hours. For most bone scans, you will lie on the imaging table with the camera positioned above or below you. Several images may be taken or the camera may move slowly, imaging the entire length of your body. Although the imaging session takes a long time, it is extremely important that you remain as still as possible so that the scan results are accurate.

For children, the procedure is the same as for adults, except that after the tracer injection, the child may be given a sedative. If the child is given a sedative, he or she will have to remain in the nuclear medicine department until they are fully awake. After the test, the child should be able to resume daily activities, and there are no restrictions about eating, drinking, or contact with others. If the child has been sedated, you may wish to let him or her rest for a day before resuming normal play activity.

Renal Imaging in Children

This test allows the physician to monitor the flow of urine, the degree of any blockage, and assess the amount of scarring in the kidney tissue.

Test Preparation

Preparation will depend on several factors, including the child's age and the medical problem being diagnosed. The child may need to:

- be sedated, particularly children under three years of age.
- be given a diuretic intravenously.
- have a catheter inserted to keep the bladder free of urine.
- discontinue taking current medications.

Exam Procedure

Radionuclide Cystography, a test used to detect the flow of urine from the bladder back into the kidney. In Direct Radionuclide Cystography, a catheter is inserted as well as an intravenous solution with enough fluid to encourage urination (voiding). Multiple images are taken as the child voids. For Indirect Radionuclide Cystography, no catheter is inserted, and images are obtained after the tracer injection.

Diuretic Renal Scintigraphy, a test used to detect kidney blockage. After a catheter is inserted, the tracer and fluid to encourage voiding are injected intravenously. Multiple images are then obtained.

Cortical Renal Scintigraphy, a test used to determine the absence of renal tissue. The tracer is administered intravenously. Two hours after the injection, multiple pictures are taken.

Liver and Hepatobiliary Imaging

Liver scans help diagnose disorders such as cirrhosis, hepatitis, tumors, and other problems in the digestive tract. Gallbladder scans are used to evaluate upper abdominal pain, determine causes of jaundice, and identify obstruction in the gallbladder.

Test Preparation

For the liver scan, no special preparation is required. If you are having a liver/spleen test, however, do not have any gastrointestinal tests with barium within 24 hours prior to the liver test.

For the gallbladder scan, you may be asked to:

- Not eat or drink for two to four hours before the test because contents in the stomach will alter the test results.
- Stop taking current medications because certain drugs affect how the tracer flows through the biliary tract.
- Remove metal accessories as they may interfere with the study.

Exam Procedure

Liver Scan: After an injection of tracer into your arm, you will wait 10 to 15 minutes for the tracer to be absorbed by the liver. You will then lie on your back on the table, and pictures will be taken of your abdomen from several positions.

Liver/Spleen Scan: Tracer is injected in your arm. Ten to 15 minutes after the injection, you will lie on your back and images from different positions will be taken of your liver and spleen.

Gallbladder Scan: After tracer injection (in the arm), you will lie on your back on the imaging table and multiple images of the abdominal area will be taken. For this test, the images are taken immediately after the tracer injection. Imaging takes one to two hours (or longer) because it is not possible to determine how long it will take your liver to excrete the tracer or when your gallbladder will be visible to the camera.

Gallbladder Scan in Children: The procedure is the same as for adults, except that children under age 3 may require sedation. Also, the imaging time for children is not as long, lasting 45 minutes to 1 hour.

Brain Imaging

A brain scan may be necessary to investigate problems within the brain itself or in blood circulation to and from the brain (perfusion imaging).

Test Preparation

Generally, no special preparation is needed. If special preparation is required, your doctor will let you know.

Exam Procedure

Perfusion Imaging: After relaxing in a dimly lit room, the tracer is injected in the arm. Thirty to 60 minutes after the injection, you will lie on your back under the camera and pictures of your brain will be taken for 30 to 60 minutes. You will be asked not to move, touch your head, or cough while the pictures are being taken.

Stress/Rest Test: Most brain scans are taken while the patient is resting, but some medical conditions require evaluation of different activity levels of the brain during active and rest periods. This test is performed using a special drug or while doing certain tasks that activate brain function. The test is performed in two parts: first, a rest image is obtained, and the next day, the necessary stress test is performed.

Cisternography: This test determines if there is abnormal flow of cerebral spinal fluid around or in the brain. The tracer is injected into the lower back region by a doctor. After the injection, you will lie still for a few hours. It usually takes two to three days to complete the images.

Part Seven

Electrical Tests

Chapter 45

Electrocardiogram (EKG)

What Is an Electrocardiogram?

ECG, EKG, or electrocardiogram all refer to the same test, which is a simple and painless test that records the changes in the electrical activity of the heart on graph paper.

An electrocardiogram helps identifies heart rhythm abnormalities and imbalances of the salts of the body. It can also tell about the size or thickness of the heart chambers and the relative position of the heart in the chest.

How the Electrocardiogram Test Is Done

An electrocardiogram can be done on hospital inpatients or outpatients. After registration, an electrocardiogram technician or nurse will take the patient into a room and have the patient take off his/her shirt and lie down on an examination table or bed. Twelve stickers called electrodes are attached to the chest, shoulders, and each leg. A wire will then be attached to each electrode.

After the patient is very still and relaxed, the technician will press a button on the electrocardiogram machine and the recording will be done. The recording generally takes less than a minute.

This information is reprinted with permission from the Heart Center Encyclopedia, Cincinnati Children's Hospital Medical Center website, http://www.cincinnatichildrens.org/health/heart-encyclopedia/default.htm. © 2003 Cincinnati Children's Hospital Medical Center. All rights reserved.

Does an Electrocardiogram Hurt?

No, an electrocardiogram is painless. In fact, the most painful part of the process is removing the electrodes which are less sticky than even adhesive bandages.

How Long Will an Electrocardiogram Take?

The whole procedure usually takes about five minutes. The quicker the patient can be still and relaxed the sooner it will be completed.

When and Where Will the Results Provided?

A cardiologist will review the electrocardiogram and record their interpretation, generally within 24 hours. Results will be sent to the referring physician in 24–48 hours.

The Cardiology Department is not able to give results to patients or their families, only to the referring physician.

Preparation before an Electrocardiogram

Please do not use baby oil or lotion before the test. It does not allow the electrodes to stick properly.

Are There Any Risks Involved?

The only risk to the test is a skin allergy to the adhesive of the electrodes that may result in temporary redness and irritation of the skin where the electrodes are applied.

Chapter 46

Electroencephalogram (EEG)/Brain Wave Test

Alternative names: Electroencephalogram; brain wave test.

Definition: An electroencephalogram (EEG) is a test to detect abnormalities in the electrical activity of the brain.

How the Test Is Performed

Brain cells communicate by producing tiny electrical impulses. In an EEG, electrodes are placed on the scalp over multiple areas of the brain to detect and record patterns of electrical activity and check for abnormalities.

The test is performed by an EEG technician in a specially designed room that may be in your health care provider's office or at a hospital. You will be asked to lie on your back on a table or in a reclining chair.

The technician will apply between 16 and 25 flat metal discs (electrodes) in different positions on your scalp. The discs are held in place with a sticky paste. The electrodes are connected by wires to an amplifier and a recording machine.

The recording machine converts the electrical signals into a series of wavy lines that are drawn onto a moving piece of graph paper. You will need to lie still with your eyes closed because any movement can alter the results.

This chapter includes "EEG," © 2003 A.D.A.M., Inc. Reprinted with permission; and "Brain Wave Monitor," Image courtesy of A.D.A.M., Inc. Reprinted with permission.

You may be asked to do certain things during the recording, such as breathe deeply and rapidly for several minutes or look at a bright flickering light.

How to Prepare for the Test

You will need to wash your hair the night before the test. Do not use any oils, sprays, or conditioner on your hair before this test.

Your health care provider may want you to discontinue some medications before the test. Do not change or stop medications without first consulting your health care provider.

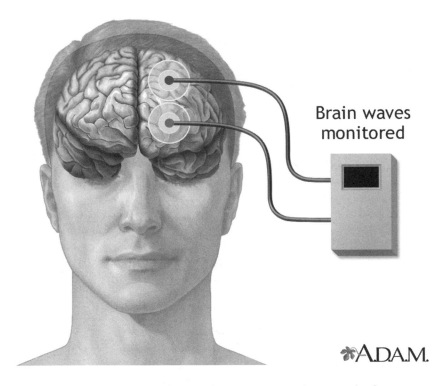

Brain waves
monitored

❀A.D.A.M.

Figure 46.1. Brain Wave Monitor. The brainstem auditory evoked response test (BAER), is performed to help diagnose nervous system abnormalities, hearing losses (especially in low-birth weight newborns), and to assess neurologic functions. The test focuses on changes and responses in brain waves. The brain waves are stimulated by a clicking sound to evaluate the central auditory pathways of the brainstem. (Source: Courtesy of A.D.A.M. © 2002, reprinted with permission)

You should avoid all foods containing caffeine for 8 hours before the test.

Sometimes it is necessary to sleep during the test, so you may be asked to reduce your sleep time the night before.

Infants and Children

The physical and psychological preparation you can provide for this or any test or procedure depends on your child's age, interests, previous experiences, and level of trust.

How the Test Will Feel

This test causes no discomfort. Although having electrodes pasted onto your skin may feel strange, they only record activity and do not produce any sensation.

Why the Test Is Performed

EEG is used to help diagnose the presence and type of seizure disorders, to look for causes of confusion, and to evaluate head injuries, tumors, infections, degenerative diseases, and metabolic disturbances that affect the brain.

It is also used to evaluate sleep disorders and to investigate periods of unconsciousness. The EEG may be done to confirm brain death in a comatose patient.

EEG cannot be used to read the mind, measure intelligence, or diagnose mental illness.

Normal Values

Brain waves have normal frequency and amplitude, and other characteristics are typical.

What Abnormal Results Mean

Abnormal findings may indicate the following:

- Seizure disorders (such as epilepsy or convulsions)
- Structural brain abnormality (such as a brain tumor or brain abscess)
- Head injury, encephalitis (inflammation of the brain)

- Hemorrhage (abnormal bleeding caused by a ruptured blood vessel)
- Cerebral infarct (tissue that is dead because of a blockage of the blood supply)
- Sleep disorders (such as narcolepsy)

EEG may confirm brain death in someone who is in a coma.

Additional conditions under which the test may be performed:

- Arteriovenous malformation (cerebral)
- Benign positional vertigo
- Cerebral aneurysm
- Complicated alcohol abstinence (delirium tremens)
- Creutzfeldt-Jacob disease
- Delirium
- Dementia
- Dementia due to metabolic causes
- Febrile seizure (children)
- Generalized tonic-clonic seizure
- Hepatic encephalopathy
- Hepatorenal syndrome
- Insomnia
- Labyrinthitis
- Ménière's disease
- Metastatic brain tumor
- Multiple sclerosis
- Optic glioma
- Partial (focal) seizure
- Partial complex seizure
- Petit mal seizure
- Pick's disease
- Senile dementia (Alzheimer's type)
- Shy-Drager syndrome
- Syphilitic aseptic meningitis
- Temporal lobe seizure

What the Risks Are

The procedure is very safe. If you have a seizure disorder, a seizure may be triggered by the flashing lights or hyperventilation. The health care provider performing the EEG is trained to take care of you if this happens.

Chapter 47

Electromyography (EMG) and Nerve Conduction Velocities

Diagnosis of neuromuscular disease hinges on a doctor's ability to identify a specific defect of neuromuscular function. Sometimes, a doctor can infer this functional defect—and the disease associated with it—by giving a physical exam, doing a blood test, or looking at the anatomy of nerves and muscles.

But other times, the doctor may have to directly evaluate the functions of nerves and muscles and the connections between them by using two complementary techniques—nerve conduction velocity testing (NCV) and electromyography (EMG).

Action Potentials

Both NCV and EMG rely on the fact that the activity of nerves and muscles produces electrical signals called action potentials. A nerve is actually a bundle of axons, cables that conduct action potentials from one end of a nerve cell (or neuron) to the other.

In motor neurons (neurons that connect to muscle), these action potentials travel toward the muscle, where they cause release of a chemical called acetylcholine. Acetylcholine opens tiny pores in the muscle, and the flow of sodium and potassium ions through these pores creates action potentials in the muscle, leading to contraction.

"Electromyography and Nerve Conduction Velocities," *Quest*, Volume 7, Number 5, October 2000. Reprinted by permission of the Muscular Dystrophy Association. For additional information, call the Muscular Dystrophy Association toll-free at 800-572-1717, or visit their website at www.mdausa.org.

In NCV and EMG, these tiny electrical events are amplified electronically, then visualized on a TV-like monitor called an oscilloscope and are even heard using audio equipment.

NCV and Axons

NCV measures action potentials conducted by axons, so doctors use it for diagnosing diseases that primarily affect nerve function, such as different forms of Charcot-Marie-Tooth disease (CMT).

It is done by placing surface electrodes (similar to those used for electrocardiograms) on the skin at various points over a nerve. One electrode delivers a mild electrical shock to the nerve, stimulating it to generate an action potential. The other electrodes record the action potential as it is conducted through the nerve.

Doctors often use NCV to determine the speed of nerve conduction (hence, its name). Conduction speed is influenced by a coating around axons, called myelin. Myelin insulates each axon and normally forces action potentials to jump quickly from one end of the axon to the other. If the myelin breaks down (as in CMT1), the action potential travels more slowly.

NCV also can measure the strength of the action potential in the nerve, which is proportional to the number of axons that contribute to it. If axons degenerate (as in amyotrophic lateral sclerosis) or become clogged with debris (as in CMT2), the action potential becomes smaller.

EMG and Muscle

An electromyogram measures the action potentials produced by muscles, and is therefore useful for diagnosing diseases that primarily affect muscle function, including the muscular dystrophies. Also, some EMG data can reveal defects in nerve function.

In EMG, the doctor inserts a needle-like electrode into a muscle. The electrode records action potentials that occur when the muscle is at rest and during voluntary contractions directed by the doctor.

While a healthy muscle appears quiet at rest, spontaneous action potentials are seen in damaged muscles or muscles that have lost input from nerve cells (as in ALS or myasthenia gravis). During voluntary contraction, dystrophic (wasted) muscles show very small action potentials, and myotonic (stiff) muscles show prolonged trains of action potentials. Altered patterns of muscle action potentials can indicate defects in nerve function.

A Little Discomfort

Though NCV and EMG are valuable tools for doctors, they can be distressing for patients. Some people find the electric shocks of the NCV or the needle penetration of the EMG uncomfortable or even painful. Young children might struggle during the tests, making it difficult for doctors to carefully monitor nerve and muscle activity. To ease discomfort, topical anesthetic can be applied to the skin—but it won't prevent muscle pain during the EMG. Sometimes sedating medications are needed to keep a child calm.

Partly because of these factors, NCV and EMG are generally used when it is not possible to gather the right information from other diagnostic tests. Muscle biopsy (excising and examining muscle tissue) can reveal hallmark anatomical features of some neuromuscular diseases, making EMG and NCV unnecessary. Genetic tests are now available for diagnosing some diseases, and in those cases, EMG and NCV usually can be bypassed.

Nonetheless, NCV and EMG remain the gold standards for evaluating the function of nerve and muscle. So, when a doctor suspects that a patient has a neuromuscular disease that is not clearly associated with anatomical or genetic defects (like some types of CMT, or myasthenia gravis), NCV and EMG are among the most valuable diagnostic tools.

Chapter 48

Exercise Stress Tests

Chapter Contents

Section 48.1

Stress Test Introduction

Reprinted with permission from www.heartsite.com. © 2003 A.S.M. Systems, Inc. All rights reserved. For additional information, visit www.heartsite.com.

Patients with coronary artery blockages may have minimal symptoms and an unremarkable or unchanged EKG while at rest. Alternatively, patients with no heart disease may have fairly convincing symptoms and a suspicious EKG. Both groups may benefit from a cardiac stress test during which exercise or a chemical substance is used to stress the heart and expose hidden heart disease or to help rule it out.

The heart may be stressed by having a patient exercise on a treadmill or a stationary bicycle. If the patient is unable to exercise secondary to physical limitations such as severe arthritis, artificial limbs, generalized weakness, paralysis, or unsteady gait, the physician may choose a pharmacological or chemical form of stress test. In the latter case, a medication is given intravenously to perform a nearly comparable degree of cardiac stress. If possible, some form of pharmacological stress testing may be combined with a brief period of treadmill exercise.

Stress testing, particularly those employing exercise, help reveal the following:

1. The length of exercise demonstrates physical tolerance and conditioning.

2. Extreme and inappropriate shortness of breath, chest discomfort, dizziness, and unexpected weakness may suggest underlying heart disease.

3. The blood pressure is recorded at intervals during stress (in the beginning and usually at three minute intervals, if stable). It may be checked more frequently if the patient's blood pressure response to exercise is abnormal.

4. High blood pressure during exercise may provide an early clue or indication about this problem. Normally, the systolic (upper

reading) blood pressure may rise up to 200 during extreme or peak exercise, while the diastolic (lower reading) remains below 90. Patients with inadequately controlled high blood pressure usually display high diastolic readings during exercise.

5. A drop in blood pressure during exercise may indicate heart disease.

6. Exercise may provoke arrhythmias (pronounced a-rhyth-me-yaz) or irregular heart rhythm which may not be seen at rest and may or may not point to heart disease.

7. The EKG is constantly monitored during exercise, recorded on paper at intervals (usually every minute), and compared to the EKG obtained at rest. Changes in the ST segment and T waves may indicate heart disease.

Labs may be equipped with a treadmill or a stationary bicycle. The EKG monitor and paper recorder plus the blood pressure cuff are used for stress tests. There are few risks with cardiac stress testing. However, since it is carried out in patients with known or suspected heart disease, almost every lab is also equipped with emergency cardiac drugs and resuscitative equipment, but these precautionary measures are rarely needed.

Preparation

The following recommendations are generic for all types of cardiac stress tests:

- Do not eat or drink for three hours prior to the procedure. This reduces the likelihood of nausea that may accompany strenuous exercise after a heavy meal. Diabetics, particularly those who use insulin, will need special instructions from the physician's office.

- Specific heart medicines may need to be stopped one or two days prior to the test. Such instructions are generally provided when the test is scheduled by the doctor's office. Call if you have any questions.

- Wear comfortable clothing and shoes that are suitable for exercise.

- An explanation of the test is provided and the patient is asked to sign a consent form.

Procedures

A trained technician or nurse will place small sticky patches on your chest. These are known as electrodes and are attached to wires that transmit the electrical activity of your heart to the EKG monitor and recorder. A wrap may be placed around your waist to hold the cables in place.

An EKG is then recorded on paper. This is known as the resting EKG and serves as a baseline. Additional recordings will be made during and following exercise. The physician will pay particular attention to changes in the pattern of the EKG (ST segments, T waves, heart rate, and the presence of an abnormal heart rhythm).

During stress testing, the heart rhythm is constantly displayed on a heart monitor. This allows the physician to keep an eye on the patient's heart rate, and to watch out for telltale EKG changes or irregular heart rhythms.

When a treadmill or stationary bicycle stress test is conducted, it is continued until the patient achieves a target heart rate (based upon age). However, it may be stopped early if the patient develops significant symptoms (chest pain, extreme shortness of breath, weakness, leg fatigue, or dizziness), serious irregular heart rhythm, or marked elevation of blood pressure. The majority of patients do not develop these problems. Fatigue, as would be expected after a good workout, is the only residual complaint.

Section 48.2

Chemical Stress Test

Reprinted with permission from www.heartsite.com. © 2003 A.S.M. Systems, Inc. All rights reserved. For additional information, visit www.heartsite.com.

How Does an Isotope Stress Test Work? How Does a Chemical Stress Test Work?

A chemical or pharmacological stress test combines an intravenous medication with an imaging technique (isotope imaging or echocardiography) to evaluate the left ventricle (LV). In these cases, the medication serves the purpose of increasing the heart load instead of using exercise. Stress causes normal coronary arteries to dilate, while the blood flow in a blocked coronary artery is reduced. This reduced blood flow may decrease the movement of the affected wall (as seen by echo), or have reduced isotope uptake in a nuclear scan. Agents that are commonly used in pharmacologic stress testing include dipyridamole, dobutamine, and Adenosine™.

When Is a Chemical Stress Test Performed?

Treadmill stress testing is the test of choice when a patient is able to exercise because of the physiologic effect that exercise has on the blood pressure and heart rate. It also helps give the physician an idea about the patient's exercise tolerance, and whether or not exertion has any adverse effects on the patient's symptoms or irregular heart beats. Additionally, one does not have to contend with any potential side-effects of chemical stress, even if they are usually minor.

However, exercise may not be possible because of physical limitations like back trouble, joint disease, marked fatigue, unsteady gait, prior stroke, dizziness, or shortness of breath. In such cases, chemical stress testing is employed. In other words, pharmacologic or chemical stress test is performed in situations where patients are unable to perform more than moderate exercise due to severe arthritis, prior injury, reduced exercise tolerance (as a result of debilitating illnesses), or in patients who are unable to increase the heart rate (as in some with heart pacemakers or with certain diseases that keep the heart from speeding up).

How Is a Chemical Stress Test Performed?

The imaging portion of the test is identical to that used during stress echocardiography or isotope stress testing (depending upon the technique employed), and is performed either in a cardiologist's office, a satellite lab, or the hospital. An intravenous line is started in the arm, the blood pressure is checked, and an EKG recorded. The EKG is also constantly monitored on the screen. If stress echo is being performed, an echocardiogram is obtained before and immediately after administration of the stress producing medication. In cases of stress isotope testing, the resting images may be obtained before or approximately two hours after the stress (depending upon the lab and the employed isotope). The stress-producing medication is given intravenously. In cases of dobutamine, the drug is given as a continuous drip with a gradual increase in the rate (at three minute intervals). The patient's heart rate accelerates and the isotope is given when 85% of the target heart rate is achieved. In cases of dipyridamole, the medication is usually given over four minutes, through the IV line. When there is a drop in the diastolic (lower number) blood pressure, the isotope is administered.

If a patient is able to perform mild exercise, he or she may be asked to walk on a treadmill for a minute or so after the injection of dipyridamole.

How Long Does the Entire Test Take?

A patient should allow two to four hours for the entire test, including the preparation. Dual isotope and technetium stress testing takes less time than thallium. The first part of the test generally takes an hour. The second part takes anywhere from 15 to 30 minutes. Between the two parts of a thallium test, you will be allowed to leave the lab and get a light snack or lunch.

How Safe Is a Chemical Stress Test?

The patient is exposed to a very small amount of radiation and the risk is minimal, if any. The risk of the chemical stress portion of the test is very small and similar to what you would expect from any strenuous form of exercise (jogging in your neighborhood or running up a flight of stairs) Experienced medical staff are in attendance to manage the rare complications like sustained irregular heart beats, unrelieved chest pain, or even a heart attack. In such cases, the patient is better off having the problem in the presence of experienced staff, rather than have it happen when they are exercising alone. Also, the stress medicine like dobutamine can be immediately stopped if there are problems. The effects of dipyridamole (which can occasionally cause nausea or a headache) can be reversed by aminophylline (an anti-asthma medication). Please also see the caution about asthma in the section on preparing for a stress test.

What Is the Reliability of a Chemical Isotope Stress Test?

If a patient is able to achieve the target heart rate in cases of dobutamine or an appropriate drop in the diastolic blood pressure with dipyridamole, and if good quality images are obtained, an isotope treadmill stress test is capable of diagnosing important disease in approximately 80% of patients with coronary artery disease. Approximately 10% of patients may have a false-positive test (when the results are falsely abnormal in a patient without coronary artery disease). Technical problems can occur when a patient is markedly overweight. Women may have an abnormality in the front portion of the heart because of overlying breast tissue. Some men may demonstrate an inferior wall abnormality because of a prominent diaphragm (muscular partition that separates the chest cavity from the abdomen). Patients who have a left bundle branch block on their EKG may also have a false abnormal test.

How Quickly Will I Get the Results and What Will It Mean?

The physician performing the stress test can give you a preliminary report about the EKG and echo (if it is used) portion of your test. However, the official result from the isotope scans may take a few days to complete. The results may influence your physician's decision to change your treatment or recommend additional testing such as cardiac catheterization.

Section 48.3

Echo Stress Test

Reprinted with permission from www.heartsite.com. © 2003 A.S.M. Systems, Inc. All rights reserved. For additional information, visit www.heartsite.com.

How Does Stress Echo Work?

Patients with coronary artery blockages may have minimal or no symptoms during rest. However, symptoms and signs of heart disease may be unmasked by exposing the heart to the stress of exercise. During exercise, healthy coronary arteries dilate (develop a more open channel) more than an artery with a blockage. This unequal dilation causes more blood to be delivered to heart muscle supplied by the normal artery. In contrast, narrowed arteries end up supplying reduced flow to their area of distribution. This reduced flow causes the involved muscle to starve during exercise. The starvation may produce symptoms (chest discomfort or inappropriate shortness of breath), EKG abnormalities, and reduced movement of the heart muscle. The latter can be recognized by examining the movement of the walls of the left ventricle (the major pumping chamber of the heart) by echocardiography.

How Is a Stress Echo Performed?

An echo stress test can be obtained in a physician's office or in the hospital. Imaging tests are generally obtained when a physician wishes to confirm or rule out the presence of coronary artery disease. A stress echo test is also performed in patients who have disease involving the heart muscle or valve, or if a patient is having inappropriate shortness of breath and a cardiac cause is suspected.

The patient is brought to the echo laboratory where a resting study is performed. This provides a baseline examination, and demonstrates the size and function of various chambers of the heart. Particular attention is paid to the movement of all walls of the left ventricle (LV). Similar to a regular echo test, sticky patches or electrodes are attached to the chest and shoulders and connected to electrodes or wires to record the electrocardiogram (EKG or ECG). The EKG helps in the timing of various cardiac events (filling and emptying of chambers).

A colorless gel is then applied to the chest and the echo transducer is placed on top of it. The echo technologist then makes recordings from different parts of the chest to obtain several views of the heart. You may be asked to move from your back and to the left side. Instructions may also be given for you to breathe slowly or to hold your breath. This helps to obtain higher quality pictures. The images are constantly viewed on the monitor. It is also recorded on photographic paper, on videotape, and on a computer disk.

Twelve leads of the EKG are recorded on paper and the blood pressure is taken. Exercise is then initiated using a treadmill (most common) or a stationary bicycle. In patients who are unable to complete a high level of exercise because of physical limitations, stress to the heart is provided by pharmaceutical or chemical stimulation of the heart. Stress echo is made up of three parts: a resting echo study, stress test, and a repeat echo while the heart is still beating fast.

Exercise stress testing usually employs the "Bruce" or a similar protocol. Exercise is started at a slower warm-up speed. The speed of the treadmill and its slope or inclination are increased every 3 minutes. The treadmill is abruptly stopped when the patient exceeds 85% of the target rate (based upon the patient's age). Exercise may be stopped earlier if the patient develops alarming symptoms (chest discomfort, marked shortness of breath, weakness, or dizziness), if there is dangerous elevation or drop in the blood pressure, significant EKG changes, or a potentially dangerous irregular heart rhythm. Please remember that you have a physician in attendance (although an experienced assistant may perform the test). The problems mentioned are uncommon and you are far safer if they occur in the presence of an experienced medical team rather than having them happen while you are exercising in a spa, jogging, or running up a flight of office stairs.

EKG recordings are made during every minute of exercise and then again after exercise is stopped. The blood pressure is recorded at three minute intervals during exercise and then again at rest. Immediately after stopping the treadmill, the patient moves directly to the examination table and lies on their left side. The echo examination is immediately repeated. Images are stored and then played back by the computer. A video clip of multiple views of the resting and exercise study are compared side-by-side. They are analyzed by the physician. Normally, one expects an increased EF or ejection fraction (a measure of how well the heart is pumping). Also, the LV walls do not show any exercise-induced abnormal movement. In contrast, a drop in EF and/ or a new wall motion abnormality is an indicator of disease.

How Long Does the Entire Test Take?

A patient should allow one and one-half to two hours for the entire test, including the preparation, echo imaging, and stress test.

How Safe Is a Stress Echo Test?

There are no known adverse effects from the ultrasound used during echo imaging. The risk of the stress portion of the test is rare and similar to what you would expect from any strenuous form of exercise (jogging in your neighborhood or running up a flight of stairs). Experienced medical staff are in attendance to manage any rare complications like sustained abnormal heart rhythm, unrelieved chest pain, or even a heart attack. These problems could have occurred if the same patient performed an equivalent level of exercise at home or on a jogging track.

What Is the Reliability of Stress Echo?

If a patient is able to achieve the target heart rate and if the echo images are of good technical quality, a stress echo is capable of diagnosing important disease in more than 85% of patients with coronary artery disease. Also, it can exclude important disease in more than 90% of cases when the test is absolutely normal.

How Quickly Will I Get the Results and What Will It Mean?

The physician conducting the test will be able to give you the preliminary results before you leave the stress echo laboratory. However, the official result may take a few days to complete. The results of the test may help confirm or rule out a diagnosis of heart disease. In patients with known coronary artery disease (prior heart attack, known coronary blockages, previous treatment with angioplasty, stents, or bypass surgery), the study will help confirm that the patient is in a stable state, or that a new blockage is developing. The results may influence your physician's decision to change your treatment or recommend additional testing such as cardiac catheterization.

Section 48.4

Isotope Stress Test

Reprinted with permission from www.heartsite.com. © 2003 A.S.M. Systems, Inc. All rights reserved. For additional information, visit www.heartsite.com.

How Does an Isotope Stress Test Work?

An isotope stress test is also known as a nuclear, thallium, Cardiolite, Myoview, or dual isotope stress test, depending upon the method used. During exercise, healthy coronary arteries dilate (develop a more open channel) more than an artery that has a blockage. This unequal dilation causes more blood to be delivered to heart muscle supplied by the normal artery. In contrast, narrowed arteries end up supplying reduced flow to its area of distribution. This reduced flow causes the involved muscle to starve during exercise. The starvation may produce symptoms (like chest discomfort or inappropriate shortness of breath), and EKG abnormalities. When a perfusion tracer (a nuclear isotope that travels to heart muscle with blood flow) is injected intravenously, it is extracted by the heart muscle in proportion to the flow of blood.

The amount of tracer uptake helps differentiate normal muscle (which receives more of the tracer) from the reduced uptake demonstrated by muscle that is supplied by a narrowed coronary artery. In other words, areas of the heart that have adequate blood flow quickly pick up the tracer material. In contrast, muscle with reduced blood flow picks up the tracer slowly or not at all. Analysis of the images of the heart (taken by a scanning camera) can help identify the location, severity, and extent of reduced blood flow to the heart. The reduced blood flow is known as ischemia (pronounced is-keem-ya).

How Is an Isotope or Nuclear Stress Test Performed?

The test is actually divided into three parts: a treadmill stress test, imaging at rest, and imaging after exercise. There are two common types of isotope used in the U.S., thallium and technetium (which are

505

marketed under the trade names Cardiolite and Myoview). Some laboratories use a dual isotope technique, where thallium is used for the resting images and technetium is used for the stress pictures. Depending upon the isotope and protocol for the laboratory, resting images may be obtained either before stress or two to four hours after stress. The preparation for the test and the treadmill procedure is similar to that described in Section 48.1. In patients who are unable to complete a high level of exercise because of physical limitations, stress to the heart is provided by pharmaceutical or chemical stimulation.

The patient is brought to the exercise laboratory where the heart rate and blood pressure are recorded at rest. Sticky electrodes are attached to the chest, shoulders and hips and connected to the EKG portion of the stress test machine. A 12-lead EKG is recorded on paper. Each lead of the EKG represents a different portion of the heart, with adjacent leads representing a single wall. The treadmill is then started at a relatively slow, warm-up speed. The treadmill speed and its slope or inclination are increased every three minutes according to a preprogrammed protocol. Bruce is the most common protocol in the U.S., but several other protocols are perfectly acceptable. It is the protocol that dictates the precise speed and slope. Each three minute interval is known as a stage (stage 1, stage 2, and stage 3). Thus, a patient completing stage 3 has exercised for 3 x 3 = 9 minutes. The patient's blood pressure is recorded during the second minute of each stage. However, it may be recorded more frequently if the patient's blood pressure is too high or too low.

The EKG is constantly displayed on the monitor. It is also recorded on paper at one minute intervals. The physician pays particular attention to the heart rate, blood pressure, changes in the EKG pattern, irregular heart rhythm, and the patient's appearance and symptoms. The treadmill is stopped when the patient achieves a target heart rate (this is 85% of the maximal heart rate predicted for the patient's age). However, if the patient is doing extremely well at peak exercise, the treadmill test may be continued further. The test may be stopped prior to achievement of the target heart rate if the patient develops significant chest discomfort, shortness of breath, dizziness, or unsteady gait, if the EKG shows alarming changes, or serious abnormal heart rhythm. It may also be stopped if the blood pressure (BP) rises or falls beyond acceptable limits.

Approximately 1 to 1 1/2 minutes prior to termination of exercise, the perfusion tracer or isotope is injected into the intravenous plug that had been placed in the forearm or hand. This is followed by a flush injection of saline (salt water) to make sure that the entire tracer is pushed into the blood circulation. After a brief waiting phase (that allows the tracer to be taken up by the heart muscle), the patient is placed under a scanning camera.

Two sets of isotope images are obtained. One at rest and one following exercise. Depending upon the isotope used and the protocol for a particular laboratory, the resting images may be obtained before the stress test, or a few hours later. The scanning camera rotates around the patient's chest, stopping to take individual pictures. The patient needs to lay flat and still during the scanning period which takes approximately 11 to 20 minutes, depending upon the type of scanning camera. Patients with severe claustrophobia should notify their physician (a mild tranquilizer before the test may minimize discomfort). The pictures or images are fed into a computer, which reconstructs them as slices of a three dimensional heart. These slices are presented in three views (vertical long axis or VLA, horizontal long axis or HLA, and short axis or SA). It also computes the data and presents an aggregate picture that compares the information to a data base of known normal cases. Areas that fall outside the expected normal range are presented as blacked out areas. In other words, your physician has an opportunity to view a three dimensional representation of your heart, examine individual slices, and then compare the findings against those computed by the computer as blackout plots. By comparing one wall against another, the physician can identify disease and assess its magnitude.

The physician can separate a normal left ventricle from ischemia (live muscle with flow that is compromised only during exercise) and the scar tissue of a heart attack.

How Long Does the Entire Test Take?

A patient should allow approximately two to four hours for the entire test, including the preparation. Dual isotope and technetium stress testing takes less time than thallium. You will be allowed to leave the lab and get a light snack or lunch in cases of thallium stress testing.

How Safe Is an Isotope Treadmill Stress Test?

The patient is exposed to a very small amount of radiation and the risk is minimal, if any. The risk of the stress portion of the test is very small and similar to what you would expect from any strenuous form of exercise (jogging in your neighborhood or running up a flight of stairs). Experienced medical staff are in attendance to manage rare complications like sustained abnormal heart rhythm, unrelieved chest pain, or even a heart attack. In such cases, the patient is better off having the problem in the presence of experienced staff, rather than have it happen when they are exercising alone.

What Is the Reliability of an Isotope Stress Test?

If a patient is able to achieve the target heart rate and good quality images are obtained, an isotope treadmill stress test is capable of diagnosing important disease in approximately 85% of patients with coronary artery disease. Approximately 10% of patients may have a false-positive test (when the result is falsely abnormal in a patient without coronary artery disease). Technical problems can occur when a patient is markedly overweight. Women may have an abnormality in the front portion of the heart because of overlying breast tissue. Some men may demonstrate an inferior wall abnormality because of a prominent diaphragm (muscular partition that separates the chest cavity from the abdomen). Patients who have a left bundle branch block on their EKG may also have a false abnormal test.

How Quickly Will I Get the Results and What Will It Mean?

The physician performing the stress test can give you a preliminary report about the EKG portion of your test. However, the official result from the isotope scans may take a few days to complete. The results may influence your physician's decision to change your treatment or recommend additional testing such as cardiac catheterization, or a change in your medications.

Chapter 49

Holter Monitor

What is a Holter monitor?

Λ Holter monitor is a continuous tape recording of a patient's EKG for 24 hours. Since it can be worn during the patient's regular daily activities, it helps the physician correlate symptoms of dizziness, palpitations (a sensation of fast or irregular heart rhythm), or black outs. Since the recording covers 24 hours, on a continuous basis, Holter monitoring is much more likely to detect an abnormal heart rhythm when compared to the EKG which lasts less than a minute. It can also help evaluate the patient's EKG during episodes of chest pain, during which time there may be telltale changes to suggest ischemia (pronounced is-keem-ya) or reduced blood supply to the muscle of the left ventricle.

How do I prepare for the test?

The only requirement is that the patient wear loose-fitting clothes. Buttons down the front of a shirt or blouse are preferable. This makes it convenient to apply the EKG electrodes, and also comfortably carry the monitor in a relatively discreet manner.

How is the test performed?

The chest is cleansed with an alcohol solution to ensure good attachment of the sticky EKG electrodes. Men who have a hairy chest

Reprinted with permission from www.heartsite.com © 2003 A.S.M. Systems, Inc. All rights reserved. For additional information, visit www.heartsite.com.

may require small areas to be shaved. The EKG electrodes are applied to the chest. Thin wires are then used to connect the electrodes to a small tape recorder. The tape recorder is secured to the patient's belt or it can be slung over the shoulder and neck with the use of a disposable pouch. The recorder is worn for 24 hours and the patient is encouraged to continue his or her daily activities. To avoid getting the equipment wet and damaging the recorder, the patient will not be able to shower for the duration of the test. A diary or log is provided so that the patient can record activity (walking the dog, upset at neighbor, etc.) and symptoms (skipped heartbeats, chest discomfort, or dizziness) together with the time. The Holter monitor has an internal clock which stamps the time on the EKG strips. These can be used to correlate the heart rhythm with symptoms or complaints. After 24 hours, the Holter monitor needs to be returned to the laboratory and can be removed by the staff. However, if you live out of town or need to take a shower before leaving the house, the monitor can be disconnected from the electrodes and sent back to the laboratory, together with the completed diary.

After returning the Holter monitor to the doctor's office, satellite clinic, or hospital lab, the tape is removed from the recorder and scanned by a technician. Multiple EKG strips are recorded on paper together with a computer-generated summary that provides details about the patient's heart rate and rhythm during the recording. This information is then provided to your doctor.

How long does it take?

It takes approximately 10 to 15 minutes to apply the monitor and less than 5 minutes to remove it. The patient will also receive directions. Many monitors are equipped with an event button. Pressing the button during a symptom (dizziness, for example) will help the technician print an ECG from that precise time.

How safe is the test?

Holter monitoring is extremely safe and no different than carrying around a small tape recorder for 24 hours. Some patients are sensitive to the electrode adhesive, but no serious allergic reactions have been reported.

When will I get the results?

The report is provided to the physician, together with multiple EKG strips after the tape has been scanned by the technician. If the technician sees a rhythm that is life-threatening or potentially dangerous, the physician is informed immediately. Otherwise, it may take a few days before you get the official results from your physician's office. At that time, you may also receive additional recommendations based upon the results of the test. For example, a pacemaker may be recommended if a patient has blackouts and the Holter monitor shows a seriously slow heart beat during the test.

Chapter 50

Sleep Studies

What Is a Sleep Study?

A sleep study, or polysomnogram, is an overnight recording of sleep patterns and behaviors associated with sleep. It is necessary to determine what stages of sleep an individual achieves and whether any sleep-related abnormalities are present. A variety of sensors are applied with paste or tape to the body's surface to record brain waves, eye movements, muscle tone, body movements, heart rate, and breathing. Audiovisual recordings are made also. None of the sensors used are painful or invasive—even the oxygen content of the blood is measured non-invasively with a simple clip on the index finger. There are connecting wires to the sensors, but you are free to get up and walk about as needed.

During the study, every attempt is made to allow for a normal night's sleep. Some people typically sleep better or worse when away from home, but in either case this does not usually affect the value of the sleep study. The sleep laboratory has a homey, bedroom-like atmosphere with a television/VCR. You wear your own bedclothes and you can bring your favorite pillow and shower in the morning. A trained sleep technologist explains all of the recording sensors during application. He or she is stationed outside the bedroom all night to both monitor the sleep recording and make sure you are comfortable.

Reprinted with permission from the St. Joseph Sleep Disorders Center, St. Joseph Hospital, Orange, California, http://www.sjhsleepcenter.com. © 2001 St. Joseph Sleep Disorders Center.

Following the sleep study, an accredited sleep specialist interprets the recording. The findings are integrated with your sleep history to determine a diagnosis and to make treatment recommendations. A sleep study report is sent to your physician, who reviews the results with you at your follow-up office visit.

Description of Procedures

Sleep Consultation

During the initial sleep consultation, a sleep specialist will interview you about your sleep habits. The specialist uses your history to evaluate symptoms such as difficulty falling asleep, difficulty staying asleep, daytime sleepiness, daytime fatigue, breathing problems in sleep, restless legs at night, and other troublesome behaviors. The sleep specialist may recommend an overnight sleep test, known as a polysomnogram, to further evaluate your complaints.

Polysomnogram (PSG)

The diagnosis of many sleep disorders requires that you sleep overnight in the laboratory. A polysomnogram, or PSG, is an overnight test that measures your sleep patterns. Sensors are applied to the surface of your skin using paste and tape. These sensors measure your brain waves, eye movements, muscle tone, breathing patterns, and blood oxygen levels. The sleep rooms are private with a comfortable double bed in a hotel-like atmosphere. The technologist is specially trained to operate the sleep diagnostic equipment and remains all night in an adjacent control room. An intercom system is installed in each sleep room so you and the technologist may communicate. None of the monitoring procedures are painful, and the technologist is immediately available to see to your needs throughout the study.

1/2 Polysomnogram (PSG) 1/2 Continuous Positive Airway Pressure (CPAP)

In some cases, both diagnosis and treatment of a breathing problem can be accomplished in a single night. As during the polysomnogram (PSG), sensors that measure brain waves, eye movements, muscle tone, breathing patterns, and blood oxygen levels are applied to your skin using paste and tape. Once you are asleep in your private, hotel-like sleep room, the technologist carefully monitors the sleep diagnostic equipment for any sign of disrupted breathing during sleep.

If interruptions in your breathing (known as sleep apnea) are seen, the technologist will apply Continuous Positive Airway Pressure (CPAP) during the second half of the test. CPAP is the most effective and widely used method of treating sleep apnea. While you sleep, this system gently delivers air into your airway through a specially designed mask that fits over your nose and mouth. This creates enough pressure to keep the airway open and produce immediate relief from sleep apnea and snoring. The CPAP device does not breathe for you. You can breathe at a normal rate. Most people find they get used to the mask after a few minutes and have little difficulty sleeping with it. The technologist is trained in using the CPAP apparatus and can answer most questions and concerns that may arise during your study.

Multiple Sleep Latency Test (MSLT)

Some people experience excessive daytime sleepiness or fall asleep at inappropriate times. If you suffer from these symptoms, your physician may send you to the sleep disorders center for the MSLT. The MSLT, or Multiple Sleep Latency Test, consists of five scheduled nap recordings during which you will be allowed to sleep for a brief period. The MSLT is conducted on the day following an overnight polysomnogram (PSG). During the PSG, sensors are applied to your skin with paste and tape to measure brain waves, eye movements, muscle tone, breathing patterns, and blood oxygen levels. On the morning after your PSG some of these sensors will be removed, and you will have the opportunity to change your clothes and freshen up before your first scheduled nap recording. The naps are scheduled 2 hours apart, with the first one occurring approximately 2 hours after you get up. During the naps, the technologist will monitor your sleep/wake patterns. In between naps you will be free to move about, although you will be asked to stay awake. A television/VCR and some magazines are available in the sleep center, and you may wish to bring along something elsc to do such as letter writing, needlework, homework, a radio or cassette tape for listening, or a book for reading. Generally, the last nap is completed before 7:00 p.m.

CPAP Titration Study

If you've had a previous polysomnogram (PSG) and have been diagnosed with sleep apnea (OSA), your physician may have you return to the sleep disorders center for a sleep study with CPAP. Sleep apnea is a sleep disorder characterized by interruptions in breathing. CPAP is the most effective and widely used method of treating sleep apnea. While you sleep, this system gently delivers air into your airway through a specially designed mask that fits over your nose and mouth. This creates enough pressure to keep the airway open and produce immediate relief from sleep apnea and snoring. The CPAP does not breathe for you. You can breathe at a normal rate. Most people find they get used to the CPAP apparatus after a few minutes and have little difficulty sleeping with it in place. At the start of a CPAP study, sensors will once again be applied to your skin and the technologist will monitor your brain waves, eye movements, muscle tone, breathing patterns, and blood oxygen levels using special diagnostic sleep equipment. Before you fall asleep the technologist will fit you with the CPAP device. The technologist is trained in using the CPAP apparatus and can answer most questions and concerns that may arise during your study.

For Additional Information

St. Joseph Sleep Disorders Center
1310 W. Stewart Dr., Suite 403
Orange, CA 92868
Toll-Free: 888-766-7363
Phone: 714-771-8950
Website: www.sjhsleepcenter.com

Chapter 51

Tilt Test

What is a tilt test?

A tilt table test (TTT), or tilt test, is widely used in making the diagnosis of neurally (pronounced new-rully) mediated syncope (pronounced syn-cup-ee) or NMS.

What is neurally mediated syncope (NMS) and why do these patients pass out?

NMS is a condition that can occur in a wide range of people, many of whom do not have any other associated cardiovascular problems. These patients give a history of repeatedly having syncope (passing out spells) over the course of several years. Some of these spells may be preceded by a hot sensation or nausea, but many happen without any warning. The patient may fall to the ground and recover consciousness quickly and without any further problems. The episodes of syncope may occur at church, in the grocery store, while a blood specimen is being drawn, or while sitting quietly at home. Surprisingly, the majority of the patients never sustain serious injuries, and the diagnosis may go undetected for decades. Patients get used to fainting and life goes on. The availability of the tilt test, its wide success in establishing the diagnosis of NMS, and effective treatment for NMS has resulted in the well deserved popularity of the test.

Reprinted with permission from www.heartsite.com © 2003 A.S.M. Systems, Inc. All rights reserved. For additional information, visit www.heartsite.com.

To understand this phenomenon, we must first examine how the nervous system of the body functions. During our daily activities, our heart rate (HR) and blood pressure (BP) constantly rise and fall to meet the needs of the body. The HR and BP are lower at rest, while the HR picks up and BP is elevated during emotional stress and exercise. The control of the HR and BP are under the domain of the sympathetic (pronounced sim-pa-thetic) and parasympathetic nervous systems. The former increases the HR and BP while the latter reduces them. To simplify this concept, let us imagine that the body is an automobile. Pressing the accelerator pedal would make the car work harder and go faster. In contrast, pressing the brake pedal would slow the car down. Thus, the sympathetic nervous system behaves like an accelerator for the body, while the parasympathetic system functions like a braking system.

Normally, the sympathetic and parasympathetic nervous systems work together in a very efficient and cooperative manner. Just like a good driver, the accelerator and brake pedals are used efficiently (one being slowly pressed while the other is smoothly released). The car slows down and speeds up so smoothly that one does not recognize the change. Similarly, our HR and BP goes up and down without us being aware of it. From time to time, this system breaks down in people with NMS. It is almost as if the accelerator pedal remains in the control of the car driver while the braking system is occasionally turned over to an extremely nervous back seat driver. This spells trouble. If the car accelerates too rapidly (HR and BP goes up), the back seat driver panics and slams the brake. The HR and BP (either singly or together) drop suddenly and severely. This reduces blood supply to the brain and the patient passes out. The back seat driver then steps off the brake pedal, the HR and BP increase, blood flow is restored, and the patient awakens.

How is the tilt test performed?

The patient is hooked to an EKG machine and a BP monitor. The HR and BP are constantly monitored during the procedure. An intravenous (IV) line is placed in the arm. Large patches are also applied to the patient's chest. These patches are connected to an external pacemaker and turned on if the patient's HR slows down and does not pick right up (in the majority of cases the slow HR is transient and the external pacemaker is only a precautionary measure).

The patient lies on a swivel table in a flat position. Safety straps are applied across the chest and legs to hold the patient in place.

After obtaining the baseline HR and BP, the motorized table is tilted up to an angle of 80 degrees. This simulates going from a flat (supine) to a standing or upright position. The change in position causes the HR and BP to rise and the patient's response is noted. Depending upon the physician and the protocol of a given laboratory, the duration of time spent in the supine and upright position can vary from 5 to 30 minutes.

If nothing happens, the table is returned to the flat position and an intravenous infusion of isoproterenol (trade name, Isuprel) is started. This medicine increases the HR and BP. This effect is similar to that produced by our own natural adrenaline release. As you may have gathered, the test is now simulating what happens when the sympathetic nervous system is stimulated and the accelerator is pressed. The tilt table is then raised back up to 80 degrees and the IV medication continued.

A stop clock in the room is used to keep track of time. If an abnormal result is not seen, the table is lowered and then raised back up after increasing the dose of the IV medicine. In patients with NMS, the increase in HR and BP is usually sufficient to cause panic in the back seat driver (parasympathetic nervous system). When this happens, the HR, BP, or both drop suddenly and dramatically as the parasympathetic system slams the brake pedal. The patient gets dizzy and passes out. Thus, TTT succeeds in simulating a real life situation and establishes the cause of recurrent black out spells. With the above changes, the test is considered positive. The IV medicine is immediately stopped, and the patient returned to the flat or supine position. Within a few seconds, the patient regains consciousness and both the HR and BP return to normal. The patient is observed for 10 to 20 minutes and then disconnected from the equipment.

How to prepare for the tilt test?

Check with your physician to see if any of your medications need to be held. You should not eat or drink after midnight to reduce the risk of nausea and vomiting during the test. Try and wear a blouse or shirt to expedite preparation for the test.

How long does the tilt test take?

The test generally takes a total of one and a half hours. This includes preparation, the actual test, and the recovery phase. Please make sure that someone can drive you home after the test.

Medical Tests Sourcebook, Second Edition

How safe is a tilt test?

The test is fairly safe, although it can be dramatic for the patient if the test is positive and causes a black out spell. However, the patient needs to recognize that this denotes a positive response, and opens the door to the addition of extremely effective medications that may dramatically reduce or totally eliminate the patient's recurrent black out spells. In rare cases, the test may produce persistent abnormal heart rhythm, and patients with coronary artery disease may occasionally experience lingering chest discomfort. Experienced staff and equipment are on hand to handle these potential complications.

What information is provided by the tilt test?

The tilt test helps to confirm the diagnosis of NMS. This is extremely important because there is effective treatment for the condition which can either totally eradicate or dramatically reduce the frequency and intensity of symptoms (dizziness and black out spells). Recent research studies have also shown a correlation between chronic fatigue syndrome (CFS) and NMS. Treatment aimed at NMS has been shown to be beneficial in many patients with CFS (if they have a positive tilt test). The use of beta-blockers is commonly employed in the treatment of NMS. The beta-blockers act as a governor on a carburetor. The motor does not rev up as much (HR and BP does not increase drastically), and the back seat driver (parasympathetic system) remains calm and does not slam on the brakes. Other drugs that have shown benefit include aminophylline, disopyramide, and certain anti-depressants serotonin-uptake inhibitors.

How quickly will I get the results of the tilt test?

The tilt test results are generally provided to you as soon as it is completed. Changes in your medications, if indicated by the results of the test, may be discussed at the same time or during a subsequent office visit.

520

Part Eight

Scope Tests

Chapter 52

Bronchoscopy

Editor's Note: This information may not apply to all patients. Please discuss it with your health care provider.

What is a bronchoscopy?

Bronchoscopy is a routine diagnostic procedure that lets your doctor see inside your lungs and possibly get tissue to examine. The procedure uses a bronchoscope: a small, narrow, tube with a light and lens at the tip.

Who might have a bronchoscopy?

People who have symptoms of a lung problem may have a bronchoscopy to help make an exact diagnosis. Patients with known lung disease may need this test to check the status of their disease. For comparison, bronchoscopy may also be done on people with normal lungs.

How do I prepare for bronchoscopy?

Before the procedure, you will have a chest x-ray, pulmonary function test, physical exam, blood work, and an electrocardiogram. Also,

This chapter includes "Bronchoscopy," Warren Grant Magnuson Clinical Center, National Institutes of Health (NIH), 6/2001; and "Bronchoscope Image," Courtesy of A.D.A.M., Inc. © 2002, reprinted with permission.

you will be asked to sign an informed consent, which will also be signed by your doctor. Do not eat or drink anything 8 hours before the procedure. The morning of the procedure, a small, intravenous tube (catheter) will be put into one of your arm veins. This will be used to give you fluids and medication to help you relax. You may get an injection of medications into your muscle to help control coughing and secretions in your mouth.

What happens during a bronchoscopy?

When you are in the bronchoscopy suite, the nurse will attach patches to your chest to monitor your heart, a blood pressure cuff to

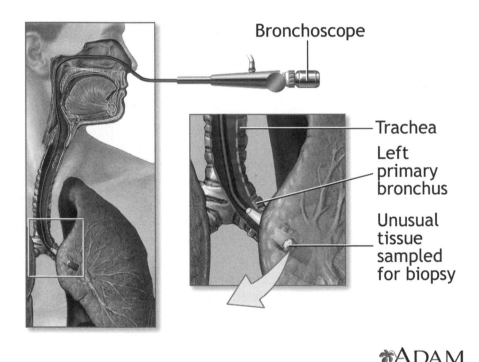

Figure 52.1. *Bronchoscope. Lung or bronchial biopsy (tissue samples taken to diagnose or rule out disease) may be done with the use of a flexible bronchoscope, an instrument with a small light and camera which is inserted through the nose or mouth. When a suspicious area is seen, an instrument is channeled through the bronchoscope to take a sample for analysis. (Source: Image courtesy of A.D.A.M. © 2002, reprinted with permission.)*

monitor your blood pressure, and a clip on your finger to check how much oxygen is in your blood.

After this, you will breathe a mist of topical anesthesia (numbing medication) through your mouth. You will breathe this mist from a tube attached to an oxygen flowmeter. You will be asked to breathe through your mouth until this mist is gone.

The nurse will give you a topical anesthetic to gargle or the back of your throat will be sprayed with anesthetic. A small amount of lidocaine (numbing medication) will be put into one of your nostrils to let the bronchoscopy tube pass through.

What are the side effects?

Because of the sedatives you may have received, you may feel groggy for several hours. Your mouth may feel dry during, and shortly after, the procedure. Some people also have a slight sore throat, blood-tinged saliva, or a low fever.

What happens afterwards?

When the procedure is over, the nurse will take you back to your room. Your vital signs (temperature, heartbeat, and blood pressure) will be monitored. Your nurse will also ask you to take deep breaths and cough gently. This helps clear your lungs of the fluid used during the procedure.

Because your throat and gag reflex will be numb, do not eat or drink for at least 2 hours after the bronchoscopy. In 2 hours, your nurse will check your gag reflex. If it has returned, you may try to drink; then eat.

Are there special instructions to follow after the procedure?

If you develop a fever higher than 100 degrees Fahrenheit, take Tylenol every 4 hours as recommended by your doctor or nurse practitioner. If your fever lasts longer than 24 hours, call your doctor.

If you have a sore throat, take throat lozenges as needed. If you have any of the following, go to the nearest emergency room:

- difficulty catching your breath
- bleeding from your nose
- coughing up blood
- chest pain or chest discomfort.

Chapter 53

Cardiac Catheterization

What is cardiac catheterization?

Cardiac catheterization is a diagnostic procedure which is performed in order to detect problems with the heart and its blood supply. A long, thin tube (a catheter) is inserted into the heart, with it, the doctor measures pressures, injects dye, and x-ray pictures are taken. It will help your physician determine which treatment is most appropriate for you.

The catheterization procedure will provide a great deal of information about your heart function. It shows the heart's pumping ability, the pressure within the various heart chambers, detailed structural information about the heart and blood vessels, and the pattern of flow within the heart and major blood vessels.

Tell your doctor about allergies. Because an iodine-related dye is injected into your bloodstream during the procedure, please advise your doctor if you have a history of being allergic to shellfish, medications, x-ray dye, or IVP dye.

How long does the procedure take? Are there any other tests involved? Will I have to stay overnight in the hospital?

The catheterization itself normally takes one to two hours; however, prior to your procedure you will need to have some blood tests, chest

"When You Need to Have a Cardiac Catheterization: A Patient Guide," is reprinted with permission from Cardiology Associates, P.C., www.cardioassoc.com. © 2002 Cardiology Associates. All rights reserved.

x-rays, and an ECG (electrocardiogram) performed either before, or the day of the catheterization. Heart catheterization is often an outpatient procedure.

Will this take place in the operating room?

Generally, cardiac catheterization takes place in a specialized cardiac catheterization laboratory. This is a sterile environment (all medical personnel will wear gowns, masks, and gloves), and there is equipment present which is specific to this type of procedure. Some of the specialized equipment includes an x-ray movie camera which takes pictures of your chest from various angles; there will also be a television monitor present that will allow the doctors to see your heart as it functions. Your heart and blood pressure will be monitored throughout the procedure.

Where and how do they insert the catheter? Will I be under general anesthetic? Does it hurt?

The normal points of entry are either the groin area or the forearm. The immediate skin area is numbed with a local anesthetic, which is administered through a needle. You will feel an initial pin prick as the needle is inserted, and then a burning sensation as the anesthetic is injected. You may also feel pressure when the catheter itself is inserted, and/or exchanged with other catheters during the procedure.

Once the initial needle is inserted, a guide wire is passed through the needle and the needle itself is removed. Next, a small plastic tube (catheter) is threaded over the wire and guided through the vessel and into the chambers of the heart. The doctor uses an x-ray to confirm the desired location of the catheter tip, and then removes the guide wire. The catheter is connected to special equipment that records pressures in the different heart chambers.

You will be awake throughout the entire procedure; in fact, the physicians will require your cooperation at various times during the testing, to perform certain basic functions (e.g., exhale, cough, hold your breath).

You may be given a mild drug to make you sleepy (mild sedation).

There will be several periods when x-ray sensitive contrast dye will be injected, via catheter, into your bloodstream. At these moments (approximately 30–60 seconds each) you will probably feel a warm sensation that spreads from head to toe.

Once the testing is complete, the catheters will be removed and pressure will be applied for approximately 15 minutes. You will then be taken back to your room.

How long does recovery take?

It is likely you will be allowed to go home the same day or the next day; however, the first few hours after the procedure are very important, and you must follow the hospital staff's directions very closely.

If the point of insertion was your groin: You will be required to lay flat on your back for a minimum of four hours once you are returned to your hospital room. It is important that you pay careful attention to your doctor's instructions not to sit up or bend your legs in order to minimize the chances of bleeding. After a few hours, if there has not been any bleeding at the site of catheter insertion, the hospital staff will assist you in turning onto your side. You will probably be allowed out of your bed in a few hours.

If the point of insertion was your arm: You will be permitted to get out of bed within two hours; however, you must keep your arm straight using a stiff armboard.

Your blood pressure and pulse will be taken frequently by the nursing staff, and the site of insertion will be checked for bleeding.

You will be encouraged to take in many fluids, first intravenously and then orally.

If you experience any back pain or discomfort during recovery, ask your nurse for pain medication. If you feel any pain in your chest or see any bleeding at the point of insertion, notify the hospital staff immediately.

The first time you get out of your hospital bed you will require assistance from a nurse as you may feel light-headed.

If there are no further complications, you will be permitted to go home.

When will I know the results of the catheterization?

Your doctor will be able to discuss the findings of the test either the same afternoon or the day after your procedure; a plan of therapy can then be discussed.

Chapter 54

Colonoscopy

Colonoscopy (koh-luh-NAH-skuh-pee) lets the physician look inside your entire large intestine, from the lowest part, the rectum, all the way up through the colon to the lower end of the small intestine. The procedure is used to look for early signs of cancer in the colon and rectum. It is also used to diagnose the causes of unexplained changes in bowel habits. Colonoscopy enables the physician to see inflamed tissue, abnormal growths, ulcers, and bleeding.

For the procedure, you will lie on your left side on the examining table. You will probably be given pain medication and a mild sedative to keep you comfortable and to help you relax during the exam. The physician will insert a long, flexible, lighted tube into your rectum and slowly guide it into your colon. The tube is called a colonoscope (koh-LON-oh-skope). The scope transmits an image of the inside of the colon, so the physician can carefully examine the lining of the colon. The scope bends, so the physician can move it around the curves of your colon. You may be asked to change position occasionally to help the physician move the scope. The scope also blows air into your colon, which inflates the colon and helps the physician see well.

If anything abnormal is seen in your colon, like a polyp or inflamed tissue, the physician can remove all or part of it using tiny instruments passed through the scope. That tissue (biopsy) is then sent to

National Institute of Diabetes and Digestive and Kidney Diseases (NIDDK), NIH Publication No. 02-4331, February 2002.

a lab for testing. If there is bleeding in the colon, the physician can pass a laser, heater probe, or electrical probe, or inject special medicines through the scope and use it to stop the bleeding.

Bleeding and puncture of the colon are possible complications of colonoscopy. However, such complications are uncommon.

Colonoscopy takes 30 to 60 minutes. The sedative and pain medicine should keep you from feeling much discomfort during the exam. You will need to remain at the endoscopy facility for 1 to 2 hours until the sedative wears off.

Preparation

Your colon must be completely empty for the colonoscopy to be thorough and safe. To prepare for the procedure you may have to follow a

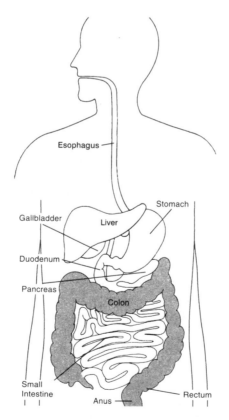

Figure 54.1. *The Digestive System*

liquid diet for 1 to 3 days beforehand. A liquid diet means fat-free bouillon or broth, strained fruit juice, water, plain coffee, plain tea, or diet soda. Gelatin or popsicles in any color but red may also be eaten. You will take one of several types of laxatives the night before the procedure. Also, you must arrange for someone to take you home afterward—you will not be allowed to drive because of the sedatives. Your physician may give you other special instructions. Inform your physician of any medical conditions or medications that you take before the colonoscopy.

Additional Information

American College of Gastroenterology (ACG)
P.O. Box 3099
Arlington, VA 22302
Phone: 703-820-7400
Fax: 703-931-4520
Website: www.acg.gi.org

International Foundation for Functional Gastrointestinal Disorders (IFFGD)
P.O. Box 170864
Milwaukee, WI 53217-8076
Toll-Free: 888-964-2001
Phone: 414-964-1799
Fax: 414-964-7176
Website: www.iffgd.org
E-mail: iffgd@iffgd.org

National Digestive Diseases Information Clearinghouse
2 Information Way
Bethesda, MD 20892-3570
Toll-Free: 800-891-5389
Phone: 301-654-3810
Fax: 301-907-8906
Website: http://digestive.niddk.nih.gov
E-mail: nddic@info.niddk.nih.gov

Chapter 55

Colposcopy and Cervical Biopsy

What Is Colposcopy?

Colposcopy is an easy office procedure that allows the practitioner to see the surface of the cervix with greater clarity than can be achieved just by looking with the naked eye. It utilizes an instrument called a colposcope which looks like and performs like a pair of binoculars to magnify the cervix.

Having colposcopy done is just like having a routine pelvic exam done, except that the practitioner looks through the colposcope. The instrument does not touch the body.

Why Is Colposcopy Done?

Most commonly, colposcopy is recommended when a Pap smear shows some changes. This is to obtain more information on what such changes represent, and how extensive they are so that appropriate follow-up may be planned.

Having an abnormal Pap smear can feel scary, but it's important to note that the majority of abnormal Paps are not cancer. The real value of Pap smears is that they can identify pre-cancerous changes long before invasive cancer develops. Pap smears and colposcopy are two tests that give complementary information, and are used hand-in-hand as a preventative measure to keep healthy people healthy.

"Colposcopy," reprinted with permission from the Hall Health Primary Care Center, University of Washington–Seattle. © 2002. All Rights Reserved.

What If the Colposcopy Shows Abnormalities?

Your practitioner will look at the cervix carefully, concentrating on a portion known as the squamo-columnar junction which is where the two types of cells of the cervix meet. If changes occur, they are most likely to arise in this area.

A small amount of a dilute vinegar solution is applied to the cervix to aid in differentiating the cell types and making abnormal areas more easily visible.

If there are abnormal areas seen, the location and extent of the areas is considered, along with the Pap smear findings, and then a decision can be made as to whether further attention is necessary. Sometimes just re-doing the Pap at yearly or more frequent intervals is all that is necessary, and sometimes further assessment with biopsies is helpful.

How Are Cervical Biopsies Done?

With the aid of the colposcope to identify the abnormal areas, a tiny portion of tissue (biopsy specimen) can be removed from the cervix. It is also necessary to sample the cells just inside the cervical canal to make sure there are no abnormalities out of sight inside the canal. This is called endocervical curettage (ECC) and is usually done in conjunction with the biopsies.

What Will I Experience during the Biopsy?

The degree of discomfort varies from person to person. Some people feel very little discomfort. Some people describe menstrual-like cramping, especially during the ECC. Some people describe a brief pinching sensation during the biopsies. A local numbing medication similar to Novocain can be used.

Bleeding can occur from the biopsy site, but this is usually minimal and can be easily stopped. You will be given a mini-pad in case there is spotting.

Feeling faint can occur, as with any medical procedure, but resting for a few minutes is usually all that is necessary.

What Happens after the Biopsy?

The cervix heals very promptly and since only very small samples are removed, the surface of the cervix usually looks normal within several days.

It is recommended that you abstain from sexual intercourse for 48 hours after the procedure, to allow for healing and prevent infection.

After the procedure, the specimens are sent to the laboratory for careful analysis. The results are sent to your practitioner in 2–3 days. Subsequent treatment is then planned according to the findings:

1. If the changes are minimal, you and your practitioner may elect just to monitor the cervix with more frequent Pap smears and not treat at that time.

2. If significant dysplasia (a descriptive term for a kind of cell change that potentially can be pre-cancerous) is found, treatment is indicated.

What Kinds of Treatment Are Available?

Treatment choices depend on the particular anatomy of your cervix and the location of the abnormal areas.

If areas of dysplasia are small and do not involve the canal, the abnormal cells can be frozen. This procedure is called cryocautery. It takes only minutes to do in the office. Healing takes about 3 weeks, during which time there is a watery vaginal discharge.

If dysplasia is very extensive, if it extends into the cervical canal, or if cancer is found, referral to an outside specialist is necessary. Treatment by LEEP (Loop Electrosurgical Excision Procedure), laser, or cone biopsy may be recommended depending on the findings in your particular situation. If referral is necessary, this will be discussed with you further.

Preparations for Colposcopy

1. Schedule your appointment when you are not menstruating.

2. Do not douche, use tampons, use vaginal medication, or have intercourse for 2 days prior to your appointment.

3. Inform the staff if you faint easily or bleed readily.

Chapter 56

Cystoscopy and Ureteroscopy

When you have a urinary problem, your doctor may use a cysto-scope to see the inside of your bladder and urethra. The urethra is the tube that carries urine from the bladder to the outside of the body. The cystoscope has lenses like a telescope or microscope. These lenses let the doctor focus on the inner surfaces of the urinary tract. Some cystoscopes use optical fibers (flexible glass fibers) that carry an image from the tip of the instrument to a viewing piece at the other end. The cystoscope is as thin as a pencil and has a light at the tip. Many cystoscopes have extra tubes to guide other instruments for proce-dures to treat urinary problems. Your doctor may recommend cystos-copy for any of the following conditions:

- Frequent urinary tract infections
- Blood in your urine (hematuria)
- Loss of bladder control (incontinence) or overactive bladder
- Unusual cells found in urine sample
- Need for a bladder catheter
- Painful urination, chronic pelvic pain, or interstitial cystitis
- Urinary blockage such as prostate enlargement, stricture, or narrowing of the urinary tract

This chapter includes "Cystoscopy and Ureteroscopy," National Institute of Diabetes and Digestive and Kidney Diseases (NIDDK), NIH Publication No. 01-4800, April 2001; and "Cystoscopy Image," © 2002 Courtesy of A.D.A.M., Inc., reprinted with permission

- Stone in the urinary tract
- Unusual growth, polyp, tumor, or cancer

If you have a stone lodged higher in your urinary tract, the doctor may extend the cystoscope through the bladder and up into the ureter. The ureter is the tube that carries urine from the kidney to the bladder. When used to view the ureters, the cystoscope is called a ureteroscope. The doctor can then see the stone and remove it with a small basket at the end of a wire inserted through an extra tube in the ureteroscope. The doctor may also use the extra tube in the cystoscope to extend a flexible fiber that carries a laser beam to break the stone into smaller pieces that can then pass out of the body in your urine.

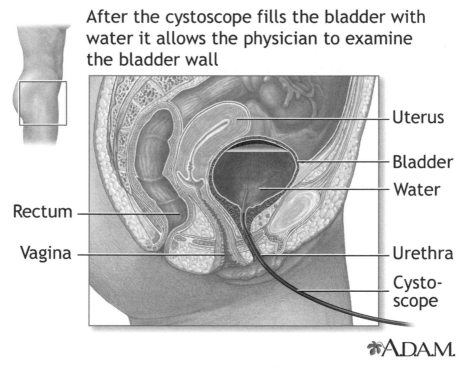

After the cystoscope fills the bladder with water it allows the physician to examine the bladder wall

Uterus

Bladder

Water

Rectum

Vagina

Urethra

Cysto-scope

✿A.D.A.M.

Figure 56.1. *Cytoscopy. Cystoscopy is a procedure that uses a flexible fiber optic scope inserted through the urethra into the urinary bladder. The physician fills the bladder with water and inspects the interior of the bladder. The image seen through the cystoscope may also be viewed on a color monitor and recorded on videotape for later evaluation. (Source: Image reprinted with permission, courtesy of A.D.A.M., © 2002.)*

Preparation

Ask your doctor whether he or she has any special instructions. In most cases, you will be able to eat normally and return to normal activities after the test. Since any medical procedure has a small risk of injury, you will need to sign a consent form before the test. Do not hesitate to ask your doctor about any concerns you might have.

You may be asked to give a urine sample before the test to check for infection. Avoid urinating for an hour before this part of the test.

You will wear a hospital gown for the examination, and the lower part of your body will be covered with a sterile drape. In most cases, you will lie on your back with your knees raised and apart. A nurse or technician will clean the area around your urethral opening and apply a local anesthetic.

If you are going to have a ureteroscopy, you may receive a spinal or general anesthetic. If you know this is the case, you will want to arrange a ride home after the test.

Test Procedures

The doctor will gently insert the tip of the cystoscope into your urethra and slowly glide it up into the bladder. Relaxing your pelvic muscles will help make this part of the test easier. A sterile liquid (water or saline) will flow through the cystoscope to slowly fill your bladder and stretch it so that the doctor has a better view of the bladder wall. As your bladder reaches capacity, you will feel some discomfort and the urge to urinate. You will be able to empty your bladder as soon as the examination is over. The time from insertion of the cystoscope to removal may be only a few minutes, or it may be longer if the doctor finds a stone and decides to remove it. Taking a biopsy (a small tissue sample for examination under a microscope) will also make the procedure last longer. In most cases, the entire examination, including preparation, will take about 15 to 20 minutes.

After the Test

You may have a mild burning feeling when you urinate, and you may see small amounts of blood in your urine. These problems should not last more than 24 hours. Tell your doctor if bleeding or pain is severe or if problems last more than a couple of days. To relieve discomfort, drink two 8-ounce glasses of water each hour for 2 hours. Ask your doctor if you can take a warm bath to relieve the burning feeling.

If not, you may be able to hold a warm, damp washcloth over the urethral opening.

Your doctor may give you an antibiotic to take for 1 or 2 days to prevent an infection. If you have signs of infection—including pain, chills, or fever—call your doctor.

Additional Information

American Foundation for Urologic Disease
1000 Corporate Blvd., Suite 410
Linthicum, MD 21090
Toll-Free: 800-828-7866
Phone: 410-689-3990
Fax: 410-689-3998
Website: www.afud.org
E-mail: admin@afud.org

Interstitial Cystitis Association of America, Inc.
110 N. Washington St., Suite 340
Rockville, MD 20850
Toll-Free: 800-HELP-ICA
Phone: 301-610-5300
Fax: 301-610-5398
Website: www.ichelp.org
E-mail: icamail@ichelp.org

National Kidney and Urologic Diseases Information Clearinghouse
3 Information Way
Bethesda, MD 20892-3580
Toll-Free: 800-891-5390
Phone: 301-654-4415
Fax: 301-907-8906
Website: http://kidney.niddk.nih.gov
E-mail: nkudic@info.niddk.nih.gov

Chapter 57

Endoscopic Retrograde Cholangiopancreatography (ERCP)

Your doctor has recommended that you have a medical procedure called an ERCP. This chapter will help you understand why ERCP is performed and what you can expect from the procedure.

ERCP is short for—Endoscopic, Retrograde, Cholangio, Pancreatography.

Endoscopic refers to the use of an instrument called an endoscope—a thin, flexible tube with a tiny video camera and light on the end. The endoscope is used by a highly trained subspecialist, the gastroenterologist, to diagnose and treat various problems of the GI tract. The GI tract includes the stomach, intestine, and other parts of the body that are connected to the intestine, such as the liver, pancreas, and gallbladder.

Retrograde refers to the direction in which the endoscope is used to inject a liquid enabling x-rays to be taken of the parts of the GI tract called the bile duct system and pancreas.

The process of taking these x-rays is known as cholangiopancreatography. Cholangio refers to the bile duct system, pancrea to the pancreas.

ERCP may be useful in diagnosing and treating problems causing jaundice (a yellowing of the whites of the eyes) or pain in the abdomen.

"What Is ERCP?" is reprinted with permission from the American Gastroenterological Association. © 2002. All rights reserved. For additional information on digestive health, visit http://www.gastro.org/public.html.

To understand how ERCP can help, it's important to know more about the pancreas and the bile duct system.

Bile is a substance made by the liver that is important in the digestion and absorption of fats. Bile is carried from the liver by a system of tubes known as bile ducts. One of these, the cystic duct, connects the gallbladder to the main bile duct. The gallbladder stores the bile between meals and empties back into the bile duct when food is consumed. The common bile duct then empties into a part of the small intestine called the duodenum. The common bile duct enters the duodenum through a nipple-like structure called the papilla.

Joining the common bile duct to pass through the papilla is the main duct from the pancreas. This pathway allows digestive juices from the pancreas to mix with food in the intestine. Problems that affect the pancreas and bile duct system can, in many cases, be diagnosed and corrected with ERCP.

For example, ERCP can be helpful when there is a blockage of the bile ducts by gallstones, tumors, scarring, or other conditions that cause obstruction or narrowing (stricture) of the ducts. Similarly, blockage of the pancreatic ducts from stones, tumors, or stricture can also be evaluated or treated by ERCP, which is useful in assessing causes of pancreatitis (inflammation of the pancreas).

Problems with the bile ducts or pancreas may first show up as jaundice or pain in the abdomen, although not always. Also, there may be changes in blood tests that show abnormalities of the liver or pancreas.

Other special exams that take pictures using x-rays or sound waves may provide important information to use along with that obtained from ERCP.

How to Prepare for the Procedure

Prior to having ERCP, there are a number of things you will need to remember:

- First, do not eat or drink anything for at least six hours beforehand or after midnight if your ERCP is scheduled for first thing in the morning.

- Be sure to tell your doctor all the medication you are taking, including aspirin, aspirin-containing drugs, or blood thinners.

- Identify any allergies or any reactions you have had to drugs, particularly antibiotics or pain medications.

- Follow all of your doctor's instructions regarding preparation for the procedure.

ERCP can be done either as an outpatient procedure or may require hospitalization, depending on the individual case. Your doctor will explain the procedure and its benefits and risks, and you will be asked to sign an informed consent form. This form verifies that you agree to have the procedure and understand what's involved.

What Can You Expect During an ERCP?

Everything will be done to ensure your comfort. Your blood pressure, pulse, and the oxygen level in your blood will be carefully monitored. A sedative will be given through a vein in your arm. You will feel drowsy, but will remain awake and able to cooperate during the procedure.

Although general anesthesia is usually not required, you may have the back of your throat sprayed with a local anesthetic to minimize discomfort as the endoscope is passed down your throat into your esophagus (the swallowing tube), and through the stomach into your duodenum.

The doctor will use it to inspect the lining of your stomach and duodenum. You should not feel any pain, but you may have a sense of fullness, since air may be introduced to help advance the scope.

In the duodenum, the instrument is positioned near the papilla, the point at which the main ducts empty into the intestine. A small tube known as a cannula is threaded down through the endoscope and can be directed into either the pancreatic or common bile duct. The cannula allows a special liquid contrast material, a dye, to be injected backwards—that is, retrograde—through the ducts.

X-ray equipment is then used to examine and take pictures of the dye outlining the ducts. In this way, widening, narrowing, or blockage of the ducts can be pinpointed.

Some of the problems that may be identified during ERCP can also be treated through the endoscope. For example, if a stone is blocking the pancreatic or common bile duct, it is usually possible to remove it.

First, the opening in the papilla is cut open and enlarged. Then, a special device can be inserted to retrieve the stone. Narrowing or obstruction can also have other causes, such as scarring or tumors. In some cases, a plastic or metal tube (called a stent), can be inserted to provide an opening. If necessary, a tissue sample or biopsy can be obtained, or a narrow area dilated.

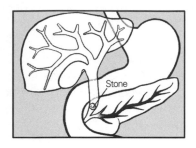

Figure 57.1. Your doctor may determine that a stone is blocking a common duct.

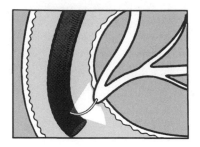

Figure 57.2. An endoscope will be lowered down your esophagus, through the stomach, and into the duodenum. A small tube will be threaded down into the duct.

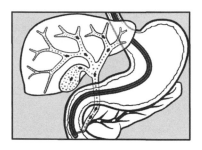

Figure 57.3. A dye will be injected backwards through the ducts, allowing x-rays to be taken.

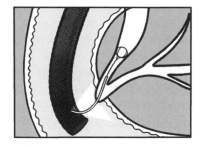

Figure 57.4. Your doctor will be able to remove the stone that is blocking the duct with the endoscope.

What Are the Possible Complications from an ERCP?

Thanks to ERCP, these kinds of procedures may help you avoid surgery. Depending on the individual and the types of procedures performed, ERCP does have a five to ten percent risk of complications. In rare cases, severe complications may require prolonged hospitalization.

Mild to severe inflammation of the pancreas is the most common complication and may require hospital care, even surgery. Bleeding can occur when the papilla has to be opened to remove stones or put in stents. This bleeding usually stops on its own, but occasionally, transfusion may be required or the bleeding may be directly controlled with endoscopic therapy.

A puncture or perforation of the bowel wall or bile duct is a rare problem that can occur with therapeutic ERCP. Infection can also result, especially if the bile duct is blocked and bile cannot drain. Treatment for infection requires antibiotics and restoring drainage. Finally, reactions may occur to any of the medications used during ERCP, but fortunately these are usually minor.

Be sure to discuss any specific concerns you may have about the procedure with your doctor.

What Can You Expect after Your ERCP?

When your ERCP is completed on an outpatient basis, you will need to remain under observation until your doctor or health care team has decided you can return home. Sometimes, admission to the hospital is necessary.

When you do go home, be sure you have arranged for someone to drive you, since you are likely to be sleepy from the sedative you received. Also, this means that you should avoid operating machinery for a day, and not drink any alcohol.

Your doctor will tell you when you can take fluids and meals. Usually, it is within a few hours after the procedure.

Because of the air used during ERCP, you may continue to feel full and pass gas for awhile, and it is not unusual to have soft stool or other brief changes in bowel habits. However, if you notice bleeding from your rectum or black, tarry stools, call your doctor.

You should also report vomiting, severe abdominal pain, weakness or dizziness, and fever over 100 degrees. Fortunately, these problems are not common.

ERCP is an effective and useful procedure for evaluating or treating a number of different problems of the GI tract.

Chapter 58

Flexible Sigmoidoscopy

Flexible sigmoidoscopy (SIG-moy-DAH-skuh-pee) enables the physician to look at the inside of the large intestine from the rectum through the last part of the colon, called the sigmoid or descending colon. Physicians may use the procedure to find the cause of diarrhea, abdominal pain, or constipation. They also use it to look for early signs of cancer in the descending colon and rectum. With flexible sigmoidoscopy, the physician can see bleeding, inflammation, abnormal growths, and ulcers in the descending colon and rectum. Flexible sigmoidoscopy is not sufficient to detect polyps or cancer in the ascending or transverse colon (two-thirds of the colon).

For the procedure, you will lie on your left side on the examining table. The physician will insert a short, flexible, lighted tube into your rectum and slowly guide it into your colon. The tube is called a sigmoidoscope (sig-MOY-duh-skope). The scope transmits an image of the inside of the rectum and colon so the physician can carefully examine the lining of these organs. The scope also blows air into these organs which inflates them and helps the physician see well.

If anything unusual is in your rectum or colon, like a polyp or inflamed tissue, the physician can remove a piece of it using instruments inserted into the scope. The physician will send that piece of tissue (biopsy) to the lab for testing.

Bleeding and puncture of the colon are possible complications of sigmoidoscopy. However, such complications are uncommon.

National Institute of Diabetes and Digestive and Kidney Diseases (NIDDK), NIH Publication No. 02-4332, February 2002.

Flexible sigmoidoscopy takes 10 to 20 minutes. During the procedure, you might feel pressure and slight cramping in your lower abdomen. You will feel better afterward when the air leaves your colon.

Preparation

The colon and rectum must be completely empty for flexible sigmoidoscopy to be thorough and safe, so the physician will probably tell you to drink only clear liquids for 12 to 24 hours beforehand. A liquid diet means fat-free bouillon or broth, gelatin, strained fruit juice, water, plain coffee, plain tea, or diet soda. The night before or right before the procedure, you may also be given an enema, which is a liquid solution that washes out the intestines. Your physician may give you other special instructions.

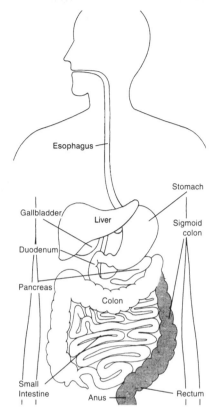

Figure 58.1. The Digestive System

Additional Information

International Foundation for Functional Gastrointestinal Disorders (IFFGD)
P.O. Box 170864
Milwaukee, WI 53217
Toll-Free: 888-964-2001
Phone: 414-964-1799
Fax: 414-964-7176
Website: www.iffgd.org
E-mail: iffgd@iffgd.org

National Digestive Diseases Information Clearinghouse
2 Information Way
Bethesda, MD 20892-3570
Toll-Free: 800-891-5389
Phone: 301-654-3810
Fax: 301-907-8906
Website: http://digestive.niddk.nih.gov
E-mail: nddic@info.niddk.nih.gov

Chapter 59

Laparoscopy

Diagnostic Laparoscopy

Patients may be referred to surgeons because of an undiagnosed abdominal problem. If your surgeon has recommended a diagnostic laparoscopy, this chapter will:

* help you understand what laparoscopy is,
* show how it helps to find out what the problem is, and
* explain what complications can occur with the procedure.

What Is Diagnostic Laparoscopy?

A laparoscope is a telescope designed for medical use. It is connected to a high intensity light and a high resolution television camera so that the surgeon can see what is happening inside of you. The laparoscope is put into the abdominal cavity through a hollow tube and the image of inside your abdomen is seen on the television screen. In most cases, this procedure (operation) will be able to diagnose or help discover what the abdominal problem is.

Laparoscopes are made in different sizes. The smaller laparoscopes are called mini- or micro-laparoscopes. Your surgeon will decide on an appropriately sized laparoscope for your condition.

"Patient Information for Diagnostic Laparoscopy," is reprinted with permission from the Society of American Gastrointestinal Endoscopic Surgeons (SAGES). For additional information, contact SAGE, 11300 West Olympic Blvd., Suite 600, Los Angeles, CA 90064, 310-437-0544, or visit www.sages.org.

What Are the Typical Reasons for Diagnostic Laparoscopy?

Abdominal Pain

Laparoscopy has a role in the diagnosis of both acute and chronic abdominal pain. There are many causes of abdominal pain. Some of these causes include appendicitis, adhesions or intra-abdominal scar tissue, pain mapping, pelvic infections, endometriosis, abdominal bleeding, and, less frequently, cancer. It is used in patients with irritable bowel disease to exclude other causes of abdominal pain. Surgeons can often diagnose the cause of the abdominal pain, and during the same procedure, correct the problem.

Abdominal Mass

A patient may have a lump (mass or tumor) which can be felt by the doctor or maybe by the patient him/herself. Other times, an x-ray may identify a lump. Most masses require a definitive diagnosis before appropriate therapy or treatment can be recommended. Laparoscopy is one of the techniques available to your physician to look directly at the mass and obtain tissue to discover the diagnosis.

Ascites

The presence of fluid in the abdominal cavity is called ascites. Sometimes the cause of this fluid accumulation cannot be found without looking into the abdominal cavity, which can often be accomplished with laparoscopy.

Liver Disease

Non-invasive x-ray imaging techniques (sonogram, CT scan, and MRI) may discover a mass inside or on the surface of the liver. If the non-invasive x-ray cannot give your physician enough information to find out the cause of your problems, a liver biopsy may be needed to confirm the diagnosis. Diagnostic laparoscopy is one of the safest and most accurate ways to obtain tissue for diagnosis. In other words, it is an accurate way to collect a biopsy to sample the liver or mass without actually opening the abdomen.

Second Look Procedure or Cancer Staging

Your doctor may need information regarding the status of a previously treated disease, such as cancer. This may occur after treatment with some forms of chemotherapy or before more chemotherapy is started. Also, information may be provided by diagnostic laparoscopy before planning a formal exploration of the abdomen, chemotherapy, or radiation therapy. This procedure is almost always performed in a hospital setting, as open, traditional surgery may often follow.

Other

There are other reasons to undergo a diagnostic laparoscopy which cannot all be listed here. This should be reviewed and discussed with your surgeon.

What Tests Are Necessary before Laparoscopy?

Ultrasound may be ordered by your doctor as a non-invasive diagnostic test. In many cases, information is provided which will allow your surgeon to have a better understanding of the problem inside your abdomen. This test is not painful and is very safe. It can improve the effectiveness of the diagnostic laparoscopy.

CT Scan is an x-ray that uses computers to visualize the intra-abdominal contents. In certain circumstances, it is accurate in making the diagnosis of abdominal disease. It will allow your surgeon to have a road map to the inside of your abdomen. Often times a CT scan will be used by a radiologist to place a needle or marker into something inside your abdomen and this is known as a CT guided needle biopsy. This will often be done before a diagnostic laparoscopy to decide if laparoscopy is appropriate for your condition.

MRI (magnetic resonance imaging) uses magnets, x-rays, and computers to view the inside of the abdominal cavity. It is not required for most abdominal problems, but it may be necessary for some.

Standard, routine blood test analysis, urinalysis, and possible chest x-ray or electrocardiogram may be needed before diagnostic laparoscopy. Your surgeon or physician will decide which tests are necessary, and will need to know the results of those tests which have already been performed.

What Type of Anesthesia Is Used?

Diagnostic laparoscopy is performed either under local anesthesia with sedation or with general anesthesia. With your help, your surgeon and an anesthesiologist will decide on a method of anesthesia to perform safe and successful surgery.

Local anesthesia can be injected into the skin of the abdominal wall to completely numb the area and allow safe placement of a laparoscope. Most patients feel a short-lived bee sting that lasts a second or two. Small doses of intravenous sedation are given at the same time allowing the patient to experience what is known as twilight sleep in which you are arousable but asleep. Once an adequate depth of sleep is reached and local anesthesia administered, gas is placed into the abdominal cavity. This is called a pneumoperitoneum. The patient may experience a bloated feeling. The gas is removed at the end of the operation. The two most common gases used are nitrous oxide (laughing gas) or carbon dioxide. There is very little risk of ill-effects of the gas.

General anesthesia is given to those patients who are not candidates for twilight sleep or who want to be completely asleep. General anesthesia may be preferable in patients who are young, who cannot lay still on the operating table, or have a medical condition that is safer to perform in this manner. Some patients end up having a general anesthesia even though they prefer local anesthesia with sedation, as the appropriate anesthesia for laparoscopy differs from patient to patient.

What Complications Can Occur?

Any procedure may have complications associated with it. The most frequent complications of any operation are bleeding and infection. There is a small risk of other complications that include, but are not limited to, injury to the abdominal organs, intestines, urinary bladder, or blood vessels. If you suffer with ascites, the ascites may leak from one of the operative sites, temporarily, before stopping. If a complication occurs, it must be attended to immediately. This may mean an additional operation with a larger incision to either stop bleeding or repair an injury that cannot be fixed through a laparoscope, or this may mean a general anesthesia instead of a local anesthesia. In experienced hands, complications may occur but are not frequent. Patient safety is your surgeon's strongest concern.

What Should I Expect before the Operation?

- Most diagnostic laparoscopy procedures are performed in an outpatient setting, meaning you will go home the same day as the procedure was performed.

- You should have nothing to eat or drink for six to eight hours before the procedure.

- Standard blood, urine, or x-ray testing may be required before your operative procedure. This will depend on your age and medical conditions.

- You may shower the evening before or the day of your operation. Cleaning your umbilicus (belly button) with soap, water, and a Q-tip is a good idea.

- Report to the hospital at the correct time, which is usually 1–2 hours earlier than your scheduled surgery.

- If you take medication on a daily basis, discuss this with your surgeon as you may need to take some or all of the medication on the day of surgery with a sip of water. If you take aspirin, blood thinners, or arthritis medication, discuss this with your surgeon so they can be stopped at the proper time before your surgery.

- You will need to ask your surgeon or his/her office staff what specifically is required in preparation for your surgery.

What Should I Expect after the Operation?

Following the operation, you will be transferred to the recovery room, where you will be monitored carefully until all the sedatives and anesthetics have worn off. Even though you may feel fully awake, the effects of any anesthetic may persist for a few hours or as long as a day. Once you are able to walk and get out of bed unassisted, you may be discharged. Because the effects of anesthesia can linger for many hours, it is recommended to have someone accompany you to the office or hospital and drive you home after the procedure.

You can expect some soreness around any incision site; this is normal. Your pain should improve every day, even though you may need to take a pain reliever. Your surgeon will instruct you on the use of pain relievers and may give you a prescription for a stronger pain medication.

Most patients are able to shower the day after surgery and begin all normal activities within a week. Your surgeon can answer any specific restrictions that apply to you.

If you have fever, chills, vomiting, are unable to urinate, develop increasing redness at an incision site, or your pain is worsening and not controlled by medication, you should contact your surgeon promptly.

You should call and schedule a follow-up appointment within two weeks after your procedure.

This chapter is not intended to take the place of a discussion with your surgeon about your need for a diagnostic laparoscopy. If you have any questions about your need for a diagnostic laparoscopy, alternative tests, the cost of the procedure, billing, or insurance coverage, do not hesitate to ask your surgeon or the office staff about it. If you have questions about your surgeon's qualifications or subsequent follow-up, please discuss them with your surgeon before or after your operation.

Additional Information

Society of American Gastrointestinal Endoscopic Surgeons (SAGES)
11300 W. Olympic Blvd., Suite 600
Los Angeles, CA 90064
Phone: 310-437-0544
Fax: 310-437-0585
Website: www.sages.org
E-mail: sagesweb@sages.org

Chapter 60

Upper Gastrointestinal (GI) Endoscopy

Your doctor has recommended that you have a medical procedure called upper GI endoscopy to evaluate or treat your condition. This chapter will help you understand how upper GI endoscopy can benefit you and what you can expect before, during, and after this procedure.

What Is Upper GI Endoscopy?

The term endoscopy refers to a special technique for looking inside a part of the body. Upper GI is the portion of the gastrointestinal tract, the digestive system that includes the esophagus, the swallowing tube leading to the stomach, which is connected to the duodenum, the beginning of the small intestine. The esophagus carries food from the mouth for digestion in the stomach and duodenum.

Upper GI endoscopy is a procedure performed by a gastroenterologist, a well-trained subspecialist who uses the endoscope to diagnose, and, in some cases, treat problems of the upper digestive system. The endoscope is a long, thin, flexible tube with a tiny video camera and light on the end. By adjusting the various controls on the endoscope, the gastroenterologist can safely guide the instrument to carefully examine the inside lining of the upper digestive system.

"What is Upper GI Endoscopy?" is reprinted with permission from the American Gastroenterological Association. © 2002. All rights reserved. For additional information on digestive health, visit http://www.gastro.org/public.html.

The high quality picture from the endoscope is shown on a TV monitor; it gives a clear, detailed view. In many cases, upper GI endoscopy is a more precise examination than x-ray studies. Upper GI endoscopy can be helpful in the evaluation or diagnosis of various problems, including difficult or painful swallowing, pain in the stomach or abdomen, bleeding, ulcers, and tumors.

How Do I Prepare for the Procedure?

Regardless of the reason upper GI endoscopy has been recommended for you, there are important steps you can take to prepare for and participate in the procedure. First, be sure to give your doctor a complete list of all the medicines you are taking and any allergies you have to drugs or other substances.

Your medical team will also want to know if you have heart, lung, or other medical conditions that may need special attention before, during, or after upper GI endoscopy. You will be given instructions in advance that will outline what you should and should not do in preparation for the upper GI endoscopy. Be sure to read and follow these instructions.

One very important step in preparing for upper GI endoscopy is that you should not eat or drink within eight to ten hours of your procedure. Food in the stomach will block the view through the endoscope, and it could cause vomiting.

Upper GI endoscopy can be done in either a hospital or outpatient office. You will be asked to sign a form that verifies that you consent

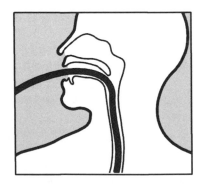

Figure 60.1. The endoscope is inserted in your mouth and gently edged down your esophagus.

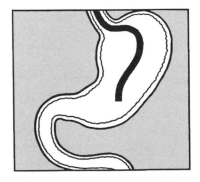

Figure 60.2. The endoscope will be inserted until it reaches your stomach.

to having the procedure and that you understand what is involved. If there is anything you do not understand, ask for more information.

What Can You Expect During an Upper GI Endoscopy?

During the procedure, everything will be done to help you be as comfortable as possible. Your blood pressure, pulse, and the oxygen level in your blood will be carefully monitored. Your doctor may give you a sedative medication; the drug will make you relaxed and drowsy, but you will remain awake enough to cooperate.

You may also have your throat sprayed or be asked to gargle with a local anesthetic to help keep you comfortable as the endoscope is passed. A supportive mouthpiece will be placed to help you keep your mouth open during the endoscopy. Once you are fully prepared, your doctor will gently maneuver the endoscope into position.

As the endoscope is slowly and carefully inserted, air is introduced through it to help your doctor see well. During the procedure, you should feel no pain and it will not interfere with your breathing.

Your doctor will use the endoscope to look closely for any problems that may require evaluation, diagnosis, or treatment.

In some cases, it may be necessary to take a sample of tissue, called a biopsy, for later examination under the microscope. This, too, is a painless procedure. In other cases, this endoscope can be used to treat a problem such as active bleeding from an ulcer.

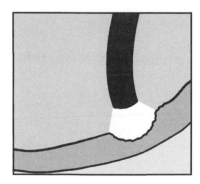
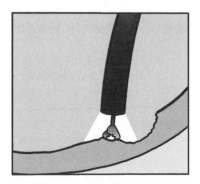

Figure 60.3. Once in the stomach, your doctor will look closely for any problem areas.

Figure 60.4. If anything suspicious is found, your doctor will take a sample for biopsy.

What Are the Possible Complications from an Upper GI Endoscopy?

Years of experience have proven that upper GI endoscopy is a safe procedure. Typically, it takes only 15–20 minutes to perform.

Complications rarely occur. These include perforation—a puncture of the intestinal wall, which could require surgical repair, and bleeding, which could require transfusion. Again, these complications are unlikely. Be sure to discuss any specific concerns you may have with your doctor.

When your endoscopy is completed you will be cared for in a recovery area until most of the effects of the medication have worn off. Your doctor will inform you about the results of the procedure and provide any additional information you need to know.

What Can I Expect after My Upper GI Endoscopy?

You will be given instructions regarding how soon you can eat and drink, plus other guidelines for resuming your normal activity.

Occasionally, minor problems may persist, such as mild sore throat, bloating, or cramping; these should disappear in 24 hours or less.

By the time you are ready to go home, you will feel stronger and more alert. Nevertheless, you should plan on resting for the remainder of the day. This means not driving, so you will need to have a family member or friend take you home.

In a few days, you will hear from your doctor with additional information such as results of the biopsy, or you may have questions you want to ask the doctor directly.

How Endoscopy Works

Upper GI endoscopy is a proven technique—an effective way to help you maintain your digestive health.

Part Nine

Genetic Testing

Chapter 61

A Brief Primer on Genetic Testing

An Introduction to Genetics and Genetic Testing

What do you know about your family tree? Have any of your relatives had health problems that tend to run in families? Which of these problems affected your parents or grandparents? Which ones affect you or your brothers or sisters now? Which problems might you pass on to your children?

Thanks to advances in genetics, doctors now have the tools to understand how certain illnesses, or increased risks for certain illnesses, pass from generation to generation. According to some health experts, the definition of an inherited or genetic illness should be expanded beyond the classic inherited disorders (like hemophilia and sickle cell anemia) to include many types of cancer, Alzheimer's disease, and other illnesses. They look toward a future where genetic test results are an important part of every healthy person's medical file.

Genes and Chromosomes

Each person has a unique set of chemical blueprints that determines how his or her body looks and functions. These blueprints are contained in a complex chemical called deoxyribonucleic acid (DNA),

This information was provided by KidsHealth, one of the largest resources online for medically reviewed health information written for parents, kids, and teens. For more articles like this one, visit www.KidsHealth.org, or www.TeensHealth.org. © 2003 The Nemours Center for Children's Health Media, a division of The Nemours Foundation.

a long, spiral-shaped molecule that is found inside each body cell. DNA carries the codes for genetic information and is made of linked subunits called nucleotides. Each nucleotide contains a phosphate molecule, a sugar molecule (deoxyribose), and one of four coding molecules called bases (adenine, guanine, cytosine, or thymine). The sequence of these four bases determines the genetic code.

Specific segments of DNA that contain the instructions for making specific body proteins are called genes. Right now, scientists believe that human DNA carries up to 30,000 genes. Some genes direct the formation of structural proteins that eventually determine physical features such as brown eyes or curly hair. Others provide the instructions for the body to produce important chemicals called enzymes. Sometimes, depending on the codes of a specific gene, even a small error within the DNA structure can mean serious problems for the entire body. Sometimes, an error in just one gene can result in a life that is shortened or physically difficult.

Genes are found in specific segments along the length of human DNA, neatly packaged within structures called chromosomes. Every human cell contains 46 chromosomes, arranged as 23 pairs, with one member of each pair inherited from each parent at the time of conception. After conception, these 46 chromosomes duplicate again and again to pass on the same genetic information to each new cell in the developing child. Human chromosomes are large enough to be seen with a high-powered microscope, and the 23 pairs can be identified according to differences in their size, shape, and the way they pick up special laboratory dyes.

Genetic Problems

Abnormal Numbers of Chromosomes (Trisomies and Monosomies)

Genetic problems can happen for many different reasons. Sometimes a mistake occurs during cell division, causing an error in chromosome number either before or shortly after conception. The developing embryo then grows from cells that have either too many chromosomes or too few. In trisomy, for example, there are three copies of one particular chromosome instead of the normal two (one from each parent). Down syndrome, trisomy 18 (Edwards) syndrome, and trisomy 13 (Patau) syndrome are all examples of this type of genetic problem. In monosomy, another form of number error, one member of a chromosome pair is missing. There are too few chromosomes rather than too many.

Deletions, Translocations, and Inversions

Sometimes it's not the number of chromosomes that's the problem. Instead, one or more chromosomes are incomplete or abnormally shaped. In both deletions and microdeletions, for example, some small part of a chromosome is missing. In a microdeletion, the missing part of a chromosome is usually so small that it amounts to a single gene or only a few genes. Some important genetic disorders caused by deletions and microdeletions include: Wolf-Hirschhorn syndrome (affects chromosome 4); Cri-du-chat syndrome (chromosome 5); DiGeorge syndrome (chromosome 22); and Williams syndrome (chromosome 7).

In translocations, bits of chromosomes shift from one chromosome to another, whereas in inversions, small parts of the DNA code seem to be snipped out and reinserted flipped over.

Sex Chromosomes

Genetic problems also occur when abnormalities affect the sex chromosomes. Normally, a child will be a male if he inherits one X chromosome from his mother and one Y chromosome from his father. A child will be a female if she inherits a double dose of X (one from each parent) and no Y. Sometimes, however, children are born with only one sex chromosome (usually a single X) or with an extra X or Y. Turner syndrome is the name of the disorder affecting girls born with only one X chromosome, whereas boys with Klinefelter syndrome are born with XXY or XXXY.

Sometimes, too, a genetic problem is X-linked, meaning that it is carried by the X chromosome. Fragile X syndrome, which causes mental retardation in boys, is one such disorder. Other diseases that are carried by genes on the X chromosome include hemophilia and Duchenne muscular dystrophy. Females may be carriers of these diseases, but because they also inherit a normal X chromosome, the abnormal X may be canceled out. Males, on the other hand, only have one X chromosome and are almost always the ones who have the disease.

Gene Mutations

Some genetic problems are caused by a single gene that is present but altered in some way. Such changes in genes are called mutations. When this is the case, chromosome number and appearance are often entirely normal. To pinpoint the defective gene, scientists use sophisticated DNA screening techniques. Some examples of genetic illnesses caused by a single problem gene include: cystic fibrosis, sickle cell anemia, Tay-Sachs disease, and achondroplasia (a type of dwarfism).

Although experts originally believed that no more than 3% of all human diseases were caused by errors in a single gene, new research suggests that this may be an underestimate. Within the last 2 years, scientists have discovered genetic links to many different diseases that were not originally thought of as genetic, including several different types of cancer.

Oncogenes (Cancer-Causing Genes)

Researchers have identified 20 to 30 cancer-susceptibility genes that greatly increase a person's odds of getting some form of malignancy. For example, a gene has been identified on chromosome number 9 that may be linked to a common skin cancer called basal cell carcinoma. This gene, labeled PTC or patched, may someday be important in screening for the cancer. Another gene, called HNPCC, is carried by one out of every 300 Americans and may greatly increase an individual's chance of getting colon cancer. And the doubly dangerous gene called BRCA-1 seems to give women an 85% chance of developing breast cancer, as well as a 50% chance of ovarian tumors.

Other Genetically Linked Diseases

Altered genes may play a role in the development of many other devastating illnesses. Parkinson's disease, for example, may be linked to a gene on chromosome number 4, and multiple sclerosis may be linked to alterations in a gene on chromosome number 6. Alzheimer's disease, linked to a gene on chromosome 19, can already be diagnosed (in some cases) by screening for that altered gene, although such screening is viewed by many as controversial.

Although heart disease and diabetes appear to be related to simultaneous changes in many different genes, the first of these may already have been identified. According to American Heart Association, this gene may be an artery-clogging gene that almost doubles the risk of fatty deposits blocking the coronary arteries. Having the gene may also triple someone's changes of getting adult-onset diabetes. Like heart disease, depression and other mental illnesses may be the result of alterations in several genes at once. Although no specific genes have yet been found, doctors estimate that 48% to 75% of depression is inherited, and they believe that they will find the exact genetic mechanism very soon.

It is important to note that much of the newest information from genetic research has not yet been translated into useful screening tests. However, experts predict that this will soon change, and they estimate that the number of available genetic tests will increase tenfold in the next decade.

Genetic Testing

At one time doctors could only diagnose genetic problems by karyotyping—checking the number, shape, and dye stains in chromosomes. Now genetic testing has developed enough so that doctors can pinpoint missing or defective genes. The type of genetic test needed to make a specific diagnosis depends on the particular genetic illness that a doctor suspects. If he or she suspects a trisomy, for example, a simple chromosome check will probably be enough. If the problem is a single problem gene, however, more high-tech DNA screening will usually be necessary. For genetic testing in children before birth, chorionic villus sampling or amniocentesis is usually performed.

Many different types of body fluids and tissues can be used in genetic testing. For DNA screening, only a very tiny bit of blood, skin, bone, or other tissue is needed. Even the small amount of tissue at the bottom end of a human hair is usually enough. That's why DNA testing is often successfully used by forensic scientists to identify human remains or as part of criminal investigations.

When Do Doctors Recommend Genetic Testing?

A doctor may recommend genetic counseling or testing for any of the following reasons:

- **A couple is planning to start a family and one of them or a close relative has an inherited illness.** Some people are carriers of genetic illnesses, even though they do not show, or manifest, the illness themselves. This happens because some genetic illnesses are recessive—they are only expressed if a person inherits two of the problem gene, one from each parent. Someone who inherits one problem gene from one parent but a normal gene from the other parent will not have symptoms of a recessive illness, but will have a 50-50 chance of someday passing the problem gene to their own children.

- **An individual already has one child with a severe birth defect.** Not all children who have birth defects have genetic problems. Sometimes birth defects are caused by exposure to a toxin (poison), infection, or physical trauma before birth. Even if a child does have a genetic problem, there is always a chance that it was not inherited and that it happened because of some spontaneous error in the child's cells, not the parents' cells.

- **A woman has had two or more miscarriages.** Severe chromosome problems in the fetus can sometimes lead to a spontaneous miscarriage. Several miscarriages may point to a genetic problem.

- **A woman has delivered a stillborn child with physical signs of a genetic illness.** Many serious genetic illnesses cause specific physical abnormalities that give an affected child a very distinctive appearance.

- **A woman is pregnant and over age 34.** Chances of having a child with a chromosomal problem (such as trisomy) increase dramatically when a pregnant woman is older.

- **A child has medical problems that might be genetic.** When a child has medical problems involving more than one body system, genetic testing may be recommended to identify the cause and make a diagnosis.

- **A child has medical problems that are recognized as a specific genetic syndrome.** Genetic testing is performed to confirm the diagnosis. In some cases, it also may aid in identifying the specific type or severity of a genetic illness, which can help identify the most appropriate treatment.

A Word of Caution

Although advances in genetic testing have created a revolution in the way that doctors diagnose and treat certain illnesses, there are still some limits that parents need to recognize. First, although genetic tests can identify a particular problem gene, they cannot always predict how severely that gene will affect the person who carries it. In cystic fibrosis, for example, finding a problem gene on chromosome number 7 cannot necessarily predict whether a child will have serious lung problems or milder respiratory symptoms.

Second, because many illnesses develop from a deadly mix of high-risk genes and unhealthy lifestyle (for example, a smoker with a family history of heart disease), simply having problem genes is only half the story. Knowing that you carry high-risk genes may actually be an advantage, if it gives you the chance to modify your lifestyle to avoid becoming sick.

Third, there are ethical issues associated with the use of genetic testing. Some people fear that testing for the presence of specific genes could eventually lead to discrimination by employers or insurance companies, to privacy and disclosure disputes, and even to the possibility that parents may one day be able to preselect certain genetic characteristics for their children.

The Future of Genetic Testing

Every day researchers are finding new evidence that people who have specific genes are at a greater risk for illnesses like cancer, heart disease, psychiatric disorders, and many other medical problems. The next step is to discover just how these problem genes work. Once we learn this, it may be possible to develop specific types of gene therapy to prevent some of humanity's major killer diseases.

Right now, gene therapy is already being used with limited success to treat cystic fibrosis and ADA deficiency (an immune deficiency). Sickle cell anemia, thalassemias, and other blood disorders may be the next targets for a genetic cure. Although genetic treatments for major killers, like cancer, may be a long way off, there is still great hope that many more genetic cures will be found. In less than 10 years, scientists working on the Human Genome Project will have finished identifying and mapping out all of the genes (up to 30,000) carried in our human chromosomes. The map will be just a beginning, but it's a very hopeful beginning.

Glossary

Amniocentesis: Amniocentesis is a test performed on a pregnant woman, usually between her sixteenth and eighteenth week of pregnancy. The doctor inserts a hollow needle into the woman's abdomen to remove a small amount of amniotic fluid from around the developing fetus. This fluid can be tested to check for genetic problems and to determine the sex of the child. When there is risk of cesarean section or premature birth, amniocentesis may also be done to see how far the child's lungs have matured. Like chorionic villus sampling, amniocentesis carries a slight risk of inducing a miscarriage.

Chorionic villus sampling: Chorionic villus sampling (CVS) is a test performed on a pregnant woman, usually between the tenth and twelfth weeks of pregnancy. In CVS, the doctor removes a small piece of the placenta to check for genetic problems in a child before birth.

Because chorionic villus sampling is an invasive test, there is a small risk that it can induce a miscarriage.

Deletions: A deletion happens when part of a chromosome is missing. Several different syndromes have been linked to deletions of specific parts of chromosomes 4, 5, 7, 13, 18, and 22. For example, Wolf-Hirschhorn syndrome is caused by a deletion of part of chromosome 4. Children born with this syndrome can have abnormalities of the head and face, malformations of the heart, and mental retardation.

DNA screening: In DNA screening, laboratories use molecular probes to check for a specific coding sequence along the length of a person's DNA molecule. This specific coding sequence is usually one that has been linked to causing an inherited disease.

Enzymes: Enzymes are proteins that act as natural catalysts. They help to direct and control the chemical reactions that happen within the body.

Inversions: In a chromosome inversion, a small portion of a chromosome breaks off, then reinserts flipped over. Inversions affect about one out of every 100 newborns and typically cause no malformations or developmental problems in the children who have them. However, when these children grow to adulthood and wish to become parents, they may have an increased risk of miscarriage or chromosome abnormalities in their own children.

Karyotyping: Karyotyping is a laboratory test that shows chromosome number and appearance. In karyotyping, a photo is taken of a person's chromosomes as they appear under a microscope.

Translocations: In translocations, small bits of chromosomes shift from one chromosome to another. Translocations may either be inherited from a parent or arise spontaneously in a child's own chromosomes. They affect one out of every 500 newborns. Translocations typically cause no malformations or developmental problems in the children who have them. However, when these children grow to adulthood and wish to become parents, they may have an increased risk of miscarriage or chromosome abnormalities in their own children.

Trisomy 13 (Patau) syndrome: Trisomy 13 syndrome affects one out of every 20,000 newborns. This syndrome causes cleft lip, flexed fingers with extra digits, hemangiomas (blood vessel malformations) of the face and neck, and many different structural abnormalities of the skull and face. It can also cause malformations of the ribs, heart, abdominal organs, and sex organs. Long-term survival is unlikely but possible.

Trisomy 18 (Edwards) syndrome: Trisomy 18 syndrome affects one out of every 8,000 newborns. Children with this syndrome have a low birth weight and a small head, mouth, and jaw. Their hands typically form closed fists with abnormal finger positioning. They may also have malformations involving the hips and feet, heart and kidney problems, and mental retardation. Only about 5% of these children live longer than 1 year.

Chapter 62

Uses of Genetic Testing

Clinically applicable genetic tests may be used for:

- Diagnostic testing
- Predictive testing
- Carrier testing
- Prenatal testing
- Preimplantation testing
- Newborn screening

Research tests generally do not give clinically applicable results.

Diagnostic Testing

Diagnostic testing is used to confirm or rule out a known or suspected genetic disorder in a symptomatic individual.

Points to Consider

- DNA testing may yield diagnostic information at a lower cost and with less risk than other procedures.

- Diagnostic testing is appropriate in symptomatic individuals of any age.

- Confirming a diagnosis may alter medical management for the individual.

Gene Tests: Medical Genetics Information Resource (database online). Educational Materials: Uses of Gene Tests. Copyright, University of Washington and Children's Health System, Seattle. 1993-2003. Available at http://www.genetests.org. Accessed November 14, 2003. Reprinted with permission.

- Diagnostic testing of an individual may have reproductive or psychosocial implications for other family members as well.

- Establishing a diagnosis may require more than one type of genetic test.

- DNA testing may not always be the best way to establish a clinical diagnosis.

Predictive Testing

Predictive testing is offered to asymptomatic individuals with a family history of a genetic disorder. Predictive testing is of two types: presymptomatic (eventual development of symptoms is certain when the gene mutation is present, e.g., Huntington disease), and predispositional (eventual development of symptoms is likely but not certain when the gene mutation is present, e.g., breast cancer).

Points to Consider

- Predictive testing is *medically indicated* if early diagnosis allows interventions which reduce morbidity or mortality.

- Even in the absence of medical indications, predictive testing can influence life planning decisions.

- Because predictive testing can have psychological ramifications, careful patient assessment, counseling, and follow-up are important.

- Many laboratories will not proceed with predictive testing without proof of informed consent and genetic counseling.

- Identification of the specific gene mutation in an affected relative or establishment of linkage within the family should precede predictive testing.

- Predictive testing of asymptomatic children at risk for adult onset disorders is strongly discouraged when no medical intervention is available.

Carrier Testing

Carrier testing is performed to identify individuals who have a gene mutation for a disorder inherited in an autosomal recessive or X-linked recessive manner. Carriers usually do not themselves have symptoms related to the gene mutation. Carrier testing is offered to individuals who have family members with a genetic condition, family members of an identified carrier, and individuals in ethnic or racial groups known to have a higher carrier rate for a particular condition.

Points to Consider

- Identifying carriers allows reproductive choices.

- Genetic counseling and education should accompany carrier testing because of the potential for personal and social concerns.

- Molecular genetic testing of an affected family member may be required to determine the disease-causing mutation(s) present in the family.

- In some situations, DNA testing may not be the primary way of determining carrier status.

- Carrier testing can improve risk assessment for members of racial and ethnic groups more likely to be carriers for certain genetic conditions.

Prenatal Testing

Prenatal testing is performed during a pregnancy to assess the health status of a fetus. Prenatal diagnostic tests are offered when there is an increased risk of having a child with a genetic condition due to maternal age, family history, ethnicity, a suggestive multiple marker screen, or fetal ultrasound examination. Routine prenatal diagnostic test procedures are amniocentesis and chorionic villus sampling (CVS). More specialized procedures include placental biopsy, periumbilical blood sampling (PUBS), and fetoscopy with fetal skin biopsy.

Points to Consider

- A laboratory that performs the disease-specific test of interest must be identified before any prenatal diagnostic test procedure is offered.

- All prenatal diagnostic test procedures have an associated risk to the fetus and the pregnancy; therefore, informed consent is required, most often in conjunction with genetic counseling.

- In most cases, before prenatal diagnosis using molecular genetic testing can be offered, specific gene mutation(s) must be identified in an affected relative or carrier parent(s).

- Prenatal testing for adult-onset conditions is controversial. Individuals seeking prenatal diagnosis for these conditions should be referred to a professional trained in genetic counseling for a complete discussion of the issues.

Preimplantation Testing (Preimplantation Genetic Diagnosis)

Preimplantation testing is performed on early embryos resulting from in vitro fertilization in order to decrease the chance of a particular genetic condition occurring in the fetus. It is generally offered to couples with a high chance of having a child with a serious disorder. Preimplantation testing provides an alternative to prenatal diagnosis and termination of affected pregnancies.

Points to Consider

- Preimplantation testing is only performed at a few centers and is only available for a limited number of disorders.

- Preimplantation testing is not possible in some cases due to difficulty in obtaining eggs or early embryos and problems with DNA analysis procedures.

- Due to possible errors in preimplantation diagnosis, traditional prenatal diagnostic methods are recommended to monitor these pregnancies.

- The cost of preimplantation testing is very high and is usually not covered by insurance.

Newborn Screening

Newborn screening identifies individuals who have an increased chance of having a specific genetic disorder so that treatment can be started as soon as possible.

Points to Consider

- Newborn screening programs are usually legally mandated and vary from state to state.

- Newborn screening is performed routinely at birth, unless specifically refused by the parents in writing.

- Screening tests are not designed to be diagnostic, but to identify individuals who may be candidates for further diagnostic tests.

- Many parents do not realize that newborn screening has been done (or which tests were included), even if they signed a consent form when their child was born.

- Education is necessary with positive screening results in order to avoid misunderstandings, anxiety, and discrimination.

Chapter 63

Ordering Genetic Testing

Genetic tests may be ordered by a medical geneticist or genetic counselor as part of a genetic consultation, or they may be ordered by a primary or specialty care provider. Considerations when ordering a genetic test include:

- Choosing a laboratory
- Pretest counseling and informed consent
- Sample logistics and supporting documentation
- Test result interpretation and follow-up

Choosing a Laboratory

Gene Tests (available at www.genetests.org on the Internet) was created to simplify the search for genetic testing laboratories, which may be difficult to locate. For many diseases, there may be only one laboratory providing genetic testing. U.S. patents have been issued covering diagnostic testing for some genetic disorders. A given laboratory may or may not be the exclusive licensee to such a patent. If there is a choice of laboratories, the following factors should be considered.

Gene Tests: Medical Genetics Information Resource (database online). Educational Materials: Ordering Genetic Testing. Copyright, University of Washington and Children's Health System, Seattle. 1993-2003. Available at http://www.genetests.org. Accessed November 14, 2003. Reprinted with permission.

579

Laboratory Personnel

Genetics laboratory personnel have two major roles: processing patient samples (technologists), and interfacing with referring clinicians regarding their patients (clinical consultants). Lab personnel, who are usually certified in their specialty, may include lab directors, supervisors, technologists, and genetic counselors.

Compatibility

The test offered by the laboratory must match the specific clinical need.

- Clinical testing gives a result which can be used in patient care; research testing usually does not. If only research testing is available, the patient or family may choose to defer testing until a clinical test is available.

- The test methodology must be suited to the testing purpose (e.g., Prader-Willi syndrome can be diagnosed with methylation testing, but other tests are required for recurrence risk counseling).

- Some diseases are caused by mutations in more than one gene. It is important to be sure that the lab selected is testing the appropriate gene(s).

- Different kinds of DNA tests are available. The laboratory selected should offer what is most appropriate for a specific clinical situation. For instance:

  - A specific gene mutation (e.g., if the familial mutation has been identified)

  - A panel of mutations (e.g., the Ashkenazi Jewish BRCA1 panel of 3 mutations)

  - The complete gene sequence

Reliability

Direct contact with the laboratory is needed to assess the laboratory's experience and qualifications.

- Does the laboratory have any other certification? (Laboratories with clinical listings in Gene Tests at www.genetests.org have CLIA certification.)

- Is the laboratory associated with a reputable company or university?

- Is the laboratory director board-certified?

- Is the laboratory's work published in the medical literature?

- What is the laboratory's experience with the specific test being ordered?

Ease of Communication

- What professionals are on staff to help assess the appropriateness of testing, determine the best testing paradigm for the family, and interpret test results?

- Does the laboratory have information on tests offered and logistics of sample collection and shipping easily available by phone, fax, or Internet?

- What information is contained in the test result report (e.g., raw data, interpretation, references, sensitivity, and specificity information)?

Geographical Location

- Some states have restrictions on insurance coverage, or, as is the case in New York, additional regulatory restrictions.

- Samples shipped outside of the U.S. must go through customs, which requires that hazard identification and a statement of value accompany the sample. Language barriers and time zones can also be an issue.

Turn-Around Time

Time from sample receipt to test result report may vary.

- Clinical laboratories generally have similar turn-around times for tests performed using the same methodology.

- A shorter turn-around time is advantageous only when it can be determined that quality control and thoroughness are not compromised. Test results for pregnancy management (prenatal diagnosis) are considered urgent due to restrictions on options late in pregnancy. Pregnancy dating should be included with all prenatal samples.

- The laboratory should be notified in advance of any sample that is *stat* (rush), as the sample processing may be different.

Cost

The cost may vary from less than $100 to more than $2000 based on several factors.

- Test methodology: Low complexity tests (e.g., single gene mutation) are less expensive than high complexity tests (e.g., full gene sequencing).

- Laboratory testing strategy: Some labs test for a large number of mutations all at once; other labs test in stepwise fashion, beginning with the most common mutations.

- Number of individuals tested: Several family members may need to be tested to obtain a meaningful test result.

- Contractural agreements: Hospitals, insurers, and laboratories negotiate contracts to set the price of testing and amount of reimbursement.

- Specimen handling: Some cell types require culturing or other special handling before testing.

- Additional services: Genetic consultation or counseling is usually recommended and sometimes required before genetic testing is performed. These fees should be considered in the total cost.

Pretest Counseling and Informed Consent

If genetic testing is clinically available and useful for a particular patient, the patient needs to understand why it is being offered and its implications for medical management and psychosocial well-being. If a competent patient (or parent/guardian) agrees to the proposed genetic test after full disclosure, this constitutes informed consent. Informed consent may be verbal or written. Some laboratories require written documentation of informed consent.

Pretest counseling includes:

- Assessing the patient's risk perception, expectations, and support systems.

- Explaining the implications of testing versus not testing for medical management and reproductive options.

- Describing the methods used to obtain specimens and associated risks.

- Reviewing test accuracy (sensitivity and specificity).

- Estimating the chance that the test will be positive based on available information (e.g., family history, clinical symptoms).

- Discussing any out-of-pocket costs to the patient.

- Establishing a plan for conveying test results. Depending on the circumstances, results may be given:
  - in person
  - by phone, with or without a follow-up appointment
  - by mail (negative results only)
  - only when positive (e.g., newborn screening)

Results should be revealed only to the individual tested, or his/her parent or guardian, unless explicit permission has been granted to share results.

Additional issues relevant in some testing situations:

- Need to clarify biological relationships (parentage, zygosity) for linkage studies.

- Potential discrimination in employment, insurability, or educational opportunities, especially in predictive testing. (Some states have State Genetics Laws in place prohibiting genetic discrimination).

- Results from research testing are not generally available for patient care.

Sample Logistics and Supporting Documentation

Contact the lab directly to ask the following questions:

What Are the Sample Requirements?

- Are samples from other family members needed?
- What specimen type is needed?

- Does the specimen need to be cultured before shipping?
- What is the requested amount of specimen? Will less be accepted in hard-to-draw situations?
- What information should be included on the label?

What Supporting Documentation Is Needed?

- Does the lab have a specific requisition form?
- What clinical history should be included?
- Are medical records or test results on family members needed?
- Is family history needed for test interpretation? A pedigree is an efficient way to show family relationships.
- Is ethnicity relevant to test interpretation?
- If crossing international borders, are hazard labels and customs paperwork included?

How Should the Sample Be Transported?

- What is the correct delivery address?
- When is delivery accepted?
- Should the sample be frozen, refrigerated, or at room temperature during shipping?
- Is there a courier to the lab, or is taxicab, mail, or overnight shipping required?

Test Result Interpretation and Follow-Up

Test results are provided in writing by the laboratory to the referring clinician. The details of the lab report vary by lab, but may include:

- Raw data
- Clinical interpretation of test result
- Sensitivity and specificity information
- References

The clinician explains the meaning of the test result to the patient and to other family members as needed. Test results and follow-up should be documented in the medical record and a copy made available to the patient. For many conditions, educational materials may be available from patient support organizations.

Table 63.1. For Positive Test Results

If the test purpose was...	The interpretation is...	And follow-up includes genetic counseling[1] and...
Diagnostic Testing	Clinical diagnosis is confirmed	Medical management and treatment
Predictive Testing	The likelihood of showing disease symptoms is increased	Counseling for life planning; Medical management if available
Carrier Testing	The patient is a carrier	Testing offered to partner; Prenatal testing offered if indicated
Prenatal Testing	A fetus is diagnosed with a specific condition	Pregnancy treatment/ management or termination
Newborn Screening	Disease in a newborn is suggested; Carrier status in a newborn may be identified.	Confirmatory testing; if positive, medical management and treatment; Carrier testing offered to parents

1. Genetic counseling includes discussion of expected course of the disorder; possible interventions; underlying cause; risks to family members; reproductive options; support.

Table 63.2. For Negative Test Results (***continued on next page***)

If the test purpose was...	The interpretation is...	And follow-up may include...
Diagnostic Testing	Clinical symptoms are unexplained	Further testing and/or follow-up genetic consultation
Predictive Testing	The likelihood of showing symptoms is decreased	Counseling for survivor guilt and long-range life planning; No high-risk surveillance needed
Carrier Testing	High likelihood that the individual is not a carrier; Low risk of having a child affected with the condition in question	Testing offered to other family members if indicated

Table 63.2. For Negative Test Results (***continued***)

If the test purpose was...	The interpretation is...	And follow-up may include...
Prenatal Testing	If fetus was symptomatic (e.g., by ultrasound findings), clinical symptoms remain unexplained and may need further investigation; If fetus was not symptomatic, the chance of the condition tested for is very small	If fetus was symptomatic, further testing and/or pregnancy management; If fetus was not symptomatic, no follow-up
Newborn Screening	The newborn is not expected to have the condition tested for	No follow-up

Chapter 64

Genetic Discrimination in Health Insurance

More than a decade of research on the human genome has yielded a wealth of information. Scientists have mapped and sequenced the genome, identified individual genes or sets of genes that are associated with diseases ranging from Alzheimer's to diabetes and certain forms of cancer, and developed genetic tests to determine an individual's predisposition for some of these diseases. Developments and discoveries like these—and others likely to come in the years ahead—offer hope that many deadly illnesses can be diagnosed, treated, and perhaps even cured both earlier and with better results than is now possible.

By learning more about their genetic makeup and susceptibility to certain diseases, people now have more choices, and potentially more control, when dealing with their health and future. Genetic information may lead people to ask their physicians to screen them regularly for certain diseases, to take preventive measures earlier in life, or even to rethink their reproductive plans and choices.

But genetic information can also be misused. It can be used to discriminate against people in health insurance and employment. People known to carry a gene that increases their likelihood of developing cancer, for example, may get turned down for health insurance. Without health insurance, it may be impossible for some people to get treatment for a disease that could be fatal. This may lead some people to decide against genetic testing for fear of what the results might show,

National Human Genome Research Institute, updated 3/2002.

and who might find out about them. It also could lead some people to decline participation in biomedical research, such as studies of gene mutations associated with certain diseases that examine the history of families prone to those maladies.

Each of us probably has half a dozen or more genetic mutations that place us at risk for some disease. That does not mean that we will develop the disease, only that we are more likely to get it than people who do not have the same genetic mutations. As our knowledge of the human genome increases, more and more people will likely be identified as carriers of mutations associated with a greater risk of certain diseases. That means that virtually all people are potential victims of genetic discrimination in health insurance.

Public Concerns

As a result, Americans have become concerned about the possible misuse of genetic information, especially in health insurance and employment. A *Time* magazine/Cable News Network (CNN) poll, published in June 2000, found that 75 percent of those surveyed would not want their insurance company to have information about their genetic code. A 1998 survey released by the National Center for Genome Resources (NCGR) found that 85 percent of those polled think employers should not have access to information about their employees' genetic conditions, risks, or predispositions.

People have reason to be concerned. Employer-sponsored health insurance plans in the private sector cover more than half of all Americans. Numerous reports in the news media and from expert groups have already uncovered instances where people were denied health insurance or coverage for particular conditions based on genetic information. In one case, a young boy, who had inherited an altered gene from his mother making him susceptible to a potentially fatal heart condition, was denied coverage by a health insurer when the boy's father lost his job and group coverage, and then tried to buy new insurance.

In 1993, the Ethical, Legal, and Social Implications (ELSI) Working Group of the Human Genome Project issued a report titled "Genetic Information and Health Insurance." The report recommended that people be eligible for health insurance no matter what is known about their past, present, or future health status. Two years later, the ELSI Working Group and the National Action Plan on Breast Cancer (NAPBC) jointly developed guidelines to assist federal and state agencies in preventing genetic discrimination in health insurance.

Further, the ELSI Working Group and NAPBC recommended that health insurers be prohibited from using genetic information or an individual's request for genetic services to deny or limit health insurance coverage, establish differential rates, or have access to an individual's genetic information without that individual's written authorization. Written authorization, the groups said, should be required for each separate disclosure and should specify the recipient of the disclosed information.

Next, the National Human Genome Research Institute (NHGRI) and the United States Department of Energy, acting through the ELSI Working Group, cosponsored a series of workshops in the mid-1990s on genetic discrimination in health insurance and the workplace. The findings and recommendations of the workshop participants were published in *Science* magazine, the monthly journal of the American Association for the Advancement of Science.

Legislative Protections

Those recommendations, and earlier ones issued by the ELSI Working Group and NAPBC led, in part, to new legislation and policies at both the federal and state levels. The Health Insurance Portability and Accountability Act (HIPAA) of 1996 provided the first federal protections against genetic discrimination in health insurance. The act prohibited health insurers from excluding individuals from group coverage due to past or present medical problems, including genetic predisposition to certain diseases. It limited exclusions from group plans for preexisting conditions to 12 months, and prohibited such exclusions for people who had been covered previously for that condition for 12 months or more. And the law specifically stated that genetic information in the absence of a current diagnosis of illness did not constitute a preexisting condition.

On the other hand, HIPAA did not prohibit health insurers from charging a higher rate to individuals based on their genetic makeup, prevent insurers from collecting genetic information, or limit the disclosure of genetic information about individuals to insurers. Nor did it prevent insurers from requiring applicants to undergo genetic testing.

The next step in addressing the issue of genetic discrimination was taken by President Bill Clinton. The President had earlier supported proposed legislation that would have banned all health plans—group or individual—from denying coverage or raising premiums on the basis of genetic information. When the legislation failed to pass Congress, President Clinton issued an Executive Order in February 2000 prohibiting agencies of the federal government from obtaining genetic information about their employees or job applicants, and from using genetic information in hiring and promotion decisions. In announcing the order, President Clinton said, "We must not allow advances in genetics to become the basis of discrimination against any individual or any group. We must never allow these discoveries to change the basic belief upon which our government, our society, and our system of ethics is founded—that all of us are created equal, entitled to equal treatment under the law." Both before and since that Executive Order, a number of bills have been introduced into Congress to further deal with genetic discrimination in health insurance and employment. Nine bills were introduced in the 106th Congress (1999-2001) and four in the 107th Congress (2001-03). Meanwhile, 41 states have enacted legislation related to genetic discrimination in health insurance and 31 states have adopted laws regarding genetic discrimination in the workplace. The state laws regarding health insurance conform to HIPAA.

There continues to be a high degree of interest in these topics in state legislatures. More than one hundred bills were introduced in state legislatures in 2000 alone. Some would inaugurate protection from genetic discrimination while others would modify or clarify existing legislation.

Part Ten

Additional Information

Chapter 65

Glossary of Medical Tests Terms

Accuracy: The degree to which a measurement, or an estimate based on measurements, represents the true value of the attribute that is being measured. In the laboratory, accuracy of a test is determined when possible by comparing results from the test in question with results generated using reference standards or an established reference method.

Angiography: Radiography of vessels after the injection of a radiopaque contrast material; usually requires percutaneous insertion of a radiopaque catheter and positioning under fluoroscopic control.

Arteriography: Demonstration of an artery or arteries by x-ray imaging after injection of a radiopaque contrast medium.

Arthroscopy: Endoscopic examination of the interior of a joint.

Asymptomatic: Without symptoms, or producing no symptoms.

Audiogram: The graphic record drawn from the results of hearing tests with an audiometer, which charts the threshold of hearing at various frequencies against sound intensity in decibels.

Biopsy: Process of removing tissue from patients for diagnostic examination.

Definitions in this chapter were taken from *Stedman's Medical Dictionary, 27ᵗʰ Edition.* © 2000, Lippincott Williams & Wilkins. All rights reserved. Reprinted with permission.

Blood count: Calculation of the number of red (RBC) or white (WBC) blood cells in a cubic millimeter of blood, by means of counting the cells in an accurate volume of diluted blood.

Blood pressure (BP): The pressure or tension of the blood within the systemic arteries, maintained by the contraction of the left ventricle, the resistance of the arterioles and capillaries, the elasticity of the arterial walls, as well as the viscosity and volume of the blood; expressed as relative to the ambient atmospheric pressure.

Bronchoscope: An endoscope for inspecting the interior of the tracheobronchial tree, either for diagnostic purposes (including biopsy) or for the removal of foreign bodies. There are two types: flexible and rigid.

Cardiac telemetry: Transmission of cardiac signals (electric or pressure derived) to a receiving location where they are displayed for monitoring.

Colonoscopy: Visual examination of the inner surface of the colon by means of a colonoscope.

Complete blood count (CBC): A combination of the following determinations: red blood cell count, white blood cell count, erythrocyte indices, hematocrit, differential blood count, and sometimes platelet count.

Computed tomography (CT): Imaging anatomic information from a cross-sectional plane of the body, each image generated by a computer synthesis of x-ray transmission data obtained in many different directions in a given plane.

Diagnosis: The determination of the nature of a disease, injury, or congenital defect.

Diagnostic ultrasound: The use of ultrasound to obtain images for medical diagnostic purposes, employing frequencies ranging from 1.6 to about 10 MHz.

Diastolic pressure: The intracardiac pressure during or resulting from diastolic relaxation of a cardiac chamber; the lowest arterial blood pressure reached during any given ventricular cycle.

Doppler ultrasonography: Application of the Doppler effect in ultrasound to detect movement of scatterers (usually red blood cells) by the analysis of the change in frequency of the returning echoes. In many settings, ultrasound has supplanted x-radiography as the imaging method of choice, because it poses no known risk to patients, is non-invasive, and of moderate cost. Doppler-created ultrasound makes possible real-time viewing of tissues, blood flow, and organs that cannot be observed by any other method. It is particularly valuable in cardiology and obstetrics.

Electrocardiogram (ECG, EKG): Graphic record of the heart's integrated action currents obtained with the electrocardiograph displayed as voltage changes over time.

Electroencephalograph: A system for recording the electric potentials of the brain derived from electrodes attached to the scalp.

Endosonoscopy: A sonographic study carried out by transducers inserted into the body as miniature probes in the esophagus, urethra, bladder, vagina, or rectum.

False negative: A test result that erroneously excludes an individual from a specific diagnostic or reference group to which the individual may truly belong.

False positive: A test result that erroneously assigns an individual to a specific diagnostic or reference group, to which the individual may not truly belong, due particularly to insufficiently exact methods of testing.

Fine needle biopsy: The aspiration and removal of tissue or suspensions of cells through a small needle.

Genetic testing: Laboratory studies of human blood or other tissue for the purpose of identifying genetic disorders. Relatively large chromosomal abnormalities such as deletion or transposition are identified by microscopic examination of chromosomes from a cell undergoing mitosis (karyotyping). More subtle aberrations can be detected by DNA probes (fabricated lengths of single-stranded DNA that match parts of the known gene). Genetic testing in the broadest sense includes biochemical testing for abnormal substances, or abnormally high or low concentrations of normal substances, that serve as markers of genetic deficiency or abnormality.

Glucose tolerance test: A test for diabetes or for hypoglycemic states such as may be seen rarely in patients with insulinomas. Following ingestion of 75 g of glucose while the patient is fasting, the blood sugar promptly rises and then falls to normal within 2 hours; in diabetics, the increase is greater and the return to normal unusually prolonged;

in hypoglycemic patients, depressed glucose levels may be observed in 3-, 4-, or 5-hour measurements.

Holter monitor: A technique for long-term, continuous usually ambulatory, recording of electrocardiographic signals on magnetic tape for scanning and selection of significant but fleeting changes that might otherwise escape notice.

Laparoscopy: Examination of the contents of the abdominopelvic cavity with a laparoscope passed through the abdominal wall. The technique has become standard, in selected cases, for many routine surgical procedures formerly requiring laparotomy, such as appendectomy, cholecystectomy, inguinal herniorrhaphy, oophorectomy, a second look after excision of an ovarian tumor, and diagnostic evaluation of endometriosis and female infertility. The risk of intraoperative and postoperative complications, the cost of treatment, and hospitalization time are generally less with laparoscopic surgery than with traditional open procedures.

Lumbar puncture: A puncture into the subarachnoid space of the lumbar region to obtain spinal fluid for diagnostic or therapeutic purposes.

MR angiography (MRA): Imaging of blood vessels using special magnetic resonance (MR) sequences that enhance the signal of flowing blood and suppress that from other tissues.

Magnetic resonance imaging (MRI): A diagnostic radiologic modality, using nuclear magnetic resonance technology, in which the magnetic nuclei (especially protons) of a patient are aligned in a strong, uniform magnetic field, absorb energy from tuned radiofrequency pulses, and emit radiofrequency signals as their excitation decays. These signals, which vary in intensity according to nuclear abundance and molecular chemical environment, are converted into sets of tomographic images by using field gradients in the magnetic field, which permits 3-dimensional localization of the point sources of the signals.

Nuclear medicine: The clinical discipline concerned with the diagnostic and therapeutic uses of radionuclides, including sealed radiation sources.

Pap test: Microscopic examination of cells exfoliated or scraped from a mucosal surface after staining with Papanicolaou stain; used especially for detection of cancer of the uterine cervix.

Pathologist: A specialist in pathology; a physician who practices, evaluates, or supervises diagnostic tests, using materials removed from living or dead patients, and functions as a laboratory consultant to clinicians, or who conducts experiments or other investigations to determine the causes or nature of disease changes.

Polysomnography: Simultaneous and continuous monitoring of relevant normal and abnormal physiologic activity during sleep.

Pulmonary: Relating to the lungs, to the pulmonary artery, or to the aperture leading from the right ventricle into the pulmonary artery.

Radiography: Examination of any part of the body for diagnostic purposes by means of x-rays with the record of the findings usually impressed upon a photographic film.

Sigmoidoscopy: Inspection, through an endoscope, of the interior of the sigmoid colon.

Stress test: Any standardized procedure for assessing the effect of stress on cardiac function and myocardial perfusion; stress may be induced by physical exercise or simulated by administration of a coronary vasodilator; heart rate, blood pressure, and electrocardiogram are monitored before, during, and after the challenge; other observations sometimes made are measurement of oxygen consumption, echocardiography, impedance cardiography, appraisal of both myocardial perfusion and cardiac wall motion by radionuclide tracer, and cardiac catheterization.

Symptom: Any morbid phenomenon or departure from the normal in structure, function, or sensation, experienced by the patient and indicative of disease.

Systolic pressure: The intracardiac pressure during or resulting from systolic contraction of a cardiac chamber; the highest arterial blood pressure reached during any given ventricular cycle.

Ultrasonography: The location, measurement, or delineation of deep structures by measuring the reflection or transmission of high frequency or ultrasonic waves. Computer calculation of the distance to the sound-reflecting or absorbing surface plus the known orientation of the sound beam gives a two-dimensional image.

Upper GI series: A radiographic contrast study of the esophagus, stomach, and duodenum.

X-ray: The ionizing electromagnetic radiation emitted from a highly evacuated tube, resulting from the excitation of the inner orbital electrons by the bombardment of the target anode with a stream of electrons from a heated cathode. Syn: radiograph

Chapter 66

Directory of Resources

Government Organizations That Provide Information about Medical Tests

Agency for Healthcare Research and Quality
540 Gaither Road
Rockville, MD 20850
Toll-Free: 800-358-9295
Phone: 301-427-1364
Website: www.ahrq.gov
E-mail: info@ahrq.gov

Cancer Information Service
National Cancer Institute
P.O. Box 24128
Baltimore, MD 21227
Toll-Free: 800-4-CANCER (422-6237)
Toll-Free TTY: 800-332-8615
Website: http://cis.nci.nih.gov

Centers for Disease Control and Prevention
NIP Public Inquiries
Mailstop E-05
1600 Clifton Rd., N.E.
Atlanta, GA 30333
Toll-Free: 800-232-2522
Toll-Free Spanish: 800-232-0233
Toll-Free National STD Hotline: 800-227-8922
Toll-Free National AIDS Hotline: 800-342-AIDS
Toll-Free AIDS TTY Hotline: 800-243-7889
Toll-Free AIDS Hotline in Spanish: 800-344-7432
Fax: 888-232-3299
Website: www.cdc.gov/nip
E-mail: NIPINFO@cdc.gov

The list of resources presented in this chapter was compiled from many sources deemed reliable; contact information was verified and updated in November 2003.

Consumer Product Safety Commission
4330 East-West Highway
Washington, DC 20207-0001
Toll-Free: 800-638-CPSC (2772)
Phone: 301-504-6816
Fax: 301-504-0124
Website: www.cpsc.gov
E-mail: info@cpsc.gov

Health Resources and Services Administration (HRSA) Information Center
U.S. Department of Health and Human Services
Parklawn Building
5600 Fishers Lane
Rockville, MD 20857
Toll-Free: 888-275-4772
Website: www.ask.hrsa.gov
E-mail: ask@arsa.gov

Joint Commission on Accreditation of Healthcare Organizations
Quality Check™
One Renaissance Blvd.
Oakbrook Terrace, IL 60181
Phone: 630-792-5000
Customer Service Center: 630-792-5800
Toll-Free Office of Quality Monitoring: 800-994-6610
Website: www.jcaho.org/qualitycheck/directry/directry.asp
E-mail: complaint@jcaho.org

National Clearinghouse for Alcohol and Drug Information
11426 Rockville Pike, Suite 280
Rockville, MD 20852
Toll-Free: 800-729-6686
Website: www.health.org

National Council on Aging
300 D Street, S.W., Suite 801
Washington, DC 20024
Phone: 202-479-1200
TDD: 202-479-6674
Fax: 202-479-0735
Website: www.ncoa.org
E-mail: info@ncoa.org

National Diabetes Information Clearinghouse
1 Information Way
Bethesda, MD 20892-3560
Toll-Free: 800-860-8747
Phone: 301-654-3327
Fax: 301-907-8906
Website: http://diabetes.niddk.nih.gov
E-mail: ndic@info.niddk.nih.gov

National Digestive Diseases Information Clearinghouse
2 Information Way
Bethesda, MD 20892-3570
Toll-Free: 800-891-5389
Phone: 301-654-3810
Fax: 301-907-8906
Website: http://digestive.niddk.nih.gov
E-mail: nddic@info.niddk.nih.gov

National Heart, Lung, and Blood Institute
Information Center
P.O. Box 30105
Bethesda, MD 20824-0105
Phone: 301-592-8573
TTY: 240-629-3255
Fax: 301-592-8563
Website: www.nhlbi.nih.gov
E-mail: nhlbiinfo@rover.nhlbi
.nih.gov

National Kidney and Urologic Diseases Information Clearinghouse
3 Information Way
Bethesda, MD 20892-3580
Toll-Free: 800-891-5390
Phone: 301-654-4415
Website: http://kidney.niddk.nih
.gov/index.htm
E-mail: nkudic@info.niddk.nih
.gov

National Women's Health Information Center
Office on Women's Health
Room 730B
200 Independence Ave., S.W.
Washington, DC 20201
Toll-Free: 800-994-9662
Toll-Free TDD: 888-220-5446
Phone: 202-690-7650
Fax: 202-205-2631
Website: www.4woman.gov

U.S. Department of Health and Human Services
Public Health Service
200 Independence Avenue, S.W.
Washington, DC 20201
Toll-Free: 877-696-6775
Phone: 202-619-0257
Website: www.hhs.gov

U.S. Food and Drug Administration
Office of Consumer Affairs
5600 Fishers Lane
Rockville, MD 20857-0001
Toll-Free: 888-463-6332
Phone: 301-827-4420
Website: www.fda.gov

Vaccine Adverse Event Reporting System
P.O. Box 1100
Rockville, MD 20849-1100
Toll-Free: 800-822-7967
Website: www.vaers.org
E-mail: info@vaers.org

Private Organizations That Provide Information about Medical Tests

American Academy of Allergy, Asthma, and Immunology
611 East Wells St.
Milwaukee, WI 53202
Toll-Free: 800-822-2762
Phone: 414-272-6071
Website: www.aaaai.org
E-mail: info@aaaai.org

American Academy of Family Physicians
11400 Tomahawk Creek Pkwy.
Leawood, KS 66211-2672
Toll-Free: 800-274-2237
Phone: 913-906-6000
Website: www.aafp.org
E-mail: fp@aafp.org

American Academy of Pediatrics
141 Northwest Point Blvd.
Elk Grove Village, IL 60007-1098
Phone: 847-434-4000
Fax: 847-434-8000
Website: www.aap.org
E-mail: kidsdocs@aap.org

American College of Cardiology
Heart House
9111 Old Georgetown Rd.
Bethesda, MD 20814-1699
Toll-Free: 800-253-4636
Phone: 301-897-5400
Fax: 301-897-9745
Website: www.acc.org
E-mail: resource@aac.org

American College of Gastroenterology (ACG)
P.O. Box 3099
Arlington, VA 22302
Phone: 703-820-7400
Fax: 703-931-4520
Website: www.acg.gi.org

American College of Physicians/American Society of Internal Medicine
190 N. Independence Mall W.
Philadelphia, PA 19106-1572
Toll-Free (customer service):
800-523-1546, ext. 2600
Phone: 215-351-2600
Website: www.acponline.org

American College of Radiology
CT Accreditation Department
1891 Preston White Dr.
Reston, VA 20191-4397
Toll-Free: 800-347-7748
Phone: 703-648-8900
Fax: 703-264-2093
Website: www.acr.org
E-mail: ctaccred@acr.org

American Diabetes Association
National Service Center
1701 N. Beauregard St.
Alexandria, VA 22311
Toll-Free: 800-342-2383
Phone: 703-549-1500
Website: www.diabetes.org
E-mail: AskADA@diabetes.org

American Foundation for Urologic Disease
1128 North Charles St.
Baltimore, MD 21201
Toll-Free: 800-828-7866
Phone: 410-468-1800
Website: www.afud.org
E-mail: admin@afud.org

American Heart Association
7272 Greenville Ave.
Dallas, TX 75231
Toll-Free: 800-242-8721
Website: www.americanheart
.org

American Stroke Association
7272 Greenville Ave.
Dallas, TX 75231
Toll-Free: 888-478-7653
Website:
www.strokeassociation.org

International Foundation for Functional Gastrointestinal Disorders (IFFGD)
P.O. Box 170864
Milwaukee, WI 53217-8076
Toll-Free: 888-964-2001
Phone: 414-964-1799
Fax: 414-964-7176
Website: www.iffgd.org
E-mail: iffgd@iffgd.org

Interstitial Cystitis Association of America, Inc.
110 N. Washington St.
Suite 340
Rockville, MD 20850
Toll-Free: 800-HELP-ICA (435-7422)
Phone: 301-610-5300
Fax: 301-610-5308
Website: www.ichelp.org
E-mail: icamail@ichelp.org

Juvenile Diabetes Research Foundation International
120 Wall St.
19th Floor
New York, NY 10005-4001
Toll-Free: 800-533-2873
Phone: 212-785-9500
Website: www.jdrf.org
E-mail: info@jdrf.org

National Mental Health Association
2001 N. Beauregard St.
12th Floor
Alexandria, VA 22311
Toll-Free: 800-969-6642
Toll-Free TTY: 800-433-5959
Phone: 703-684-7722
Fax: 703-684-5968
Website: www.nmha.org

The Prostatitis Foundation
1063 30th Street
Box 8
Smithshire, IL 61478
Toll-Free: 888-891-4200
Fax: 309-325-7184
Website: www.prostate.org

Radiological Society of North America, Inc.
820 Jorie Blvd.
Oak Brook, IL 60523-2251
Toll-Free: 800-381-6660
Phone: 630-571-2670
Fax: 630-571-7837
Website: www.rsna.org or
www.radiologyinfo.org

RESOLVE
The National Infertility
Association
1310 Broadway
Somerville, MA 02144
Toll-Free: 888-623-1744
Phone: 617-623-1156
Fax: 617-623-0252
Helpline: 617-623-0744
Website: www.resolve.org
E-mail: info@resolve.org

**Society of American
Gastrointestinal
Endoscopic Surgeons
(SAGES)**
11300 W. Olympic Blvd.
Suite 600
Los Angeles, CA 90064
Phone: 310-437-0544
Fax: 310-437-0585
Website: www.sages.org
E-mail: sagesweb@sages.org

**St. Joseph Sleep Disorders
Center**
1310 W. Stewart Dr.
Suite 403
Orange, CA 92868
Toll-Free: 888-766-7363
Phone: 714-771-8950
Website: www.sjhsleepcenter
.com

**University of Pittsburgh
Medical Center**
Cancer Centers Administration
5150 Centre Avenue
Pittsburgh, PA 15232
Toll-Free: 800-237-4724
Phone: 412-647-2811
Website: www
.upmccancercenters.com
E-mail: PCI-INFO@msx.upmc
.edu

Index

Index

Health Reference Series
COMPLETE CATALOG

Adolescent Health Sourcebook

Basic Consumer Health Information about Common Medical, Mental, and Emotional Concerns in Adolescents, Including Facts about Acne, Body Piercing, Mononucleosis, Nutrition, Eating Disorders, Stress, Depression, Behavior Problems, Peer Pressure, Violence, Gangs, Drug Use, Puberty, Sexuality, Pregnancy, Learning Disabilities, and More

Along with a Glossary of Terms and Other Resources for Further Help and Information

Edited by Chad T. Kimball. 658 pages. 2002. 0-7808-0248-9. $78.

"It is written in clear, nontechnical language aimed at general readers. . . . Recommended for public libraries, community colleges, and other agencies serving health care consumers."
— American Reference Books Annual, 2003

"Recommended for school and public libraries. Parents and professionals dealing with teens will appreciate the easy-to-follow format and the clearly written text. This could become a 'must have' for every high school teacher." — E-Streams, Jan '03

"A good starting point for information related to common medical, mental, and emotional concerns of adolescents." — School Library Journal, Nov '02

"This book provides accurate information in an easy to access format. It addresses topics that parents and caregivers might not be aware of and provides practical, useable information." — Doody's Health Sciences Book Review Journal, Sep-Oct '02

"Recommended reference source."
— Booklist, American Library Association, Sep '02

AIDS Sourcebook, 3rd Edition

Basic Consumer Health Information about Acquired Immune Deficiency Syndrome (AIDS) and Human Immunodeficiency Virus (HIV) Infection, Including Facts about Transmission, Prevention, Diagnosis, Treatment, Opportunistic Infections, and Other Complications, with a Section for Women and Children, Including Details about Associated Gynecological Concerns, Pregnancy, and Pediatric Care

Along with Updated Statistical Information, Reports on Current Research Initiatives, a Glossary, and Directories of Internet, Hotline, and Other Resources

Edited by Dawn D. Matthews. 664 pages. 2003. 0-7808-0631-X. $78.

ALSO AVAILABLE: AIDS Sourcebook, 1st Edition. Edited by Karen Bellenir and Peter D. Dresser. 831 pages. 1995. 0-7808-0031-1. $78.

AIDS Sourcebook, 2nd Edition. Edited by Karen Bellenir. 751 pages. 1999. 0-7808-0225-X. $78.

"Highly recommended."
— American Reference Books Annual, 2000

"Excellent sourcebook. This continues to be a highly recommended book. There is no other book that provides as much information as this book provides."
— AIDS Book Review Journal, Dec-Jan 2000

"Recommended reference source."
— Booklist, American Library Association, Dec '99

"A solid text for college-level health libraries."
— The Bookwatch, Aug '99

Cited in Reference Sources for Small and Medium-Sized Libraries, American Library Association, 1999

Alcoholism Sourcebook

Basic Consumer Health Information about the Physical and Mental Consequences of Alcohol Abuse, Including Liver Disease, Pancreatitis, Wernicke-Korsakoff Syndrome (Alcoholic Dementia), Fetal Alcohol Syndrome, Heart Disease, Kidney Disorders, Gastrointestinal Problems, and Immune System Compromise and Featuring Facts about Addiction, Detoxification, Alcohol Withdrawal, Recovery, and the Maintenance of Sobriety

Along with a Glossary and Directories of Resources for Further Help and Information

Edited by Karen Bellenir. 613 pages. 2000. 0-7808-0325-6. $78.

"This title is one of the few reference works on alcoholism for general readers. For some readers this will be a welcome complement to the many self-help books on the market. Recommended for collections serving general readers and consumer health collections."
— E-Streams, Mar '01

"This book is an excellent choice for public and academic libraries."
— American Reference Books Annual, 2001

"Recommended reference source."
— Booklist, American Library Association, Dec '00

"Presents a wealth of information on alcohol use and abuse and its effects on the body and mind, treatment, and prevention." — SciTech Book News, Dec '00

"Important new health guide which packs in the latest consumer information about the problems of alcoholism." — Reviewer's Bookwatch, Nov '00

SEE ALSO Drug Abuse Sourcebook, Substance Abuse Sourcebook

Allergies Sourcebook, 2nd Edition

Basic Consumer Health Information about Allergic Disorders, Triggers, Reactions, and Related Symptoms, Including Anaphylaxis, Rhinitis, Sinusitis, Asthma, Dermatitis, Conjunctivitis, and Multiple Chemical Sensitivity

Along with Tips on Diagnosis, Prevention, and Treatment, Statistical Data, a Glossary, and a Directory of Sources for Further Help and Information

Edited by Annemarie S. Muth. 598 pages. 2002. 0-7808-0376-0. $78.

ALSO AVAILABLE: *Allergies Sourcebook, 1st Edition.* Edited by Allan R. Cook. 611 pages. 1997. 0-7808-0036-2. $78.

"This book brings a great deal of useful material together. . . . This is an excellent addition to public and consumer health library collections."
— *American Reference Books Annual, 2003*

"This second edition would be useful to laypersons with little or advanced knowledge of the subject matter. This book would also serve as a resource for nursing and other health care professions students. It would be useful in public, academic, and hospital libraries with consumer health collections." — *E-Streams, Jul '02*

Alternative Medicine Sourcebook, 2nd Edition

Basic Consumer Health Information about Alternative and Complementary Medical Practices, Including Acupuncture, Chiropractic, Herbal Medicine, Homeopathy, Naturopathic Medicine, Mind-Body Interventions, Ayurveda, and Other Non-Western Medical Traditions

Along with Facts about such Specific Therapies as Massage Therapy, Aromatherapy, Qigong, Hypnosis, Prayer, Dance, and Art Therapies, a Glossary, and Resources for Further Information

Edited by Dawn D. Matthews. 618 pages. 2002. 0-7808-0605-0. $78.

ALSO AVAILABLE: *Alternative Medicine Sourcebook, 1st Edition.* Edited by Allan R. Cook. 737 pages. 1999. 0-7808-0200-4. $78.

"Recommended for public, high school, and academic libraries that have consumer health collections. Hospital libraries that also serve the public will find this to be a useful resource." — *E-Streams, Feb '03*

"Recommended reference source."
— *Booklist, American Library Association, Jan '03*

"An important alternate health reference."
— *MBR Bookwatch, Oct '02*

"A great addition to the reference collection of every type of library." — *American Reference Books Annual, 2000*

Alzheimer's Disease Sourcebook, 3rd Edition

Basic Consumer Health Information about Alzheimer's Disease, Other Dementias, and Related Disorders, Including Multi-Infarct Dementia, AIDS Dementia Complex, Dementia with Lewy Bodies, Huntington's Disease, Wernicke-Korsakoff Syndrome (Alcohol-Reated Dementia), Delirium, and Confusional States

Along with Information for People Newly Diagnosed with Alzheimer's Disease and Caregivers, Reports Detailing Current Research Efforts in Prevention, Diagnosis, and Treatment, Facts about Long-Term Care Issues, and Listings of Sources for Additional Information

Edited by Karen Bellenir. 645 pages. 2003. 0-7808-0666-2. $78.

ALSO AVAILABLE: *Alzheimer's, Stroke & 29 Other Neurological Disorders Sourcebook, 1st Edition.* Edited by Frank E. Bair. 579 pages. 1993. 1-55888-748-2. $78.

ALSO AVAILABLE: *Alzheimer's Disease Sourcebook, 2nd Edition.* Edited by Karen Bellenir. 524 pages. 1999. 0-7808-0223-3. $78.

"Provides a wealth of useful information not otherwise available in one place. This resource is recommended for all types of libraries."
— *American Reference Books Annual, 2000*

"Recommended reference source."
— *Booklist, American Library Association, Oct '99*

SEE ALSO *Brain Disorders Sourcebook*

Arthritis Sourcebook

Basic Consumer Health Information about Specific Forms of Arthritis and Related Disorders, Including Rheumatoid Arthritis, Osteoarthritis, Gout, Polymyalgia Rheumatica, Psoriatic Arthritis, Spondyloarthropathies, Juvenile Rheumatoid Arthritis, and Juvenile Ankylosing Spondylitis

Along with Information about Medical, Surgical, and Alternative Treatment Options, and Including Strategies for Coping with Pain, Fatigue, and Stress

Edited by Allan R. Cook. 550 pages. 1998. 0-7808-0201-2. $78.

". . . accessible to the layperson."
— *Reference and Research Book News, Feb '99*

Asthma Sourcebook

Basic Consumer Health Information about Asthma, Including Symptoms, Traditional and Nontraditional Remedies, Treatment Advances, Quality-of-Life Aids, Medical Research Updates, and the Role of Allergies, Exercise, Age, the Environment, and Genetics in the Development of Asthma

Along with Statistical Data, a Glossary, and Directories of Support Groups, and Other Resources for Further Information

Edited by Annemarie S. Muth. 628 pages. 2000. 0-7808-0381-7. $78.

"A worthwhile reference acquisition for public libraries and academic medical libraries whose readers desire a quick introduction to the wide range of asthma information." —*Choice, Association of College & Research Libraries, Jun '01*

"Recommended reference source."
—*Booklist, American Library Association, Feb '01*

"Highly recommended." —*The Bookwatch, Jan '01*

"There is much good information for patients and their families who deal with asthma daily."
—*American Medical Writers Association Journal, Winter '01*

"This informative text is recommended for consumer health collections in public, secondary school, and community college libraries and the libraries of universities with a large undergraduate population."
—*American Reference Books Annual, 2001*

∎

Attention Deficit Disorder Sourcebook

Basic Consumer Health Information about Attention Deficit/Hyperactivity Disorder in Children and Adults, Including Facts about Causes, Symptoms, Diagnostic Criteria, and Treatment Options Such as Medications, Behavior Therapy, Coaching, and Homeopathy

Along with Reports on Current Research Initiatives, Legal Issues, and Government Regulations, and Featuring a Glossary of Related Terms, Internet Resources, and a List of Additional Reading Material

Edited by Dawn D. Matthews. 470 pages. 2002. 0-7808-0624-7. $78.

"Recommended reference source."
—*Booklist, American Library Association, Jan '03*

"This book is recommended for all school libraries and the reference or consumer health sections of public libraries." —*American Reference Books Annual, 2003*

∎

Back & Neck Disorders Sourcebook

Basic Information about Disorders and Injuries of the Spinal Cord and Vertebrae, Including Facts on Chiropractic Treatment, Surgical Interventions, Paralysis, and Rehabilitation

Along with Advice for Preventing Back Trouble

Edited by Karen Bellenir. 548 pages. 1997. 0-7808-0202-0. $78.

"The strength of this work is its basic, easy-to-read format. Recommended."
—*Reference and User Services Quarterly, American Library Association, Winter '97*

Blood & Circulatory Disorders Sourcebook

Basic Information about Blood and Its Components, Anemias, Leukemias, Bleeding Disorders, and Circulatory Disorders, Including Aplastic Anemia, Thalassemia, Sickle-Cell Disease, Hemochromatosis, Hemophilia, Von Willebrand Disease, and Vascular Diseases

Along with a Special Section on Blood Transfusions and Blood Supply Safety, a Glossary, and Source Listings for Further Help and Information

Edited by Karen Bellenir and Linda M. Shin. 554 pages. 1998. 0-7808-0203-9. $78.

"Recommended reference source."
—*Booklist, American Library Association, Feb '99*

"An important reference sourcebook written in simple language for everyday, non-technical users. "
—*Reviewer's Bookwatch, Jan '99*

∎

Brain Disorders Sourcebook

Basic Consumer Health Information about Strokes, Epilepsy, Amyotrophic Lateral Sclerosis (ALS/Lou Gehrig's Disease), Parkinson's Disease, Brain Tumors, Cerebral Palsy, Headache, Tourette Syndrome, and More

Along with Statistical Data, Treatment and Rehabilitation Options, Coping Strategies, Reports on Current Research Initiatives, a Glossary, and Resource Listings for Additional Help and Information

Edited by Karen Bellenir. 481 pages. 1999. 0-7808-0229-2. $78.

"Belongs on the shelves of any library with a consumer health collection." —*E-Streams, Mar '00*

"Recommended reference source."
—*Booklist, American Library Association, Oct '99*

SEE ALSO Alzheimer's Disease Sourcebook

∎

Breast Cancer Sourcebook

Basic Consumer Health Information about Breast Cancer, Including Diagnostic Methods, Treatment Options, Alternative Therapies, Self-Help Information, Related Health Concerns, Statistical and Demographic Data, and Facts for Men with Breast Cancer

Along with Reports on Current Research Initiatives, a Glossary of Related Medical Terms, and a Directory of Sources for Further Help and Information

Edited by Edward J. Prucha and Karen Bellenir. 580 pages. 2001. 0-7808-0244-6. $78.

"It would be a useful reference book in a library or on loan to women in a support group."
—*Cancer Forum, Mar '03*

"Recommended reference source."
Booklist, American Library Association, Jan '02

"This reference source is highly recommended. It is quite informative, comprehensive and detailed in nature, and yet it offers practical advice in easy-to-read language. It could be thought of as the 'bible' of breast cancer for the consumer." — *E-Streams, Jan '02*

"The broad range of topics covered in lay language make the *Breast Cancer Sourcebook* an excellent addition to public and consumer health library collections." — *American Reference Books Annual 2002*

"From the pros and cons of different screening methods and results to treatment options, *Breast Cancer Sourcebook* provides the latest information on the subject." — *Library Bookwatch, Dec '01*

"This thoroughgoing, very readable reference covers all aspects of breast health and cancer. . . . Readers will find much to consider here. Recommended for all public and patient health collections." — *Library Journal, Sep '01*

SEE ALSO *Cancer Sourcebook for Women, Women's Health Concerns Sourcebook*

Breastfeeding Sourcebook

Basic Consumer Health Information about the Benefits of Breastmilk, Preparing to Breastfeed, Breastfeeding as a Baby Grows, Nutrition, and More, Including Information on Special Situations and Concerns Such as Mastitis, Illness, Medications, Allergies, Multiple Births, Prematurity, Special Needs, and Adoption

Along with a Glossary and Resources for Additional Help and Information

Edited by Jenni Lynn Colson. 388 pages. 2002. 0-7808-0332-9. $78.

SEE ALSO *Pregnancy & Birth Sourcebook*

"Particularly useful is the information about professional lactation services and chapters on breastfeeding when returning to work. . . . *Breastfeeding Sourcebook* will be useful for public libraries, consumer health libraries, and technical schools offering nurse assistant training, especially in areas where Internet access is problematic." — *American Reference Books Annual, 2003*

Burns Sourcebook

Basic Consumer Health Information about Various Types of Burns and Scalds, Including Flame, Heat, Cold, Electrical, Chemical, and Sun Burns

Along with Information on Short-Term and Long-Term Treatments, Tissue Reconstruction, Plastic Surgery, Prevention Suggestions, and First Aid

Edited by Allan R. Cook. 604 pages. 1999. 0-7808-0204-7. $78.

"This is an exceptional addition to the series and is highly recommended for all consumer health collections, hospital libraries, and academic medical centers." — *E-Streams, Mar '00*

"This key reference guide is an invaluable addition to all health care and public libraries in confronting this ongoing health issue." — *American Reference Books Annual, 2000*

"Recommended reference source." — *Booklist, American Library Association, Dec '99*

SEE ALSO *Skin Disorders Sourcebook*

Cancer Sourcebook, 4th Edition

Basic Consumer Health Information about Major Forms and Stages of Cancer, Featuring Facts about Head and Neck Cancers, Lung Cancers, Gastrointestinal Cancers, Genitourinary Cancers, Lymphomas, Blood Cell Cancers, Endocrine Cancers, Skin Cancers, Bone Cancers, Sarcomas, and Others, and Including Information about Cancer Treatments and Therapies, Identifying and Reducing Cancer Risks, and Strategies for Coping with Cancer and the Side Effects of Treatment

Along with a Cancer Glossary, Statistical and Demographic Data, and a Directory of Sources for Additional Help and Information

Edited by Karen Bellenir. 1,119 pages. 2003. 0-7808-0633-6. $78.

ALSO AVAILABLE: *Cancer Sourcebook, 1st Edition.* Edited by Frank E. Bair. 932 pages. 1990. 1-55888-888-8. $78.

New Cancer Sourcebook, 2nd Edition. Edited by Allan R. Cook. 1,313 pages. 1996. 0-7808-0041-9. $78.

Cancer Sourcebook, 3rd Edition. Edited by Edward J. Prucha. 1,069 pages. 2000. 0-7808-0227-6. $78.

"This title is recommended for health sciences and public libraries with consumer health collections." — *E-Streams, Feb '01*

". . . can be effectively used by cancer patients and their families who are looking for answers in a language they can understand. Public and hospital libraries should have it on their shelves." — *American Reference Books Annual, 2001*

"Recommended reference source." — *Booklist, American Library Association, Dec '00*

Cited in *Reference Sources for Small and Medium-Sized Libraries, American Library Association, 1999*

"The amount of factual and useful information is extensive. The writing is very clear, geared to general readers. Recommended for all levels." — *Choice, Association of College & Research Libraries, Jan '97*

SEE ALSO *Breast Cancer Sourcebook, Cancer Sourcebook for Women, Pediatric Cancer Sourcebook, Prostate Cancer Sourcebook*

Cancer Sourcebook for Women, 2nd Edition

Basic Consumer Health Information about Gynecologic Cancers and Related Concerns, Including Cervical Cancer, Endometrial Cancer, Gestational Trophoblastic Tumor, Ovarian Cancer, Uterine Cancer, Vaginal Cancer, Vulvar Cancer, Breast Cancer, and Common Non-Cancerous Uterine Conditions, with Facts about Cancer Risk Factors, Screening and Prevention, Treatment Options, and Reports on Current Research Initiatives

Along with a Glossary of Cancer Terms and a Directory of Resources for Additional Help and Information

Edited by Karen Bellenir. 604 pages. 2002. 0-7808-0226-8. $78.

ALSO AVAILABLE: *Cancer Sourcebook for Women, 1st Edition.* Edited by Allan R. Cook and Peter D. Dresser. 524 pages. 1996. 0-7808-0076-1. $78.

"An excellent addition to collections in public, consumer health, and women's health libraries."
— *American Reference Books Annual, 2003*

"Overall, the information is excellent, and complex topics are clearly explained. As a reference book for the consumer it is a valuable resource to assist them to make informed decisions about cancer and its treatments." — *Cancer Forum, Nov '02*

"Highly recommended for academic and medical reference collections." — *Library Bookwatch, Sep '02*

"This is a highly recommended book for any public or consumer library, being reader friendly and containing accurate and helpful information."
— *E-Streams, Aug '02*

"Recommended reference source."
— *Booklist, American Library Association, Jul '02*

SEE ALSO *Breast Cancer Sourcebook, Women's Health Concerns Sourcebook*

■

Cardiovascular Diseases & Disorders Sourcebook, 1st Edition

SEE *Heart Diseases & Disorders Sourcebook, 2nd Edition*

■

Caregiving Sourcebook

Basic Consumer Health Information for Caregivers, Including a Profile of Caregivers, Caregiving Responsibilities and Concerns, Tips for Specific Conditions, Care Environments, and the Effects of Caregiving

Along with Facts about Legal Issues, Financial Information, and Future Planning, a Glossary, and a Listing of Additional Resources

Edited by Joyce Brennfleck Shannon. 600 pages. 2001. 0-7808-0331-0. $78.

"Essential for most collections."
— *Library Journal, Apr 1, 2002*

"An ideal addition to the reference collection of any public library. Health sciences information professionals may also want to acquire the *Caregiving Sourcebook* for their hospital or academic library for use as a ready reference tool by health care workers interested in aging and caregiving." — *E-Streams, Jan '02*

"Recommended reference source."
— *Booklist, American Library Association, Oct '01*

■

Child Abuse Sourcebook

Basic Consumer Health Information about the Physical, Sexual, and Emotional Abuse of Children, with Additional Facts about Neglect, Munchausen Syndrome by Proxy (MSBP), Shaken Baby Syndrome, and Controversial Issues Related to Child Abuse, Such as Withholding Medical Care, Corporal Punishment, and Child Maltreatment in Youth Sports, and Featuring Facts about Child Protective Services, Foster Care, Adoption, Parenting Challenges, and Other Abuse Prevention Efforts

Along with a Glossary of Related Terms and Resources for Additional Help and Information

Edited by Dawn D. Matthews. 625 pages. 2004. 0-7808-0705-7. $78.

■

Childhood Diseases & Disorders Sourcebook

Basic Consumer Health Information about Medical Problems Often Encountered in Pre-Adolescent Children, Including Respiratory Tract Ailments, Ear Infections, Sore Throats, Disorders of the Skin and Scalp, Digestive and Genitourinary Diseases, Infectious Diseases, Inflammatory Disorders, Chronic Physical and Developmental Disorders, Allergies, and More

Along with Information about Diagnostic Tests, Common Childhood Surgeries, and Frequently Used Medications, with a Glossary of Important Terms and a Resource Directory

Edited by Chad T. Kimball. 662 pages. 2003. 0-7808-0458-9. $78.

■

Colds, Flu & Other Common Ailments Sourcebook

Basic Consumer Health Information about Common Ailments and Injuries, Including Colds, Coughs, the Flu, Sinus Problems, Headaches, Fever, Nausea and Vomiting, Menstrual Cramps, Diarrhea, Constipation, Hemorrhoids, Back Pain, Dandruff, Dry and Itchy Skin, Cuts, Scrapes, Sprains, Bruises, and More

Along with Information about Prevention, Self-Care, Choosing a Doctor, Over-the-Counter Medications, Folk Remedies, and Alternative Therapies, and Including a Glossary of Important Terms and a Directory of Resources for Further Help and Information

Edited by Chad T. Kimball. 638 pages. 2001. 0-7808-0435-X. $78.

"A good starting point for research on common illnesses. It will be a useful addition to public and consumer health library collections."
— *American Reference Books Annual 2002*

"Will prove valuable to any library seeking to maintain a current, comprehensive reference collection of health resources. . . . Excellent reference."
— *The Bookwatch, Aug '01*

"Recommended reference source."
— *Booklist, American Library Association, July '01*

■

Communication Disorders Sourcebook

Basic Information about Deafness and Hearing Loss, Speech and Language Disorders, Voice Disorders, Balance and Vestibular Disorders, and Disorders of Smell, Taste, and Touch

Edited by Linda M. Ross. 533 pages. 1996. 0-7808-0077-X. $78.

"This is skillfully edited and is a welcome resource for the layperson. It should be found in every public and medical library." — *Booklist Health Sciences Supplement, American Library Association, Oct '97*

■

Congenital Disorders Sourcebook

Basic Information about Disorders Acquired during Gestation, Including Spina Bifida, Hydrocephalus, Cerebral Palsy, Heart Defects, Craniofacial Abnormalities, Fetal Alcohol Syndrome, and More

Along with Current Treatment Options and Statistical Data

Edited by Karen Bellenir. 607 pages. 1997. 0-7808-0205-5. $78.

"Recommended reference source."
— *Booklist, American Library Association, Oct '97*

SEE ALSO Pregnancy & Birth Sourcebook

■

Consumer Issues in Health Care Sourcebook

Basic Information about Health Care Fundamentals and Related Consumer Issues, Including Exams and Screening Tests, Physician Specialties, Choosing a Doctor, Using Prescription and Over-the-Counter Medications Safely, Avoiding Health Scams, Managing Common Health Risks in the Home, Care Options for Chronically or Terminally Ill Patients, and a List of Resources for Obtaining Help and Further Information

Edited by Karen Bellenir. 618 pages. 1998. 0-7808-0221-7. $78.

"Both public and academic libraries will want to have a copy in their collection for readers who are interested in self-education on health issues."
— *American Reference Books Annual, 2000*

"The editor has researched the literature from government agencies and others, saving readers the time and effort of having to do the research themselves. Recommended for public libraries."
— *Reference and User Services Quarterly, American Library Association, Spring '99*

"Recommended reference source."
— *Booklist, American Library Association, Dec '98*

■

Contagious & Non-Contagious Infectious Diseases Sourcebook

Basic Information about Contagious Diseases like Measles, Polio, Hepatitis B, and Infectious Mononucleosis, and Non-Contagious Infectious Diseases like Tetanus and Toxic Shock Syndrome, and Diseases Occurring as Secondary Infections Such as Shingles and Reye Syndrome

Along with Vaccination, Prevention, and Treatment Information, and a Section Describing Emerging Infectious Disease Threats

Edited by Karen Bellenir and Peter D. Dresser. 566 pages. 1996. 0-7808-0075-3. $78.

■

Death & Dying Sourcebook

Basic Consumer Health Information for the Layperson about End-of-Life Care and Related Ethical and Legal Issues, Including Chief Causes of Death, Autopsies, Pain Management for the Terminally Ill, Life Support Systems, Insurance, Euthanasia, Assisted Suicide, Hospice Programs, Living Wills, Funeral Planning, Counseling, Mourning, Organ Donation, and Physician Training

Along with Statistical Data, a Glossary, and Listings of Sources for Further Help and Information

Edited by Annemarie S. Muth. 641 pages. 1999. 0-7808-0230-6. $78.

"Public libraries, medical libraries, and academic libraries will all find this sourcebook a useful addition to their collections."
— *American Reference Books Annual, 2001*

"An extremely useful resource for those concerned with death and dying in the United States."
— *Respiratory Care, Nov '00*

"Recommended reference source."
— *Booklist, American Library Association, Aug '00*

"This book is a definite must for all those involved in end-of-life care." — *Doody's Review Service, 2000*

■

Dental Care & Oral Health Sourcebook, 2nd Edition

Basic Consumer Health Information about Dental Care, Including Oral Hygiene, Dental Visits, Pain Management, Cavities, Crowns, Bridges, Dental Implants, and Fillings, and Other Oral Health Concerns, Such as Gum Disease, Bad Breath, Dry Mouth, Genetic and Developmental Abnormalities, Oral Cancers, Orthodontics, and Temporomandibular Disorders

Along with Updates on Current Research in Oral Health, a Glossary, a Directory of Dental and Oral Health Organizations, and Resources for People with Dental and Oral Health Disorders

Edited by Amy L. Sutton. 609 pages. 2003. 0-7808-0634-4. $78.

ALSO AVAILABLE: Oral Health Sourcebook, 1st Edition. Edited by Allan R. Cook. 558 pages. 1997. 0-7808-0082-6. $78.

"Unique source which will fill a gap in dental sources for patients and the lay public. A valuable reference tool even in a library with thousands of books on dentistry. Comprehensive, clear, inexpensive, and easy to read and use. It fills an enormous gap in the health care literature." — Reference and User Services Quarterly, American Library Association, Summer '98

"Recommended reference source."
— Booklist, American Library Association, Dec '97

Depression Sourcebook

Basic Consumer Health Information about Unipolar Depression, Bipolar Disorder, Postpartum Depression, Seasonal Affective Disorder, and Other Types of Depression in Children, Adolescents, Women, Men, the Elderly, and Other Selected Populations

Along with Facts about Causes, Risk Factors, Diagnostic Criteria, Treatment Options, Coping Strategies, Suicide Prevention, a Glossary, and a Directory of Sources for Additional Help and Information

Edited by Karen Belleni. 602 pages. 2002. 0-7808-0611-5. $78.

"Invaluable reference for public and school library collections alike." — Library Bookwatch, Apr '03

"Recommended for purchase."
— American Reference Books Annual, 2003

Diabetes Sourcebook, 3rd Edition

Basic Consumer Health Information about Type 1 Diabetes (Insulin-Dependent or Juvenile-Onset Diabetes), Type 2 Diabetes (Noninsulin-Dependent or Adult-Onset Diabetes), Gestational Diabetes, Impaired Glucose Tolerance (IGT), and Related Complications, Such as Amputation, Eye Disease, Gum Disease, Nerve Damage, and End-Stage Renal Disease, Including Facts about Insulin, Oral Diabetes Medications, Blood Sugar Testing, and the Role of Exercise and Nutrition in the Control of Diabetes

Along with a Glossary and Resources for Further Help and Information

Edited by Dawn D. Matthews. 622 pages. 2003. 0-7808-0629-8. $78.

ALSO AVAILABLE: Diabetes Sourcebook, 1st Edition. Edited by Karen Bellenir and Peter D. Dresser. 827 pages. 1994. 1-55888-751-2. $78.

Diabetes Sourcebook, 2nd Edition. Edited by Karen Bellenir. 688 pages. 1998. 0-7808-0224-1. $78.

"An invaluable reference." — Library Journal, May '00

Selected as one of the 250 "Best Health Sciences Books of 1999." — Doody's Rating Service, Mar-Apr 2000

"This comprehensive book is an excellent addition for high school, academic, medical, and public libraries. This volume is highly recommended."
—American Reference Books Annual, 2000

"Provides useful information for the general public."
— Healthlines, University of Michigan Health Management Research Center, Sep/Oct '99

". . . provides reliable mainstream medical information . . . belongs on the shelves of any library with a consumer health collection." — E-Streams, Sep '99

"Recommended reference source."
— Booklist, American Library Association, Feb '99

Diet & Nutrition Sourcebook, 2nd Edition

Basic Consumer Health Information about Dietary Guidelines, Recommended Daily Intake Values, Vitamins, Minerals, Fiber, Fat, Weight Control, Dietary Supplements, and Food Additives

Along with Special Sections on Nutrition Needs throughout Life and Nutrition for People with Such Specific Medical Concerns as Allergies, High Blood Cholesterol, Hypertension, Diabetes, Celiac Disease, Seizure Disorders, Phenylketonuria (PKU), Cancer, and Eating Disorders, and Including Reports on Current Nutrition Research and Source Listings for Additional Help and Information

Edited by Karen Bellenir. 650 pages. 1999. 0-7808-0228-4. $78.

ALSO AVAILABLE: Diet & Nutrition Sourcebook, 1st Edition. Edited by Dan R. Harris. 662 pages. 1996. 0-7808-0084-2. $78.

"This book is an excellent source of basic diet and nutrition information." — Booklist Health Sciences Supplement, American Library Association, Dec '00

"This reference document should be in any public library, but it would be a very good guide for beginning students in the health sciences. If the other books in this publisher's series are as good as this, they should all be in the health sciences collections."
—American Reference Books Annual, 2000

"This book is an excellent general nutrition reference for consumers who desire to take an active role in their health care for prevention. Consumers of all ages who select this book can feel confident they are receiving current and accurate information." — Journal of Nutrition for the Elderly, Vol. 19, No. 4, '00

"Recommended reference source."
—Booklist, American Library Association, Dec '99

SEE ALSO Digestive Diseases & Disorders Sourcebook, Eating Disorders Sourcebook, Gastrointestinal Diseases & Disorders Sourcebook, Vegetarian Sourcebook

Digestive Diseases & Disorders Sourcebook

Basic Consumer Health Information about Diseases and Disorders that Impact the Upper and Lower Digestive System, Including Celiac Disease, Constipation, Crohn's Disease, Cyclic Vomiting Syndrome, Diarrhea, Diverticulosis and Diverticulitis, Gallstones, Heartburn, Hemorrhoids, Hernias, Indigestion (Dyspepsia), Irritable Bowel Syndrome, Lactose Intolerance, Ulcers, and More

Along with Information about Medications and Other Treatments, Tips for Maintaining a Healthy Digestive Tract, a Glossary, and Directory of Digestive Diseases Organizations

Edited by Karen Bellenir. 335 pages. 2000. 0-7808-0327-2. $78.

"This title would be an excellent addition to all public or patient-research libraries."
—*American Reference Books Annual, 2001*

"This title is recommended for public, hospital, and health sciences libraries with consumer health collections." —*E-Streams, Jul-Aug '00*

"Recommended reference source."
—*Booklist, American Library Association, May '00*

SEE ALSO Diet & Nutrition Sourcebook, Eating Disorders Sourcebook, Gastrointestinal Diseases & Disorders Sourcebook

■

Disabilities Sourcebook

Basic Consumer Health Information about Physical and Psychiatric Disabilities, Including Descriptions of Major Causes of Disability, Assistive and Adaptive Aids, Workplace Issues, and Accessibility Concerns

Along with Information about the Americans with Disabilities Act, a Glossary, and Resources for Additional Help and Information

Edited by Dawn D. Matthews. 616 pages. 2000. 0-7808-0389-2. $78.

"It is a must for libraries with a consumer health section." —*American Reference Books Annual 2002*

"A much needed addition to the Omnigraphics *Health Reference Series*. A current reference work to provide people with disabilities, their families, caregivers or those who work with them, a broad range of information in one volume, has not been available until now. . . . It is recommended for all public and academic library reference collections." —*E-Streams, May '01*

"An excellent source book in easy-to-read format covering many current topics; highly recommended for all libraries." —*Choice, Association of College and Research Libraries, Jan '01*

"Recommended reference source."
—*Booklist, American Library Association, Jul '00*

Domestic Violence Sourcebook, 2nd Edition

Basic Consumer Health Information about the Causes and Consequences of Abusive Relationships, Including Physical Violence, Sexual Assault, Battery, Stalking, and Emotional Abuse, and Facts about the Effects of Violence on Women, Men, Young Adults, and the Elderly, with Reports about Domestic Violence in Selected Populations, and Featuring Facts about Medical Care, Victim Assistance and Protection, Prevention Strategies, Mental Health Services, and Legal Issues

Along with a Glossary of Related Terms and Resources for Additional Help and Information

Edited by Dawn D. Matthews. 625 pages. 2004. 0-7808-0669-7. $78.

ALSO AVAILABLE: Domestic Violence & Child Abuse Sourcebook, 1st Edition. Edited by Helene Henderson. 1,064 pages. 2001. 0-7808-0235-7. $78.

"Interested lay persons should find the book extremely beneficial. . . . A copy of *Domestic Violence and Child Abuse Sourcebook* should be in every public library in the United States."
—*Social Science & Medicine, No. 56, 2003*

"This is important information. The Web has many resources but this sourcebook fills an important societal need. I am not aware of any other resources of this type." —*Doody's Review Service, Sep '01*

"Recommended for all libraries, scholars, and practitioners." —*Choice, Association of College & Research Libraries, Jul '01*

"Recommended reference source."
—*Booklist, American Library Association, Apr '01*

"Important pick for college-level health reference libraries." —*The Bookwatch, Mar '01*

"Because this problem is so widespread and because this book includes a lot of issues within one volume, this work is recommended for all public libraries."
—*American Reference Books Annual, 2001*

■

Drug Abuse Sourcebook

Basic Consumer Health Information about Illicit Substances of Abuse and the Diversion of Prescription Medications, Including Depressants, Hallucinogens, Inhalants, Marijuana, Narcotics, Stimulants, and Anabolic Steroids

Along with Facts about Related Health Risks, Treatment Issues, and Substance Abuse Prevention Programs, a Glossary of Terms, Statistical Data, and Directories of Hotline Services, Self-Help Groups, and Organizations Able to Provide Further Information

Edited by Karen Bellenir. 629 pages. 2000. 0-7808-0242-X. $78.

"Containing a wealth of information . . . . This resource belongs in libraries that serve a lower-division undergraduate or community college clientele as well as the general public." —*Choice, Association of College and Research Libraries, Jun '01*

"Recommended reference source."
— *Booklist, American Library Association, Feb '01*

"Highly recommended." — *The Bookwatch, Jan '01*

"Even though there is a plethora of books on drug abuse, this volume is recommended for school, public, and college libraries."
— *American Reference Books Annual, 2001*

SEE ALSO *Alcoholism Sourcebook, Substance Abuse Sourcebook*

Ear, Nose & Throat Disorders Sourcebook

Basic Information about Disorders of the Ears, Nose, Sinus Cavities, Pharynx, and Larynx, Including Ear Infections, Tinnitus, Vestibular Disorders, Allergic and Non-Allergic Rhinitis, Sore Throats, Tonsillitis, and Cancers That Affect the Ears, Nose, Sinuses, and Throat

Along with Reports on Current Research Initiatives, a Glossary of Related Medical Terms, and a Directory of Sources for Further Help and Information

Edited by Karen Bellenir and Linda M. Shin. 576 pages. 1998. 0-7808-0206-3. $78.

"Overall, this sourcebook is helpful for the consumer seeking information on ENT issues. It is recommended for public libraries."
— *American Reference Books Annual, 1999*

"Recommended reference source."
— *Booklist, American Library Association, Dec '98*

Eating Disorders Sourcebook

Basic Consumer Health Information about Eating Disorders, Including Information about Anorexia Nervosa, Bulimia Nervosa, Binge Eating, Body Dysmorphic Disorder, Pica, Laxative Abuse, and Night Eating Syndrome

Along with Information about Causes, Adverse Effects, and Treatment and Prevention Issues, and Featuring a Section on Concerns Specific to Children and Adolescents, a Glossary, and Resources for Further Help and Information

Edited by Dawn D. Matthews. 322 pages. 2001. 0-7808-0335-3. $78.

"Recommended for health science libraries that are open to the public, as well as hospital libraries. This book is a good resource for the consumer who is concerned about eating disorders." — *E-Streams, Mar '02*

"This volume is another convenient collection of excerpted articles. Recommended for school and public library patrons; lower-division undergraduates; and two-year technical program students." — *Choice, Association of College & Research Libraries, Jan '02*

"Recommended reference source." — *Booklist, American Library Association, Oct '01*

SEE ALSO *Diet & Nutrition Sourcebook, Digestive Diseases & Disorders Sourcebook, Gastrointestinal Diseases & Disorders Sourcebook*

Emergency Medical Services Sourcebook

Basic Consumer Health Information about Preventing, Preparing for, and Managing Emergency Situations, When and Who to Call for Help, What to Expect in the Emergency Room, the Emergency Medical Team, Patient Issues, and Current Topics in Emergency Medicine

Along with Statistical Data, a Glossary, and Sources of Additional Help and Information

Edited by Jenni Lynn Colson. 494 pages. 2002. 0-7808-0420-1. $78.

"Handy and convenient for home, public, school, and college libraries. Recommended."
— *Choice, Association of College and Research Libraries, Apr '03*

"This reference can provide the consumer with answers to most questions about emergency care in the United States, or it will direct them to a resource where the answer can be found."
— *American Reference Books Annual, 2003*

"Recommended reference source."
— *Booklist, American Library Association, Feb '03*

Endocrine & Metabolic Disorders Sourcebook

Basic Information for the Layperson about Pancreatic and Insulin-Related Disorders Such as Pancreatitis, Diabetes, and Hypoglycemia; Adrenal Gland Disorders Such as Cushing's Syndrome, Addison's Disease, and Congenital Adrenal Hyperplasia; Pituitary Gland Disorders Such as Growth Hormone Deficiency, Acromegaly, and Pituitary Tumors; Thyroid Disorders Such as Hypothyroidism, Graves' Disease, Hashimoto's Disease, and Goiter; Hyperparathyroidism; and Other Diseases and Syndromes of Hormone Imbalance or Metabolic Dysfunction

Along with Reports on Current Research Initiatives

Edited by Linda M. Shin. 574 pages. 1998. 0-7808-0207-1. $78.

"Omnigraphics has produced another needed resource for health information consumers."
— *American Reference Books Annual, 2000*

"Recommended reference source."
— *Booklist, American Library Association, Dec '98*

Environmental Health Sourcebook, 2nd Edition

Basic Consumer Health Information about the Environment and Its Effect on Human Health, Including the Effects of Air Pollution, Water Pollution, Hazardous Chemicals, Food Hazards, Radiation Hazards, Biological Agents, Household Hazards, Such as Radon, Asbestos, Carbon Monoxide, and Mold, and Information about Associated Diseases and Disorders, Including Cancer, Allergies, Respiratory Problems, and Skin Disorders

Along with Information about Environmental Concerns for Specific Populations, a Glossary of Related Terms, and Resources for Further Help and Information

Edited by Dawn D. Matthews. 673 pages. 2003. 0-7808-0632-8. $78.

ALSO AVAILABLE: Environmentally Induced Disorders Sourcebook, 1st Edition. Edited by Allan R. Cook. 620 pages. 1997. 0-7808-0083-4. $78.

"Recommended reference source."
— *Booklist, American Library Association, Sep '98*

"This book will be a useful addition to anyone's library." — *Choice Health Sciences Supplement, Association of College and Research Libraries, May '98*

". . . a good survey of numerous environmentally induced physical disorders . . . a useful addition to anyone's library."
— *Doody's Health Sciences Book Reviews, Jan '98*

". . . provide[s] introductory information from the best authorities around. Since this volume covers topics that potentially affect everyone, it will surely be one of the most frequently consulted volumes in the *Health Reference Series*." — *Rettig on Reference, Nov '97*

Environmentally Induced Disorders Sourcebook, 1st Edition

SEE Environmental Health Sourcebook, 2nd Edition

Ethnic Diseases Sourcebook

Basic Consumer Health Information for Ethnic and Racial Minority Groups in the United States, Including General Health Indicators and Behaviors, Ethnic Diseases, Genetic Testing, the Impact of Chronic Diseases, Women's Health, Mental Health Issues, and Preventive Health Care Services

Along with a Glossary and a Listing of Additional Resources

Edited by Joyce Brennfleck Shannon. 664 pages. 2001. 0-7808-0336-1. $78.

"Recommended for health sciences libraries where public health programs are a priority."
— *E-Streams, Jan '02*

"Not many books have been written on this topic to date, and the *Ethnic Diseases Sourcebook* is a strong addition to the list. It will be an important introductory resource for health consumers, students, health care personnel, and social scientists. It is recommended for public, academic, and large hospital libraries."
— *American Reference Books Annual 2002*

"Recommended reference source."
— *Booklist, American Library Association, Oct '01*

"Will prove valuable to any library seeking to maintain a current, comprehensive reference collection of health resources. . . . An excellent source of health information about genetic disorders which affect particular ethnic and racial minorities in the U.S."
— *The Bookwatch, Aug '01*

Eye Care Sourcebook, 2nd Edition

Basic Consumer Health Information about Eye Care and Eye Disorders, Including Facts about the Diagnosis, Prevention, and Treatment of Common Refractive Problems Such as Myopia, Hyperopia, Astigmatism, and Presbyopia, and Eye Diseases, Including Glaucoma, Cataract, Age-Related Macular Degeneration, and Diabetic Retinopathy

Along with a Section on Vision Correction and Refractive Surgeries, Including LASIK and LASEK, a Glossary, and Directories of Resources for Additional Help and Information

Edited by Amy L. Sutton. 543 pages. 2003. 0-7808-0635-2. $78.

ALSO AVAILABLE: Ophthalmic Disorders Sourcebook, 1st Edition. Edited by Linda M. Ross. 631 pages. 1996. 0-7808-0081-8. $78.

Family Planning Sourcebook

Basic Consumer Health Information about Planning for Pregnancy and Contraception, Including Traditional Methods, Barrier Methods, Hormonal Methods, Permanent Methods, Future Methods, Emergency Contraception, and Birth Control Choices for Women at Each Stage of Life

Along with Statistics, a Glossary, and Sources of Additional Information

Edited by Amy Marcaccio Keyzer. 520 pages. 2001. 0-7808-0379-5. $78.

"Recommended for public, health, and undergraduate libraries as part of the circulating collection."
— *E-Streams, Mar '02*

"Information is presented in an unbiased, readable manner, and the sourcebook will certainly be a necessary addition to those public and high school libraries where Internet access is restricted or otherwise problematic." — *American Reference Books Annual 2002*

"Recommended reference source."
— *Booklist, American Library Association, Oct '01*

"Will prove valuable to any library seeking to maintain a current, comprehensive reference collection of health resources. . . . Excellent reference."
— *The Bookwatch, Aug '01*

SEE ALSO Pregnancy & Birth Sourcebook

Fitness & Exercise Sourcebook, 2nd Edition

Basic Consumer Health Information about the Fundamentals of Fitness and Exercise, Including How to Begin and Maintain a Fitness Program, Fitness as a Lifestyle, the Link between Fitness and Diet, Advice for Specific Groups of People, Exercise as It Relates to Specific Medical Conditions, and Recent Research in Fitness and Exercise

Along with a Glossary of Important Terms and Resources for Additional Help and Information

Edited by Kristen M. Gledhill. 646 pages. 2001. 0-7808-0334-5. $78.

ALSO AVAILABLE: Fitness & Exercise Sourcebook, 1st Edition. Edited by Dan R. Harris. 663 pages. 1996. 0-7808-0186-5. $78.

"This work is recommended for all general reference collections."
— *American Reference Books Annual 2002*

"Highly recommended for public, consumer, and school grades fourth through college."
— *E-Streams, Nov '01*

"Recommended reference source." — *Booklist, American Library Association, Oct '01*

"The information appears quite comprehensive and is considered reliable. . . . This second edition is a welcomed addition to the series."
— *Doody's Review Service, Sep '01*

"This reference is a valuable choice for those who desire a broad source of information on exercise, fitness, and chronic-disease prevention through a healthy lifestyle." — *American Medical Writers Association Journal, Fall '01*

"Will prove valuable to any library seeking to maintain a current, comprehensive reference collection of health resources. . . . Excellent reference."
— *The Bookwatch, Aug '01*

Food & Animal Borne Diseases Sourcebook

Basic Information about Diseases That Can Be Spread to Humans through the Ingestion of Contaminated Food or Water or by Contact with Infected Animals and Insects, Such as Botulism, E. Coli, Hepatitis A, Trichinosis, Lyme Disease, and Rabies

Along with Information Regarding Prevention and Treatment Methods, and Including a Special Section for International Travelers Describing Diseases Such as Cholera, Malaria, Travelers' Diarrhea, and Yellow Fever, and Offering Recommendations for Avoiding Illness

Edited by Karen Bellenir and Peter D. Dresser. 535 pages. 1995. 0-7808-0033-8. $78.

"Targeting general readers and providing them with a single, comprehensive source of information on selected topics, this book continues, with the excellent caliber of its predecessors, to catalog topical information on health matters of general interest. Readable and thorough, this valuable resource is highly recommended for all libraries."
— *Academic Library Book Review, Summer '96*

"A comprehensive collection of authoritative information." — *Emergency Medical Services, Oct '95*

Food Safety Sourcebook

Basic Consumer Health Information about the Safe Handling of Meat, Poultry, Seafood, Eggs, Fruit Juices, and Other Food Items, and Facts about Pesticides, Drinking Water, Food Safety Overseas, and the Onset, Duration, and Symptoms of Foodborne Illnesses, Including Types of Pathogenic Bacteria, Parasitic Protozoa, Worms, Viruses, and Natural Toxins

Along with the Role of the Consumer, the Food Handler, and the Government in Food Safety; a Glossary, and Resources for Additional Help and Information

Edited by Dawn D. Matthews. 339 pages. 1999. 0-7808-0326-4. $78.

"This book is recommended for public libraries and universities with home economic and food science programs." — *E-Streams, Nov '00*

"Recommended reference source."
— *Booklist, American Library Association, May '00*

"This book takes the complex issues of food safety and foodborne pathogens and presents them in an easily understood manner. [It does] an excellent job of covering a large and often confusing topic."
— *American Reference Books Annual, 2000*

Forensic Medicine Sourcebook

Basic Consumer Information for the Layperson about Forensic Medicine, Including Crime Scene Investigation, Evidence Collection and Analysis, Expert Testimony, Computer-Aided Criminal Identification, Digital Imaging in the Courtroom, DNA Profiling, Accident Reconstruction, Autopsies, Ballistics, Drugs and Explosives Detection, Latent Fingerprints, Product Tampering, and Questioned Document Examination

Along with Statistical Data, a Glossary of Forensics Terminology, and Listings of Sources for Further Help and Information

Edited by Annemarie S. Muth. 574 pages. 1999. 0-7808-0232-2. $78.

"Given the expected widespread interest in its content and its easy to read style, this book is recommended for most public and all college and university libraries."
— *E-Streams, Feb '01*

"Recommended for public libraries."
— *Reference & User Services Quarterly, American Library Association, Spring 2000*

"Recommended reference source."
— *Booklist, American Library Association, Feb '00*

"A wealth of information, useful statistics, references are up-to-date and extremely complete. This wonderful collection of data will help students who are interested in a career in any type of forensic field. It is a great resource for attorneys who need information about types of expert witnesses needed in a particular case. It also offers useful information for fiction and nonfiction writers whose work involves a crime. A fascinating compilation. All levels." — *Choice, Association of College and Research Libraries, Jan 2000*

641

"There are several items that make this book attractive to consumers who are seeking certain forensic data. . . . This is a useful current source for those seeking general forensic medical answers."
—*American Reference Books Annual, 2000*

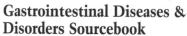

Gastrointestinal Diseases & Disorders Sourcebook

Basic Information about Gastroesophageal Reflux Disease (Heartburn), Ulcers, Diverticulosis, Irritable Bowel Syndrome, Crohn's Disease, Ulcerative Colitis, Diarrhea, Constipation, Lactose Intolerance, Hemorrhoids, Hepatitis, Cirrhosis, and Other Digestive Problems, Featuring Statistics, Descriptions of Symptoms, and Current Treatment Methods of Interest for Persons Living with Upper and Lower Gastrointestinal Maladies

Edited by Linda M. Ross. 413 pages. 1996. 0-7808-0078-8. $78.

". . . very readable form. The successful editorial work that brought this material together into a useful and understandable reference makes accessible to all readers information that can help them more effectively understand and obtain help for digestive tract problems."
— *Choice, Association of College & Research Libraries, Feb '97*

SEE ALSO *Diet & Nutrition Sourcebook, Digestive Diseases & Disorders, Eating Disorders Sourcebook*

Genetic Disorders Sourcebook, 2nd Edition

Basic Consumer Health Information about Hereditary Diseases and Disorders, Including Cystic Fibrosis, Down Syndrome, Hemophilia, Huntington's Disease, Sickle Cell Anemia, and More; Facts about Genes, Gene Research and Therapy, Genetic Screening, Ethics of Gene Testing, Genetic Counseling, and Advice on Coping and Caring

Along with a Glossary of Genetic Terminology and a Resource List for Help, Support, and Further Information

Edited by Kathy Massimini. 768 pages. 2001. 0-7808-0241-1. $78.

ALSO AVAILABLE: *Genetic Disorders Sourcebook, 1st Edition.* Edited by Karen Bellenir. 642 pages. 1996. 0-7808-0034-6. $78.

"Recommended for public libraries and medical and hospital libraries with consumer health collections."
— *E-Streams, May '01*

"Recommended reference source."
— *Booklist, American Library Association, Apr '01*

"Important pick for college-level health reference libraries."
— *The Bookwatch, Mar '01*

"Provides essential medical information to both the general public and those diagnosed with a serious or fatal genetic disease or disorder."   —*Choice, Association of College and Research Libraries, Jan '97*

Head Trauma Sourcebook

Basic Information for the Layperson about Open-Head and Closed-Head Injuries, Treatment Advances, Recovery, and Rehabilitation

Along with Reports on Current Research Initiatives

Edited by Karen Bellenir. 414 pages. 1997. 0-7808-0208-X. $78.

Headache Sourcebook

Basic Consumer Health Information about Migraine, Tension, Cluster, Rebound and Other Types of Headaches, with Facts about the Cause and Prevention of Headaches, the Effects of Stress and the Environment, Headaches during Pregnancy and Menopause, and Childhood Headaches

Along with a Glossary and Other Resources for Additional Help and Information

Edited by Dawn D. Matthews. 362 pages. 2002. 0-7808-0337-X. $78.

"Highly recommended for academic and medical reference collections."   — *Library Bookwatch, Sep '02*

Health Insurance Sourcebook

Basic Information about Managed Care Organizations, Traditional Fee-for-Service Insurance, Insurance Portability and Pre-Existing Conditions Clauses, Medicare, Medicaid, Social Security, and Military Health Care

Along with Information about Insurance Fraud

Edited by Wendy Wilcox. 530 pages. 1997. 0-7808-0222-5. $78.

"Particularly useful because it brings much of this information together in one volume. This book will be a handy reference source in the health sciences library, hospital library, college and university library, and medium to large public library."
— *Medical Reference Services Quarterly, Fall '98*

Awarded "Books of the Year Award"
— *American Journal of Nursing, 1997*

"The layout of the book is particularly helpful as it provides easy access to reference material. A most useful addition to the vast amount of information about health insurance. The use of data from U.S. government agencies is most commendable. Useful in a library or learning center for healthcare professional students."
— *Doody's Health Sciences Book Reviews, Nov '97*

Health Reference Series Cumulative Index 1999

A Comprehensive Index to the Individual Volumes of the Health Reference Series, Including a Subject Index, Name Index, Organization Index, and Publication Index

Along with a Master List of Acronyms and Abbreviations

Edited by Edward J. Prucha, Anne Holmes, and Robert Rudnick. 990 pages. 2000. 0-7808-0382-5. $78.

"This volume will be most helpful in libraries that have a relatively complete collection of the Health Reference Series." —*American Reference Books Annual, 2001*

"Essential for collections that hold any of the numerous *Health Reference Series* titles." — *Choice, Association of College and Research Libraries, Nov '00*

■

Healthy Aging Sourcebook

Basic Consumer Health Information about Maintaining Health through the Aging Process, Including Advice on Nutrition, Exercise, and Sleep, Help in Making Decisions about Midlife Issues and Retirement, and Guidance Concerning Practical and Informed Choices in Health Consumerism

Along with Data Concerning the Theories of Aging, Different Experiences in Aging by Minority Groups, and Facts about Aging Now and Aging in the Future; and Featuring a Glossary, a Guide to Consumer Help, Additional Suggested Reading, and Practical Resource Directory

Edited by Jenifer Swanson. 536 pages. 1999. 0-7808-0390-6. $78.

"Recommended reference source." —*Booklist, American Library Association, Feb '00*

SEE ALSO *Physical & Mental Issues in Aging Sourcebook*

■

Healthy Children Sourcebook

Basic Consumer Health Information about the Physical and Mental Development of Children between the Ages of 3 and 12, Including Routine Health Care, Preventative Health Services, Safety and First Aid, Healthy Sleep, Dental Care, Nutrition, and Fitness, and Featuring Parenting Tips on Such Topics as Bedwetting, Choosing Day Care, Monitoring TV and Other Media, and Establishing a Foundation for Substance Abuse Prevention

Along with a Glossary of Commonly Used Pediatric Terms and Resources for Additional Help and Information.

Edited by Chad T. Kimball. 647 pages. 2003. 0-7808-0247-0. $78.

■

Healthy Heart Sourcebook for Women

Basic Consumer Health Information about Cardiac Issues Specific to Women, Including Facts about Major Risk Factors and Prevention, Treatment and Control Strategies, and Important Dietary Issues

Along with a Special Section Regarding the Pros and Cons of Hormone Replacement Therapy and Its Impact on Heart Health, and Additional Help, Including Recipes, a Glossary, and a Directory of Resources

Edited by Dawn D. Matthews. 336 pages. 2000. 0-7808-0329-9. $78.

"A good reference source and recommended for all public, academic, medical, and hospital libraries." — *Medical Reference Services Quarterly, Summer '01*

"Because of the lack of information specific to women on this topic, this book is recommended for public libraries and consumer libraries." —*American Reference Books Annual, 2001*

"Contains very important information about coronary artery disease that all women should know. The information is current and presented in an easy-to-read format. The book will make a good addition to any library." — *American Medical Writers Association Journal, Summer '00*

"Important, basic reference." —*Reviewer's Bookwatch, Jul '00*

SEE ALSO *Heart Diseases & Disorders Sourcebook, Women's Health Concerns Sourcebook*

■

Heart Diseases & Disorders Sourcebook, 2nd Edition

Basic Consumer Health Information about Heart Attacks, Angina, Rhythm Disorders, Heart Failure, Valve Disease, Congenital Heart Disorders, and More, Including Descriptions of Surgical Procedures and Other Interventions, Medications, Cardiac Rehabilitation, Risk Identification, and Prevention Tips

Along with Statistical Data, Reports on Current Research Initiatives, a Glossary of Cardiovascular Terms, and Resource Directory

Edited by Karen Bellenir. 612 pages. 2000. 0-7808-0238-1. $78.

ALSO AVAILABLE: *Cardiovascular Diseases & Disorders Sourcebook, 1st Edition.* Edited by Karen Bellenir and Peter D. Dresser. 683 pages. 1995. 0-7808-0032-X. $78.

"This work stands out as an imminently accessible resource for the general public. It is recommended for the reference and circulating shelves of school, public, and academic libraries." —*American Reference Books Annual, 2001*

"Recommended reference source." —*Booklist, American Library Association, Dec '00*

"Provides comprehensive coverage of matters related to the heart. This title is recommended for health sciences and public libraries with consumer health collections." —*E-Streams, Oct '00*

SEE ALSO *Healthy Heart Sourcebook for Women*

■

Household Safety Sourcebook

Basic Consumer Health Information about Household Safety, Including Information about Poisons, Chemicals, Fire, and Water Hazards in the Home

Along with Advice about the Safe Use of Home Maintenance Equipment, Choosing Toys and Nursery Furni-

ture, Holiday and Recreation Safety, a Glossary, and Resources for Further Help and Information

Edited by Dawn D. Matthews. 606 pages. 2002. 0-7808-0338-8. $78.

"This work will be useful in public libraries with large consumer health and wellness departments."
— American Reference Books Annual, 2003

"As a sourcebook on household safety this book meets its mark. It is encyclopedic in scope and covers a wide range of safety issues that are commonly seen in the home." — E-Streams, Jul '02

Immune System Disorders Sourcebook

Basic Information about Lupus, Multiple Sclerosis, Guillain-Barré Syndrome, Chronic Granulomatous Disease, and More

Along with Statistical and Demographic Data and Reports on Current Research Initiatives

Edited by Allan R. Cook. 608 pages. 1997. 0-7808-0209-8. $78.

Infant & Toddler Health Sourcebook

Basic Consumer Health Information about the Physical and Mental Development of Newborns, Infants, and Toddlers, Including Neonatal Concerns, Nutrition Recommendations, Immunization Schedules, Common Pediatric Disorders, Assessments and Milestones, Safety Tips, and Advice for Parents and Other Caregivers

Along with a Glossary of Terms and Resource Listings for Additional Help

Edited by Jenifer Swanson. 585 pages. 2000. 0-7808-0246-2. $78.

"As a reference for the general public, this would be useful in any library." — E-Streams, May '01

"Recommended reference source."
— Booklist, American Library Association, Feb '01

"This is a good source for general use."
— American Reference Books Annual, 2001

Infectious Diseases Sourcebook

Basic Consumer Health Information about Non-Contagious Bacterial, Viral, Prion, Fungal, and Parasitic Diseases Spread by Food and Water, Insects and Animals, or Environmental Contact, Including Botulism, E. Coli, Encephalitis, Legionnaires' Disease, Lyme Disease, Malaria, Plague, Rabies, Salmonella, Tetanus, and Others, and Facts about Newly Emerging Diseases, Such as Hantavirus, Mad Cow Disease, Monkeypox, and West Nile Virus

Along with Information about Preventing Disease Transmission, the Threat of Bioterrorism, and Current

Research Initiatives, with a Glossary and Directory of Resources for More Information

Edited by Karen Bellenir. 600 pages. 2004. 0-7808-0675-1. $78.

Injury & Trauma Sourcebook

Basic Consumer Health Information about the Impact of Injury, the Diagnosis and Treatment of Common and Traumatic Injuries, Emergency Care, and Specific Injuries Related to Home, Community, Workplace, Transportation, and Recreation

Along with Guidelines for Injury Prevention, a Glossary, and a Directory of Additional Resources

Edited by Joyce Brennfleck Shannon. 696 pages. 2002. 0-7808-0421-X. $78.

"This publication is the most comprehensive work of its kind about injury and trauma."
— American Reference Books Annual, 2003

"This sourcebook provides concise, easily readable, basic health information about injuries. . . . This book is well organized and an easy to use reference resource suitable for hospital, health sciences and public libraries with consumer health collections."
— E-Streams, Nov '02

"Practitioners should be aware of guides such as this in order to facilitate their use by patients and their families." — Doody's Health Sciences
Book Review Journal, Sep-Oct '02

"Recommended reference source."
— Booklist, American Library Association, Sep '02

"Highly recommended for academic and medical reference collections." — Library Bookwatch, Sep '02

Kidney & Urinary Tract Diseases & Disorders Sourcebook

Basic Information about Kidney Stones, Urinary Incontinence, Bladder Disease, End Stage Renal Disease, Dialysis, and More

Along with Statistical and Demographic Data and Reports on Current Research Initiatives

Edited by Linda M. Ross. 602 pages. 1997. 0-7808-0079-6. $78.

Learning Disabilities Sourcebook, 2nd Edition

Basic Consumer Health Information about Learning Disabilities, Including Dyslexia, Developmental Speech and Language Disabilities, Non-Verbal Learning Disorders, Developmental Arithmetic Disorder, Developmental Writing Disorder, and Other Conditions That Impede Learning Such as Attention Deficit/ Hyperactivity Disorder, Brain Injury, Hearing Impairment, Klinefelter Syndrome, Dyspraxia, and Tourette Syndrome

Along with Facts about Educational Issues and Assistive Technology, Coping Strategies, a Glossary of Re-

lated Terms, and Resources for Further Help and Information

Edited by Dawn D. Matthews. 621 pages. 2003. 0-7808-0626-3. $78.

ALSO AVAILABLE: Learning Disabilities Sourcebook, 1st Edition. Edited by Linda M. Shin. 579 pages. 1998. 0-7808-0210-1. $78.

"Teachers as well as consumers will find this an essential guide to understanding various syndromes and their latest treatments. [An] invaluable reference for public and school library collections alike."
— *Library Bookwatch, Apr '03*

Named "Outstanding Reference Book of 1999."
— *New York Public Library, Feb 2000*

"An excellent candidate for inclusion in a public library reference section. It's a great source of information. Teachers will also find the book useful. Definitely worth reading."
— *Journal of Adolescent & Adult Literacy, Feb 2000*

"Readable . . . provides a solid base of information regarding successful techniques used with individuals who have learning disabilities, as well as practical suggestions for educators and family members. Clear language, concise descriptions, and pertinent information for contacting multiple resources add to the strength of this book as a useful tool." — *Choice, Association of College and Research Libraries, Feb '99*

"Recommended reference source."
— *Booklist, American Library Association, Sep '98*

"A useful resource for libraries and for those who don't have the time to identify and locate the individual publications." — *Disability Resources Monthly, Sep '98*

∎

Leukemia Sourcebook

Basic Consumer Health Information about Adult and Childhood Leukemias, Including Acute Lymphocytic Leukemia (ALL), Chronic Lymphocytic Leukemia (CLL), Acute Myelogenous Leukemia (AML), Chronic Myelogenous Leukemia (CML), and Hairy Cell Leukemia, and Treatments Such as Chemotherapy, Radiation Therapy, Peripheral Blood Stem Cell and Marrow Transplantation, and Immunotherapy

Along with Tips for Life During and After Treatment, a Glossary, and Directories of Additional Resources

Edited by Joyce Brennfleck Shannon. 587 pages. 2003. 0-7808-0627-1. $78.

∎

Liver Disorders Sourcebook

Basic Consumer Health Information about the Liver and How It Works; Liver Diseases, Including Cancer, Cirrhosis, Hepatitis, and Toxic and Drug Related Diseases; Tips for Maintaining a Healthy Liver; Laboratory Tests, Radiology Tests, and Facts about Liver Transplantation

Along with a Section on Support Groups, a Glossary, and Resource Listings

Edited by Joyce Brennfleck Shannon. 591 pages. 2000. 0-7808-0383-3. $78.

"A valuable resource."
— *American Reference Books Annual, 2001*

"This title is recommended for health sciences and public libraries with consumer health collections."
— *E-Streams, Oct '00*

"Recommended reference source."
— *Booklist, American Library Association, Jun '00*

∎

Lung Disorders Sourcebook

Basic Consumer Health Information about Emphysema, Pneumonia, Tuberculosis, Asthma, Cystic Fibrosis, and Other Lung Disorders, Including Facts about Diagnostic Procedures, Treatment Strategies, Disease Prevention Efforts, and Such Risk Factors as Smoking, Air Pollution, and Exposure to Asbestos, Radon, and Other Agents

Along with a Glossary and Resources for Additional Help and Information

Edited by Dawn D. Matthews. 678 pages. 2002. 0-7808-0339-6. $78.

"This title is a great addition for public and school libraries because it provides concise health information on the lungs."
— *American Reference Books Annual, 2003*

"Highly recommended for academic and medical reference collections." — *Library Bookwatch, Sep '02*

∎

Medical Tests Sourcebook, 2nd Edition

Basic Consumer Health Information about Medical Tests, Including Age-Specific Health Tests, Important Health Screenings and Exams, Home-Use Tests, Blood and Specimen Tests, Electrical Tests, Scope Tests, Genetic Testing, and Imaging Tests, Such as X-Rays, Ultrasound, Computed Tomography, Magnetic Resonance Imaging, Angiography, and Nuclear Medicine

Along with a Glossary and Directory of Additional Resources

Edited by Joyce Brennfleck Shannon. 654 pages. 2004. 0-7808-0670-0. $78.

ALSO AVAILABLE: Medical Tests, 1st Edition. Edited by Joyce Brennfleck Shannon. 691 pages. 1999. 0-7808-0243-8. $78.

"Recommended for hospital and health sciences libraries with consumer health collections."
— *E-Streams, Mar '00*

"This is an overall excellent reference with a wealth of general knowledge that may aid those who are reluctant to get vital tests performed."
— *Today's Librarian, Jan 2000*

"A valuable reference guide."
— *American Reference Books Annual, 2000*

Men's Health Concerns Sourcebook, 2nd Edition

Basic Consumer Health Information about the Medical and Mental Concerns of Men, Including Theories about the Shorter Male Lifespan, the Leading Causes of Death and Disability, Physical Concerns of Special Significance to Men, Reproductive and Sexual Concerns, Sexually Transmitted Diseases, Men's Mental and Emotional Health, and Lifestyle Choices That Affect Wellness, Such as Nutrition, Fitness, and Substance Use

Along with a Glossary of Related Terms and a Directory of Organizational Resources in Men's Health

Edited by Robert Aquinas McNally. 644 pages. 2004. 0-7808-0671-9. $78.

ALSO AVAILABLE: Men's Health Concerns Sourcebook, 1st Edition. Edited by Allan R. Cook. 738 pages. 1998. 0-7808-0212-8. $78.

"This comprehensive resource and the series are highly recommended."
— American Reference Books Annual, 2000

"Recommended reference source."
— Booklist, American Library Association, Dec '98

Mental Health Disorders Sourcebook, 2nd Edition

Basic Consumer Health Information about Anxiety Disorders, Depression and Other Mood Disorders, Eating Disorders, Personality Disorders, Schizophrenia, and More, Including Disease Descriptions, Treatment Options, and Reports on Current Research Initiatives

Along with Statistical Data, Tips for Maintaining Mental Health, a Glossary, and Directory of Sources for Additional Help and Information

Edited by Karen Bellenir. 605 pages. 2000. 0-7808-0240-3. $78.

ALSO AVAILABLE: Mental Health Disorders Sourcebook, 1st Edition. Edited by Karen Bellenir. 548 pages. 1995. 0-7808-0040-0. $78.

"Well organized and well written."
— American Reference Books Annual, 2001

"Recommended reference source."
— Booklist, American Library Association, Jun '00

Mental Retardation Sourcebook

Basic Consumer Health Information about Mental Retardation and Its Causes, Including Down Syndrome, Fetal Alcohol Syndrome, Fragile X Syndrome, Genetic Conditions, Injury, and Environmental Sources

Along with Preventive Strategies, Parenting Issues, Educational Implications, Health Care Needs, Employment and Economic Matters, Legal Issues, a Glossary, and a Resource Listing for Additional Help and Information

Edited by Joyce Brennfleck Shannon. 642 pages. 2000. 0-7808-0377-9. $78.

"Public libraries will find the book useful for reference and as a beginning research point for students, parents, and caregivers."
— American Reference Books Annual, 2001

"The strength of this work is that it compiles many basic fact sheets and addresses for further information in one volume. It is intended and suitable for the general public. This sourcebook is relevant to any collection providing health information to the general public."
— E-Streams, Nov '00

"From preventing retardation to parenting and family challenges, this covers health, social and legal issues and will prove an invaluable overview."
— Reviewer's Bookwatch, Jul '00

Movement Disorders Sourcebook

Basic Consumer Health Information about Neurological Movement Disorders, Including Essential Tremor, Parkinson's Disease, Dystonia, Cerebral Palsy, Huntington's Disease, Myasthenia Gravis, Multiple Sclerosis, and Other Early-Onset and Adult-Onset Movement Disorders, Their Symptoms and Causes, Diagnostic Tests, and Treatments

Along with Mobility and Assistive Technology Information, a Glossary, and a Directory of Additional Resources

Edited by Joyce Brennfleck Shannon. 655 pages. 2003. 0-7808-0628-X. $78.

Obesity Sourcebook

Basic Consumer Health Information about Diseases and Other Problems Associated with Obesity, and Including Facts about Risk Factors, Prevention Issues, and Management Approaches

Along with Statistical and Demographic Data, Information about Special Populations, Research Updates, a Glossary, and Source Listings for Further Help and Information

Edited by Wilma Caldwell and Chad T. Kimball. 376 pages. 2001. 0-7808-0333-7. $78.

"The book synthesizes the reliable medical literature on obesity into one easy-to-read and useful resource for the general public."
— American Reference Books Annual 2002

"This is a very useful resource book for the lay public."
— Doody's Review Service, Nov '01

"Well suited for the health reference collection of a public library or an academic health science library that serves the general population." — E-Streams, Sep '01

"Recommended reference source."
— Booklist, American Library Association, Apr '01

" Recommended pick both for specialty health library collections and any general consumer health reference collection." — The Bookwatch, Apr '01

Ophthalmic Disorders Sourcebook, 1st Edition

SEE *Eye Care Sourcebook, 2nd Edition*

■

Oral Health Sourcebook

SEE *Dental Care & Oral Health Sourcebook, 2nd Ed.*

■

Osteoporosis Sourcebook

Basic Consumer Health Information about Primary and Secondary Osteoporosis and Juvenile Osteoporosis and Related Conditions, Including Fibrous Dysplasia, Gaucher Disease, Hyperthyroidism, Hypophosphatasia, Myeloma, Osteopetrosis, Osteogenesis Imperfecta, and Paget's Disease

Along with Information about Risk Factors, Treatments, Traditional and Non-Traditional Pain Management, a Glossary of Related Terms, and a Directory of Resources

Edited by Allan R. Cook. 584 pages. 2001. 0-7808-0239-X. $78.

"This would be a book to be kept in a staff or patient library. The targeted audience is the layperson, but the therapist who needs a quick bit of information on a particular topic will also find the book useful."
— *Physical Therapy, Jan '02*

"This resource is recommended as a great reference source for public, health, and academic libraries, and is another triumph for the editors of Omnigraphics."
— *American Reference Books Annual 2002*

"Recommended for all public libraries and general health collections, especially those supporting patient education or consumer health programs."
— *E-Streams, Nov '01*

"Will prove valuable to any library seeking to maintain a current, comprehensive reference collection of health resources. . . . From prevention to treatment and associated conditions, this provides an excellent survey."
— *The Bookwatch, Aug '01*

"Recommended reference source."
— *Booklist, American Library Association, July '01*

SEE ALSO *Women's Health Concerns Sourcebook*

■

Pain Sourcebook, 2nd Edition

Basic Consumer Health Information about Specific Forms of Acute and Chronic Pain, Including Muscle and Skeletal Pain, Nerve Pain, Cancer Pain, and Disorders Characterized by Pain, Such as Fibromyalgia, Shingles, Angina, Arthritis, and Headaches

Along with Information about Pain Medications and Management Techniques, Complementary and Alternative Pain Relief Options, Tips for People Living with Chronic Pain, a Glossary, and a Directory of Sources for Further Information

Edited by Karen Bellenir. 670 pages. 2002. 0-7808-0612-3. $78.

ALSO AVAILABLE: *Pain Sourcebook, 1st Edition.* Edited by Allan R. Cook. 667 pages. 1997. 0-7808-0213-6. $78.

"A source of valuable information. . . . This book offers help to nonmedical people who need information about pain and pain management. It is also an excellent reference for those who participate in patient education."
— *Doody's Review Service, Sep '02*

"The text is readable, easily understood, and well indexed. This excellent volume belongs in all patient education libraries, consumer health sections of public libraries, and many personal collections."
— *American Reference Books Annual, 1999*

"A beneficial reference." — *Booklist Health Sciences Supplement, American Library Association, Oct '98*

"The information is basic in terms of scholarship and is appropriate for general readers. Written in journalistic style . . . intended for non-professionals. Quite thorough in its coverage of different pain conditions and summarizes the latest clinical information regarding pain treatment." — *Choice, Association of College and Research Libraries, Jun '98*

"Recommended reference source."
— *Booklist, American Library Association, Mar '98*

■

Pediatric Cancer Sourcebook

Basic Consumer Health Information about Leukemias, Brain Tumors, Sarcomas, Lymphomas, and Other Cancers in Infants, Children, and Adolescents, Including Descriptions of Cancers, Treatments, and Coping Strategies

Along with Suggestions for Parents, Caregivers, and Concerned Relatives, a Glossary of Cancer Terms, and Resource Listings

Edited by Edward J. Prucha. 587 pages. 1999. 0-7808-0245-4. $78.

"An excellent source of information. Recommended for public, hospital, and health science libraries with consumer health collections." — *E-Streams, Jun '00*

"Recommended reference source."
— *Booklist, American Library Association, Feb '00*

"A valuable addition to all libraries specializing in health services and many public libraries."
— *American Reference Books Annual, 2000*

■

Physical & Mental Issues in Aging Sourcebook

Basic Consumer Health Information on Physical and Mental Disorders Associated with the Aging Process, Including Concerns about Cardiovascular Disease, Pulmonary Disease, Oral Health, Digestive Disorders, Musculoskeletal and Skin Disorders, Metabolic Changes, Sexual and Reproductive Issues, and Changes in Vision, Hearing, and Other Senses

Along with Data about Longevity and Causes of Death, Information on Acute and Chronic Pain,

Descriptions of Mental Concerns, a Glossary of Terms, and Resource Listings for Additional Help

Edited by Jenifer Swanson. 660 pages. 1999. 0-7808-0233-0. $78.

"This is a treasure of health information for the layperson." — *Choice Health Sciences Supplement, Association of College & Research Libraries, May 2000*

"Recommended for public libraries."
—*American Reference Books Annual, 2000*

"Recommended reference source."
—*Booklist, American Library Association, Oct '99*

SEE ALSO Healthy Aging Sourcebook

■

Podiatry Sourcebook

Basic Consumer Health Information about Foot Conditions, Diseases, and Injuries, Including Bunions, Corns, Calluses, Athlete's Foot, Plantar Warts, Hammertoes and Clawtoes, Clubfoot, Heel Pain, Gout, and More

Along with Facts about Foot Care, Disease Prevention, Foot Safety, Choosing a Foot Care Specialist, a Glossary of Terms, and Resource Listings for Additional Information

Edited by M. Lisa Weatherford. 380 pages. 2001. 0-7808-0215-2. $78.

"Recommended reference source."
—*Booklist, American Library Association, Feb '02*

"There is a lot of information presented here on a topic that is usually only covered sparingly in most larger comprehensive medical encyclopedias."
— *American Reference Books Annual 2002*

■

Pregnancy & Birth Sourcebook, 2nd Edition

Basic Consumer Health Information about Conception and Pregnancy, Including Facts about Fertility, Infertility, Pregnancy Symptoms and Complications, Fetal Growth and Development, Labor, Delivery, and the Postpartum Period, as Well as Information about Maintaining Health and Wellness during Pregnancy and Caring for a Newborn

Along with Information about Public Health Assistance for Low-Income Pregnant Women, a Glossary, and Directories of Agencies and Organizations Providing Help and Support

Edited by Amy L. Sutton. 626 pages. 2004. 0-7808-0672-7. $78.

ALSO AVAILABLE: Pregnancy & Birth Sourcebook, 1st Edition. Edited by Heather E. Aldred. 737 pages. 1997. 0-7808-0216-0. $78.

"A well-organized handbook. Recommended."
— *Choice, Association of College and Research Libraries, Apr '98*

"Recommended reference source."
—*Booklist, American Library Association, Mar '98*

"Recommended for public libraries."
—*American Reference Books Annual, 1998*

SEE ALSO Congenital Disorders Sourcebook, Family Planning Sourcebook

■

Prostate Cancer Sourcebook

Basic Consumer Health Information about Prostate Cancer, Including Information about the Associated Risk Factors, Detection, Diagnosis, and Treatment of Prostate Cancer

Along with Information on Non-Malignant Prostate Conditions, and Featuring a Section Listing Support and Treatment Centers and a Glossary of Related Terms

Edited by Dawn D. Matthews. 358 pages. 2001. 0-7808-0324-8. $78.

"Recommended reference source."
— *Booklist, American Library Association, Jan '02*

"A valuable resource for health care consumers seeking information on the subject. . . .All text is written in a clear, easy-to-understand language that avoids technical jargon. Any library that collects consumer health resources would strengthen their collection with the addition of the *Prostate Cancer Sourcebook*."
—*American Reference Books Annual 2002*

■

Public Health Sourcebook

Basic Information about Government Health Agencies, Including National Health Statistics and Trends, Healthy People 2000 Program Goals and Objectives, the Centers for Disease Control and Prevention, the Food and Drug Administration, and the National Institutes of Health

Along with Full Contact Information for Each Agency

Edited by Wendy Wilcox. 698 pages. 1998. 0-7808-0220-9. $78.

"Recommended reference source."
— *Booklist, American Library Association, Sep '98*

"This consumer guide provides welcome assistance in navigating the maze of federal health agencies and their data on public health concerns."
—*SciTech Book News, Sep '98*

■

Reconstructive & Cosmetic Surgery Sourcebook

Basic Consumer Health Information on Cosmetic and Reconstructive Plastic Surgery, Including Statistical Information about Different Surgical Procedures, Things to Consider Prior to Surgery, Plastic Surgery Techniques and Tools, Emotional and Psychological Considerations, and Procedure-Specific Information

Along with a Glossary of Terms and a Listing of Resources for Additional Help and Information

Edited by M. Lisa Weatherford. 374 pages. 2001. 0-7808-0214-4. $78.

"An excellent reference that addresses cosmetic and medically necessary reconstructive surgeries. . . . The style of the prose is calm and reassuring, discussing the many positive outcomes now available due to advances in surgical techniques."
—*American Reference Books Annual 2002*

"Recommended for health science libraries that are open to the public, as well as hospital libraries that are open to the patients. This book is a good resource for the consumer interested in plastic surgery."
—*E-Streams, Dec '01*

"Recommended reference source."
—*Booklist, American Library Association, July '01*

■

Rehabilitation Sourcebook

Basic Consumer Health Information about Rehabilitation for People Recovering from Heart Surgery, Spinal Cord Injury, Stroke, Orthopedic Impairments, Amputation, Pulmonary Impairments, Traumatic Injury, and More, Including Physical Therapy, Occupational Therapy, Speech/ Language Therapy, Massage Therapy, Dance Therapy, Art Therapy, and Recreational Therapy

Along with Information on Assistive and Adaptive Devices, a Glossary, and Resources for Additional Help and Information

Edited by Dawn D. Matthews. 531 pages. 1999. 0-7808-0236-5. $78.

"This is an excellent resource for public library reference and health collections."
—*American Reference Books Annual, 2001*

"Recommended reference source."
—*Booklist, American Library Association, May '00*

■

Respiratory Diseases & Disorders Sourcebook

Basic Information about Respiratory Diseases and Disorders, Including Asthma, Cystic Fibrosis, Pneumonia, the Common Cold, Influenza, and Others, Featuring Facts about the Respiratory System, Statistical and Demographic Data, Treatments, Self-Help Management Suggestions, and Current Research Initiatives

Edited by Allan R. Cook and Peter D. Dresser. 771 pages. 1995. 0-7808-0037-0. $78.

"Designed for the layperson and for patients and their families coping with respiratory illness. . . . an extensive array of information on diagnosis, treatment, management, and prevention of respiratory illnesses for the general reader."
—*Choice, Association of College and Research Libraries, Jun '96*

"A highly recommended text for all collections. It is a comforting reminder of the power of knowledge that good books carry between their covers."
—*Academic Library Book Review, Spring '96*

"A comprehensive collection of authoritative information presented in a nontechnical, humanitarian style for patients, families, and caregivers."
—*Association of Operating Room Nurses, Sep/Oct '95*

SEE ALSO Lung Disorders Sourcebook

■

Sexually Transmitted Diseases Sourcebook, 2nd Edition

Basic Consumer Health Information about Sexually Transmitted Diseases, Including Information on the Diagnosis and Treatment of Chlamydia, Gonorrhea, Hepatitis, Herpes, HIV, Mononucleosis, Syphilis, and Others

Along with Information on Prevention, Such as Condom Use, Vaccines, and STD Education; And Featuring a Section on Issues Related to Youth and Adolescents, a Glossary, and Resources for Additional Help and Information

Edited by Dawn D. Matthews. 538 pages. 2001. 0-7808-0249-7. $78.

ALSO AVAILABLE: *Sexually Transmitted Diseases Sourcebook, 1st Edition.* Edited by Linda M. Ross. 550 pages. 1997. 0-7808-0217-9. $78.

"Recommended for consumer health collections in public libraries, and secondary school and community college libraries."
—*American Reference Books Annual 2002*

"Every school and public library should have a copy of this comprehensive and user-friendly reference book."
—*Choice, Association of College & Research Libraries, Sep '01*

"This is a highly recommended book. This is an especially important book for all school and public libraries." —*AIDS Book Review Journal, Jul-Aug '01*

"Recommended reference source."
—*Booklist, American Library Association, Apr '01*

"Recommended pick both for specialty health library collections and any general consumer health reference collection." —*The Bookwatch, Apr '01*

■

Skin Disorders Sourcebook

Basic Information about Common Skin and Scalp Conditions Caused by Aging, Allergies, Immune Reactions, Sun Exposure, Infectious Organisms, Parasites, Cosmetics, and Skin Traumas, Including Abrasions, Cuts, and Pressure Sores

Along with Information on Prevention and Treatment

Edited by Allan R. Cook. 647 pages. 1997. 0-7808-0080-X. $78.

". . . comprehensive, easily read reference book."
—*Doody's Health Sciences Book Reviews, Oct '97*

SEE ALSO Burns Sourcebook

Sleep Disorders Sourcebook

Basic Consumer Health Information about Sleep and Its Disorders, Including Insomnia, Sleepwalking, Sleep Apnea, Restless Leg Syndrome, and Narcolepsy

Along with Data about Shiftwork and Its Effects, Information on the Societal Costs of Sleep Deprivation, Descriptions of Treatment Options, a Glossary of Terms, and Resource Listings for Additional Help

Edited by Jenifer Swanson. 439 pages. 1998. 0-7808-0234-9. $78.

"This text will complement any home or medical library. It is user-friendly and ideal for the adult reader."
— *American Reference Books Annual, 2000*

"A useful resource that provides accurate, relevant, and accessible information on sleep to the general public. Health care providers who deal with sleep disorders patients may also find it helpful in being prepared to answer some of the questions patients ask."
— *Respiratory Care, Jul '99*

"Recommended reference source."
— *Booklist, American Library Association, Feb '99*

Sports Injuries Sourcebook, 2nd Edition

Basic Consumer Health Information about the Diagnosis, Treatment, and Rehabilitation of Common Sports-Related Injuries in Children and Adults

Along with Suggestions for Conditioning and Training, Information and Prevention Tips for Injuries Frequently Associated with Specific Sports and Special Populations, a Glossary, and a Directory of Additional Resources

Edited by Joyce Brennfleck Shannon. 614 pages. 2002. 0-7808-0604-2. $78.

ALSO AVAILABLE: Sports Injuries Sourcebook, 1st Edition. Edited by Heather E. Aldred. 624 pages. 1999. 0-7808-0218-7. $78.

"This is an excellent reference for consumers and it is recommended for public, community college, and undergraduate libraries."
— *American Reference Books Annual, 2003*

"Recommended reference source."
— *Booklist, American Library Association, Feb '03*

Stress-Related Disorders Sourcebook

Basic Consumer Health Information about Stress and Stress-Related Disorders, Including Stress Origins and Signals, Environmental Stress at Work and Home, Mental and Emotional Stress Associated with Depression, Post-Traumatic Stress Disorder, Panic Disorder, Suicide, and the Physical Effects of Stress on the Cardiovascular, Immune, and Nervous Systems

Along with Stress Management Techniques, a Glossary, and a Listing of Additional Resources

Edited by Joyce Brennfleck Shannon. 610 pages. 2002. 0-7808-0560-7. $78.

"Well written for a general readership, the *Stress-Related Disorders Sourcebook* is a useful addition to the health reference literature."
— *American Reference Books Annual, 2003*

"I am impressed by the amount of information. It offers a thorough overview of the causes and consequences of stress for the layperson. . . . A well-done and thorough reference guide for professionals and nonprofessionals alike."
— *Doody's Review Service, Dec '02*

Stroke Sourcebook

Basic Consumer Health Information about Stroke, Including Ischemic, Hemorrhagic, Transient Ischemic Attack (TIA), and Pediatric Stroke, Stroke Triggers and Risks, Diagnostic Tests, Treatments, and Rehabilitation Information

Along with Stroke Prevention Guidelines, Legal and Financial Information, a Glossary, and a Directory of Additional Resources

Edited by Joyce Brennfleck Shannon. 606 pages. 2003. 0-7808-0630-1. $78.

Substance Abuse Sourcebook

Basic Health-Related Information about the Abuse of Legal and Illegal Substances Such as Alcohol, Tobacco, Prescription Drugs, Marijuana, Cocaine, and Heroin; and Including Facts about Substance Abuse Prevention Strategies, Intervention Methods, Treatment and Recovery Programs, and a Section Addressing the Special Problems Related to Substance Abuse during Pregnancy

Edited by Karen Bellenir. 573 pages. 1996. 0-7808-0038-9. $78.

"A valuable addition to any health reference section. Highly recommended."
— *The Book Report, Mar/Apr '97*

". . . a comprehensive collection of substance abuse information that's both highly readable and compact. Families and caregivers of substance abusers will find the information enlightening and helpful, while teachers, social workers and journalists should benefit from the concise format. Recommended."
— *Drug Abuse Update, Winter '96/'97*

SEE ALSO Alcoholism Sourcebook, Drug Abuse Sourcebook

Surgery Sourcebook

Basic Consumer Health Information about Inpatient and Outpatient Surgeries, Including Cardiac, Vascular, Orthopedic, Ocular, Reconstructive, Cosmetic, Gynecologic, and Ear, Nose, and Throat Procedures and More

Along with Information about Operating Room Policies and Instruments, Laser Surgery Techniques, Hospital Errors, Statistical Data, a Glossary, and Listings of Sources for Further Help and Information

Edited by Annemarie S. Muth and Karen Bellenir. 596 pages. 2002. 0-7808-0380-9. $78.

"Invaluable reference for public and school library collections alike." — *Library Bookwatch, Apr '03*

■

Transplantation Sourcebook

Basic Consumer Health Information about Organ and Tissue Transplantation, Including Physical and Financial Preparations, Procedures and Issues Relating to Specific Solid Organ and Tissue Transplants, Rehabilitation, Pediatric Transplant Information, the Future of Transplantation, and Organ and Tissue Donation

Along with a Glossary and Listings of Additional Resources

Edited by Joyce Brennfleck Shannon. 628 pages. 2002. 0-7808-0322-1. $78.

"Along with these advances [in transplantation technology] have come a number of daunting questions for potential transplant patients, their families, and their health care providers. This reference text is the best single tool to address many of these questions. . . . It will be a much-needed addition to the reference collections in health care, academic, and large public libraries." — *American Reference Books Annual, 2003*

"Recommended for libraries with an interest in offering consumer health information." — *E-Streams, Jul '02*

"This is a unique and valuable resource for patients facing transplantation and their families." — *Doody's Review Service, Jun '02*

■

Traveler's Health Sourcebook

Basic Consumer Health Information for Travelers, Including Physical and Medical Preparations, Transportation Health and Safety, Essential Information about Food and Water, Sun Exposure, Insect and Snake Bites, Camping and Wilderness Medicine, and Travel with Physical or Medical Disabilities

Along with International Travel Tips, Vaccination Recommendations, Geographical Health Issues, Disease Risks, a Glossary, and a Listing of Additional Resources

Edited by Joyce Brennfleck Shannon. 613 pages. 2000. 0-7808-0384-1. $78.

"Recommended reference source." — *Booklist, American Library Association, Feb '01*

"This book is recommended for any public library, any travel collection, and especially any collection for the physically disabled." — *American Reference Books Annual, 2001*

■

Vegetarian Sourcebook

Basic Consumer Health Information about Vegetarian Diets, Lifestyle, and Philosophy, Including Definitions of Vegetarianism and Veganism, Tips about Adopting Vegetarianism, Creating a Vegetarian Pantry, and Meeting Nutritional Needs of Vegetarians, with Facts Regarding Vegetarianism's Effect on Pregnant and Lactating Women, Children, Athletes, and Senior Citizens

Along with a Glossary of Commonly Used Vegetarian Terms and Resources for Additional Help and Information

Edited by Chad T. Kimball. 360 pages. 2002. 0-7808-0439-2. $78.

"Organizes into one concise volume the answers to the most common questions concerning vegetarian diets and lifestyles. This title is recommended for public and secondary school libraries." — *E-Streams, Apr '03*

"Invaluable reference for public and school library collections alike." — *Library Bookwatch, Apr '03*

"The articles in this volume are easy to read and come from authoritative sources. The book does not necessarily support the vegetarian diet but instead provides the pros and cons of this important decision. The *Vegetarian Sourcebook* is recommended for public libraries and consumer health libraries." — *American Reference Books Annual, 2003*

■

Women's Health Concerns Sourcebook, 2nd Edition

Basic Consumer Health Information about the Medical and Mental Concerns of Women, Including Maintaining Health and Wellness, Gynecological Concerns, Breast Health, Sexuality and Reproductive Issues, Menopause, Cancer in Women, the Leading Causes of Death and Disability among Women, Physical Concerns of Special Significance to Women, and Women's Mental and Emotional Health

Along with a Glossary of Related Terms and Directories of Resources for Additional Help and Information

Edited by Amy L. Sutton. 748 pages. 2004. 0-7808-0673-5. $78.

ALSO AVAILABLE: *Women's Health Concerns Sourcebook, 1st Edition.* Edited by Heather E. Aldred. 567 pages. 1997. 0-7808-0219-5. $78.

"Handy compilation. There is an impressive range of diseases, devices, disorders, procedures, and other physical and emotional issues covered . . . well organized, illustrated, and indexed." — *Choice, Association of College and Research Libraries, Jan '98*

SEE ALSO *Breast Cancer Sourcebook, Cancer Sourcebook for Women, Healthy Heart Sourcebook for Women, Osteoporosis Sourcebook*

■

Workplace Health & Safety Sourcebook

Basic Consumer Health Information about Workplace Health and Safety, Including the Effect of Workplace Hazards on the Lungs, Skin, Heart, Ears, Eyes, Brain, Reproductive Organs, Musculoskeletal System, and Other Organs and Body Parts

Along with Information about Occupational Cancer, Personal Protective Equipment, Toxic and Hazardous Chemicals, Child Labor, Stress, and Workplace Violence

Edited by Chad T. Kimball. 626 pages. 2000. 0-7808-0231-4. $78.

"As a reference for the general public, this would be useful in any library."   —*E-Streams, Jun '01*

"Provides helpful information for primary care physicians and other caregivers interested in occupational medicine.... General readers; professionals."
— *Choice, Association of College & Research Libraries, May '01*

"Recommended reference source."
—*Booklist, American Library Association, Feb '01*

"Highly recommended."   —*The Bookwatch, Jan '01*

Worldwide Health Sourcebook

Basic Information about Global Health Issues, Including Malnutrition, Reproductive Health, Disease Dispersion and Prevention, Emerging Diseases, Risky Health Behaviors, and the Leading Causes of Death

Along with Global Health Concerns for Children, Women, and the Elderly, Mental Health Issues, Research and Technology Advancements, and Economic, Environmental, and Political Health Implications, a Glossary, and a Resource Listing for Additional Help and Information

Edited by Joyce Brennfleck Shannon. 614 pages. 2001. 0-7808-0330-2. $78.

"Named an Outstanding Academic Title."
—*Choice, Association of College & Research Libraries, Jan '02*

"Yet another handy but also unique compilation in the extensive Health Reference Series, this is a useful work because many of the international publications reprinted or excerpted are not readily available. Highly recommended."   —*Choice, Association of College & Research Libraries, Nov '01*

"Recommended reference source."
—*Booklist, American Library Association, Oct '01*

Teen Health Series

Helping Young Adults Understand, Manage, and Avoid Serious Illness

Cancer Information for Teens

Health Tips about Cancer Awareness, Prevention, Diagnosis, and Treatment

Including Facts about Frequently Occurring Cancers, Cancer Risk Factors, and Coping Strategies for Teens Fighting Cancer or Dealing with Cancer in Friends or Family Members

Edited by Wilma R. Caldwell. 415 pages. 2004. 0-7808-0678-6. $58.

Diet Information for Teens

Health Tips about Diet and Nutrition

Including Facts about Nutrients, Dietary Guidelines, Breakfasts, School Lunches, Snacks, Party Food, Weight Control, Eating Disorders, and More

Edited by Karen Bellenir. 399 pages. 2001. 0-7808-0441-4. $58.

"Full of helpful insights and facts throughout the book. ... An excellent resource to be placed in public libraries or even in personal collections."
— *American Reference Books Annual 2002*

"Recommended for middle and high school libraries and media centers as well as academic libraries that educate future teachers of teenagers. It is also a suitable addition to health science libraries that serve patrons who are interested in teen health promotion and education."
— *E-Streams, Oct '01*

"This comprehensive book would be beneficial to collections that need information about nutrition, dietary guidelines, meal planning, and weight control. ... This reference is so easy to use that its purchase is recommended."
— *The Book Report, Sep-Oct '01*

"This book is written in an easy to understand format describing issues that many teens face every day, and then provides thoughtful explanations so that teens can make informed decisions. This is an interesting book that provides important facts and information for today's teens."
— *Doody's Health Sciences Book Review Journal, Jul-Aug '01*

"A comprehensive compendium of diet and nutrition. The information is presented in a straightforward, plain-spoken manner. This title will be useful to those working on reports on a variety of topics, as well as to general readers concerned about their dietary health."
— *School Library Journal, Jun '01*

Drug Information for Teens

Health Tips about the Physical and Mental Effects of Substance Abuse

Including Facts about Alcohol, Anabolic Steroids, Club Drugs, Cocaine, Depressants, Hallucinogens, Herbal Products, Inhalants, Marijuana, Narcotics, Stimulants, Tobacco, and More

Edited by Karen Bellenir. 452 pages. 2002. 0-7808-0444-9. $58.

"The chapters are quick to make a connection to their teenage reading audience. The prose is straightforward and the book lends itself to spot reading. It should be useful both for practical information and for research, and it is suitable for public and school libraries."
— *American Reference Books Annual, 2003*

"Recommended reference source."
— *Booklist, American Library Association, Feb '03*

"This is an excellent resource for teens and their parents. Education about drugs and substances is key to discouraging teen drug abuse and this book provides this much needed information in a way that is interesting and factual."
— *Doody's Review Service, Dec '02*

Fitness Information for Teens

Health Tips about Exercise, Physical Well-Being, and Health Maintenance

Including Facts about Aerobic and Anaerobic Conditioning, Stretching, Body Shape and Body Image, Sports Training, Nutrition, and Activities for Non-Athletes

Edited by Karen Bellenir. 400 pages. 2004. 0-7808-0679-4. $58.

Mental Health Information for Teens

Health Tips about Mental Health and Mental Illness

Including Facts about Anxiety, Depression, Suicide, Eating Disorders, Obsessive-Compulsive Disorders, Panic Attacks, Phobias, Schizophrenia, and More

Edited by Karen Bellenir. 406 pages. 2001. 0-7808-0442-2. $58.

"In both language and approach, this user-friendly entry in the *Teen Health Series* is on target for teens needing information on mental health concerns."
— *Booklist, American Library Association, Jan '02*

"Readers will find the material accessible and informative, with the shaded notes, facts, and embedded glossary insets adding appropriately to the already interesting and succinct presentation."

—*School Library Journal, Jan '02*

"This title is highly recommended for any library that serves adolescents and parents/caregivers of adolescents." —*E-Streams, Jan '02*

"Recommended for high school libraries and young adult collections in public libraries. Both health professionals and teenagers will find this book useful."

—*American Reference Books Annual 2002*

"This is a nice book written to enlighten the society, primarily teenagers, about common teen mental health issues. It is highly recommended to teachers and parents as well as adolescents."

—*Doody's Review Service, Dec '01*

Sexual Health Information for Teens

Health Tips about Sexual Development, Human Reproduction, and Sexually Transmitted Diseases

Including Facts about Puberty, Reproductive Health, Chlamydia, Human Papillomavirus, Pelvic Inflammatory Disease, Herpes, AIDS, Contraception, Pregnancy, and More

Edited by Deborah A. Stanley. 391 pages. 2003. 0-7808-0445-7. $58.

Skin Health Information For Teens

Health Tips about Dermatological Concerns and Skin Cancer Risks

Including Facts about Acne, Warts, Hives, and Other Conditions and Lifestyle Choices, Such as Tanning, Tattooing, and Piercing, That Affect the Skin, Nails, Scalp, and Hair

Edited by Robert Aquinas McNally. 430 pages. 2003. 0-7808-0446-5. $58.

Sports Injuries Information For Teens

Health Tips about Sports Injuries and Injury Protection

Including Facts about Specific Injuries, Emergency Treatment, Rehabilitation, Sports Safety, Competition Stress, Fitness, Sports Nutrition, Steroid Risks, and More

Edited by Joyce Brennfleck Shannon. 425 pages. 2003. 0-7808-0447-3. $58.

Health Reference Series